Exploring Communication Disorders

A 21st Century Introduction through Literature and Media

Dennis C. Tanner

Northern Arizona University

Boston   New York   San Francisco
Mexico City   Montreal   Toronto   London   Madrid   Munich   Paris
Hong Kong   Singapore   Tokyo   Cape Town   Sydney

*For my wife, Jody—three decades as my companion,
collaborator, counsel, confidante, and colleague*

Editor in Chief, Social Sciences: *Paul Smith*
Executive Editor and Publisher: *Stephen D. Dragin*
Editorial Assistant: *Barbara Strickland*
Marketing Manager: *Tara Whorf*
Production Coordinator: *Susan Brown*
Composition Buyer: *Linda Cox*
Editorial Production Service: *Matrix Productions Inc.*
Electronic Composition: *Peggy Cabot, Cabot Computer Services*
Manufacturing Buyer: *JoAnne Sweeney*
Cover Administrator: *Kristina Mose-Libon*

For related titles and support materials, visit our online catalog at www.ablongman.com.

Library of Congress Cataloging-in-Publication Data

Tanner, Dennis C.
    Exploring communication disorders : a 21st century introduction through literature and media /
by Dennis C. Tanner
        p.   cm.
    Includes bibliographical references and index.
    ISBN 0-205-37360-7
        1. Communicative disorders.   I. Title.

RC423 .T264 2003
616.85'5—dc21   2002024886

Printed in the United States of America

10 9 8 7 6 5 4 3 2 1   08 07 06 05 04 03 02

Contents

4   *Articulation and Phonological Disorders*   86

Foreword

Every now and then, an idea comes along that is simply so good and makes so much sense that you feel like you thought of it yourself. Such is the case with *Exploring Communication Disorders: A 21st Century Introduction through Literature and Media*. I was there the day that Dennis Tanner proposed a new undergraduate course called Communication Disorders in Literature and Media. He wanted something that would capture the students' interest, challenge their thinking, and elevate their sensitivity for people with communication disorders. But, even more so, he wanted students to *feel* how important communication is and experience the tragedy of its loss. It was one of those moments when everyone thought to themselves, "Now there's a course I'd like to take." So we were all instantly bonded to the idea and now celebrate the publication of this outstanding text in support of it.

Exploring Communication Disorders is an innovative text. It is an incredibly thorough work that provides countless examples that stretch your imagination, warm your heart, and stir your fears. It is comprehensive, easy-to-read, well organized, and immensely appropriate for a college-level text. To that end it is also ideally designed to support a liberal studies course that examines how communication disorders are treated in literature and media. It also provides an inviting way to tell students about the discipline of communication sciences and disorders in an entertaining and engaging manner. Professionals in speech–language pathology and audiology touch the lives of children and adults in very special ways. Students also learn about these professionals, gain a deeper understanding of human communication, and may someday as a result find their way to a career in speech–language pathology or audiology.

To me, what makes this text so effective is that I grew up with so many of the examples or characters. I can relate to many of them and even remember the feelings they evoked. The importance of communication was never so real to me than it was in *Children of a Lesser God*. The book and the movie helped shape in me a deeper understanding for the struggle one can experience trying to communicate and the sense of loss that can occur as a result. I was working in a school for the deaf at the time. Needless to say, the movie had a profound impact on my clinical work. We all have these realities, so literature and the movies are both a lens and a mirror. Dennis Tanner has brought together a text that has something personal in it for everyone and something that may change students' lives as well. There is nothing more uniquely personal, more human, or more real than how we communicate. This text will help students take a critical but entertaining look at something immensely personal, and they will grow personally and professionally as a result.

From idea to concept to reality, Dennis Tanner has succeeded in developing a novel text to support a wonderful undergraduate experience. Let me commend him for this outstanding contribution. Enjoy!

Wayne A. Secord, Ph.D.
University of Cincinnati

Preface

Exploring Communication Disorders: A 21ˢᵗ Century Introduction through Literature and Media is a different kind of "intro" book. It was written for college students, typically first- and second-year students, who are shopping for a major or testing the waters to see if the discipline of communication sciences and disorders is worthy of commitment. This text uses references to books, films, television programs, and a Broadway play having characters with communication disorders. There are also references to public figures who have them.

For the professor, teaching an introduction course is both challenging and rewarding. It is challenging to motivate students who are simply trying to find a possible major, and it is rewarding to capture their interest. Having taught for more than 25 years, I find the introductory course to be one of the most exciting and stimulating courses to teach.

A professor teaching the introduction course must walk a fine line. He or she should provide substantive information so that the course is not without substance and known as a "twinkie." Today, too many college courses, particularly those dealing with pop culture and trendy issues, pander to the superficial and avoid serious academic challenges for the students. It has been my experience that students frown upon weak courses and embrace those that stimulate and engage. Most college students today, as in the past, are idealistic about education and the scholarly challenges they face. Many students are happy to defer the gratification of salaries, cars, homes, and children for the allure of education. They understand that a good education does not come easily, nor should it. Like a racquetball game, the sweetest victory requires the greatest commitment, and the postgame exhaustion is both expected and welcomed. The best courses are those that challenge, provoke, arouse, excite, stimulate, and exhaust. The best courses are those requiring the best of the student.

With that said, the professor of the intro course must take care not to alienate students with information that is beyond their interest. In an ideal world, all students, in fact all people, would have an innate interest in human communication and the myriad of disorders that can lay waste to it. Human communication encompasses the best of our noble and hard-fought evolutionary history. It is the highest cognitive and physical function that we perform. Human communication is the abstract symbolic thought used in inner speech, the marvels of motor speech programming, the vitality of respiration, and the sophistication of voicing. Dynamic articulation involves hundreds of muscles and thousands of neurological impulses per second. The study of acoustics is the exploration of the vibratory energy of the world. Sound is the physics of mechanical and hydraulic energy occurring in the middle and inner ear. And the way humans perceive and associate verbal symbols into units of meaning boggles the mind. The disorders afflicting this marvelous ability range from those that are minor and simply inconveniences to those that can render the best and brightest of our species mute, as is the case of Dr. Stephen Hawking. The courage and resourcefulness of Dr. Hawking, and people like him, are tributes to the human spirit in overcoming the adversity of a wordless world.

In a perfect world, all students would be drawn to this inherently interesting subject matter and appreciate even the smallest intricacies of human communication and the challenges of its disorders. But we do not live in a perfect world, and many first- and second-year students' interests lie elsewhere. Their interests lie in movies, television programs, novels, musicians, actors, and media personalities. Traditional first- and second-year students, like we who came before them, are products of their time, and to reach them in the classroom and during lonely pretest cramming sessions, generational and academic fences must be torn down and bridges built. It is the professor's responsibility to segue from the students' interests to the marvels of human communication and the thousands of diseases, deficiencies, disorders, defects, and deviations that can impair or destroy it. This book is an attempt at that segue.

Walking the fine line between "fluff," those classroom references to pop culture, and the "substance" of science is difficult, and some may say that fluff has no business in communication sciences and disorders. Some may say that in college, and college texts, there is no room for current or past rockers and right-wing talk-show hosts. There is no room in serious science for current or classic movies or the silly sexual advice of the limp, lisping Leon Phelps in *The Ladies Man*. But to make that assertion is to deny the real world and to disavow the need to relate to our customers: the eager and not-so-eager students whose faces brighten up the dingiest of lecture halls. So-called fluff has a place in communication sciences and disorders and in academic texts, if it bridges the gap between students and the substance of phonetics, anatomy, physiology, neurology, acoustics, and cognition. And what is fluff to one is substance to another.

Acknowledgments

Several people were instrumental in helping me conceptualize and write this book. Brooke Wonders, Cindy Dambach, Janel Matousek, and Andrea Nicole Tanner were indispensable in reviewing and editing the manuscript. Jennifer Spencer and Anastasia Gloeckler did a wonderful job researching the Internet and preparing tables and figures. The following reviewers offered helpful suggestions: Terre Blankenship, Wichita State University; James C. Cantrell, Tennessee State University; and Carolyn De Soto, University of Cincinnati. Finally, thanks to Drs. James Blagg, Wayne Secord, and William Culbertson for their encouragement, support, and help in conceptualizing this book.

Dennis C. Tanner, Ph.D.
Flagstaff, Arizona

To the Reader

In this book you will see how communication disorders are portrayed in media and literature. Movies, television programs, books, and a Broadway play, which have characters with communication disorders, are studied. There are also references to well-known people who have them. Singers, actors, politicians, writers, radio personalities, and other people in the public eye are discussed with an emphasis on their particular communication disorder. There is also a comprehensive academic review of communication disorders in which their nature, diagnosis, and treatment are discussed.

The first chapter of this book is a sociological examination of communication disorders and the power that the media and literature have in shaping public perceptions. Because this book may be used as an introductory text, the final chapter, in a question-and-answer format, addresses the clinical and educational requirements to enter the professions of speech–language pathology and audiology, salaries, job opportunities, the American Speech-Language-Hearing Association (ASHA), and so on. To better help understand the nature and type of employment opportunities in speech–language pathology and audiology, three original short stories are in Appendix B:

A Day at JFK chronicles a typical workday for a speech–language pathologist employed in a public school.

Preponderance of Evidence describes the type of work done by speech–language pathologists in a hospital setting.

Welcome to the Cyber Speech and Hearing Clinic is an account of what the practice of speech–language pathology and audiology may become in the not-so-distant future.

Throughout the text, technical terms are defined when used, and a comprehensive glossary is also included. Several books and dictionaries were consulted in creating it. Rather than have a separate chapter addressing anatomy and physiology of the speech and hearing mechanism, anatomical figures and illustrations are provided in the appropriate chapters.

There are two types of referencing in this book. The academic and scholarly references are in standard American Psychological Association (APA) style and format and are provided at the end of the book. Because of the unique nature of this book, the literature and media references and citations are dealt with in a nonstandard way. Most of the personalities discussed in this book have home pages on the World Wide Web, and some information about movies and books come from the Web, film trailers, video jackets, and critical books on films and television programs. To give proper credit to the respective authors, quoting and citations were integrated into the text in a way the reader can determine their source. The section Literature, Media, and Personality: Home Pages, Suggested Readings, References, and Resources gives the reader the informational sources to the films, television programs, and personalities referred to in this book. They are listed at the end of the book on a chapter-by-chapter basis and by the person, book, television program, or movie. The goal was to keep the academic and scholarly references separate from the books, films, and television program sources of information.

The book, television, and movie examples span several decades. To be included in this book, they must have had a main or supporting character with a communication disorder and have had wide exposure to the general public. Movies such as *One Flew Over the Cuckoo's Nest* and *Children of a Lesser God* are classic films receiving several Academy Awards. Others, like *Deuce Bigalo, Male Gigolo* and *The Ladies Man* are silly films, but they were included because they had wide distribution and increased the visibility of communication disorders. As noted above, most of the public figures included in this book have home pages that refer to their communication disorders. Efforts were taken to respect the privacy of public figures, and only those who have publicly acknowledged their communication disorder or who have had them widely publicized were included herein.

1

Communication Disorders, Literature, Media, and Society

Chapter Preview

This chapter introduces communication sciences and disorders as a discipline and the way society views people with communication disorders. To illustrate the complexities of verbal communication, a simple communicative act between two people is described. The process of verbal communication is broken down into (1) thought, (2) language, (3) motor speech programming, (4) sound production, (5) acoustic, mechanical, hydraulic, and electrochemical energy transmission, (6) auditory perception and decoding, and (7) receptive verbal and visual associations. Various ways of categorizing communication disorders are described. To show how widespread these disorders are, incidence and prevalence figures are provided. The history of the perception and treatment of people with communication disorders is examined. The American Speech-Language-Hearing Association (ASHA) is described, including its leadership in protecting and advocating for the rights and ethical treatment of people with communication disorders. The social group of people with communication disorders is discussed, including factors relating to its size, power, status, visibility, and cohesiveness. Their historical and current economic disadvantage is considered, as are recent political and technological advances that counter it. Finally, social perceptions and stereotypes of people with communication disorders are analyzed, as is the role of media and literature in dispelling or propagating them.

What do the following films, books, and public figures have in common?

Rush Limbaugh	Moses
Forrest Gump	Mel Tillis
Warner Bros. cartoon characters	*Wings:* A broadway play
Bill Clinton	Christopher Reeve
A Fish Called Wanda	*Rain Man*
Children of a Lesser God	Patricia Neal
The World According to Garp	Ronald Reagan
One Flew Over the Cuckoo's Nest	Stephen Hawking

The Sixth Sense   *Anywhere But Here*
James Brady   *The Heart Is a Lonely Hunter*
The Ladies Man   *Pearl Harbor*

The one commonality among these films, books, and public figures is a communication disorder. A communication disorder is an impairment in the ability to express, understand, and/or process thoughts and information. These disorders range from minor nuisances to ones that render a person completely unable to speak or understand the speech of others. Communication disorders can result from strokes, mental deficiency, deafness, learning, anxiety and tension, muscular degeneration, tumors, and a host of other causes. Virtually any disorder or disease that can affect the muscles, brain, or nervous system of a person can affect the ability to communicate normally. Some problems with communication, especially those seen in childhood, are temporary and diminish or disappear because of maturation. Others are permanent aspects of a person's life. Many communication disorders are aspects of larger cognitive or neurological disorders, whereas others occur independently and are disorders unto themselves. Several prominent people have communication disorders, including the politicians and movie stars noted previously, and such disorders are frequently portrayed in the movies and on television and referred to in books. As will be discussed later, the way communication disorders are dealt with in literature and media becomes part of society's assumptions, beliefs, and prejudices about people with these disorders.

The Process of Communication

In the broadest sense, human communication is the act of sharing and exchanging information between people through a variety of ways such as talking, writing, and gesturing. Communication is a marvelous ability; being able to share thoughts and feelings with other people is a wonderful part of human life. Communication allows people to share their lives with one another. Without communication, business and industry would crawl to a halt, and society as we know it would not exist. Our ability to communicate through speech and language is the highest evolved function we have—a gift allowing us to cooperate, solve problems, and build and maintain relationships. In many ways, communication is the core of our existence. We are "talking animals." From our birth cry to our last words, we are born into a world of communication and spend a large part of our lives engaging in it. It occurs on playgrounds, classrooms, dining halls, coffee shops, courtrooms, libraries, and churches. Communication takes place on many levels. For example, we greet people by asking "How's it going?"—often never expecting an answer. This is a simple act of communication. On a more complex level, we may request a reply to a marriage proposal, provide justification for a salary increase, or pray to a deity. As will be discussed later, verbal communication is an intricate and interwoven cognitive, neurological, muscular, acoustic, and sensory process.

Verbal communication is a complex cognitive ability involving the highest mental functions. The physical requirements to make sound involve hundreds of muscles and neurological impulses: taking air into the lungs, compressing it, and shaping the airstream into speech sounds. These speech sounds are also acoustic energy—sound waves that radiate outwardly from our bodies. On the receiving end of verbal communication, hearing is one of our most important senses. It allows us to detect and make sense of the air vibrations. Finally, our ability to comprehend that which was spoken brings understanding to our lives. We tend to take all of this for granted because it is done naturally and easily; it is as natural as standing upright or breathing. We are born with the innate capacity to communicate, and we live our lives immersed in acts of communication.

To introduce the intricate, complex process of communication, it is helpful to describe the cognitive, neurological, muscular, acoustic, and sensory events in a typical conversation. Breaking down the process into its components, and describing them, shows the complexity and sophistication of the process. Suppose two college students, Nick and Andrea, have just met on the first day of classes. As they walk from a classroom, they decide to go to the student union for a cup of coffee. After waiting in line, they finally get their cups of expensive Italian coffee and sit down together at a small table. Their conversation begins with emotionally neutral remarks about crisp autumn weather, crowded buses, large classes, and demanding professors. As their interest in each other builds, the conversation turns to recent summer activities. They are surprised to find that they both have taken vacations to Yellowstone National Park. Let's explore Andrea's representation and formulation of her ideas, the way her brain automatically programs them into **speech acts,** and her physical production of the sounds of language. Her thoughts and feelings about Yellowstone National Park will be transformed into acoustic, mechanical, hydraulic, and electrochemical energy as they are transmitted, received, and understood by Nick.

In Andrea's mind, her mental concept of Yellowstone National Park is primarily made up of words and images, but her memory records other sensations as well. For example, she recalls the sounds of rushing mountain rivers and the putrid, sulfur smells of geysers. Nevertheless, in Andrea's mind, her memory of the visit to Yellowstone consists primarily of what she saw and her verbal thoughts about those images. Her concept of Yellowstone includes remembered images of large lakes; tall trees, some burned by devastating fires; huge mountains stretched to

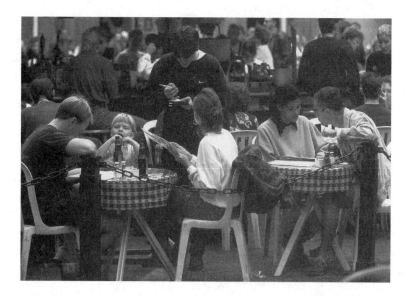

the Big Sky of Montana, Idaho, and Wyoming; Old Faithful; and bears, swans, beavers, ducks, moose, and elk. Her thoughts include inner-speech statements she makes to herself as she remembers the long traffic delays due to hundreds of tourists taking pictures of scavenging animals. Her thoughts jump to the narrow roads, expensive hot dogs and hamburgers at quaint park restaurants, and her fantasy of someday being a park ranger. Her recollections of wonderful summer days of camping, fishing, and sightseeing are coded into the structure and form of the English language, which Nick will decode. Had Andrea and Nick been Spanish, Japanese, Hopi, French, or Italian, the language code would be different, but the words would still carry the meaning.

Of course, the goings on in Andrea's "mind" are not easily discussed in terms of what is happening in her "brain." This dichotomy is sometimes called the *brain–mind leap*. The image and word thoughts in Andrea's mind are neurological impulses in the **gray** and **white matter,** shooting to and from the hemispheres, lobes, and deep structures of her brain. They result in brain waves, emissions, and magnetic characteristics, which can be detected and measured by sophisticated and sensitive machines. Thoughts and memories are electrical discharges and chemical reactions in Andrea's brain that become images and words in her mind.

Once Andrea's thoughts are coded into her native language, they go to an area of her brain that is involved with programming them into sounds and words. Here, the many movements required by the muscles and structures of her body to turn thoughts into the physical act of speech are planned. Andrea's brain automatically programs each sound, syllable, word, and sentence about Yellowstone National Park. The necessary air support, vocal cord vibrations, and tongue and lip movements to make the sounds of speech are planned, much the same way a computer's software is programmed to execute certain tasks. Then, in an instant, the speech plan is made a reality, and Andrea's body begins to utter the words *Yellowstone National Park*.

To create the sounds and words, Andrea's diaphragm contracts and her chest walls expand to allow the air in the coffee shop to rush into her lungs. Controlled relaxation and contraction of the muscles of breathing cause the compressed air flowing from her lungs to vibrate her vocal cords and to make sounds in her mouth. Her voice makes the sounds with just the right loudness to carry over the noise in the coffee shop. Fine movements of the muscles in her voice box adjust the pitch of her utterances to give interest and meaning to them. Andrea's tongue quickly moves from one position to another in her mouth, and her lips open and close, shaping the airstream into the 44 sounds of the English language. Her soft palate bounces up and down, allowing air through the nasal chambers to give the proper **nasality** to the three nasal sounds in English: /m/, /n/, and "ng" (as in tho<u>ng</u>). All the time that speech sounds are being made, her eyes, lips, hands, and body accentuate them with nonverbal descriptive and reinforcing gestures. During speech, Andrea's hands describe Old Faithful's burst of heat and energy, and her eyes, lips, and fist reinforce her passion in watching one of nature's marvels. Her speech and body movements reflect the excitement of her trip to Yellowstone.

The movements made by Andrea's vocal cords, lower jaw, tongue, lips, teeth, and soft palate create disruptions in the air. The billions and billions of air molecules surrounding her and Nick vibrate in response, Andrea's interrupting and constricting of the airstream in her throat, nose, and mouth. The molecules of air vibrate, creating sound waves that move outward from her. Like waves of water, sound waves are high and low points of pressure that radiate away from the source of their disruptions. Because Nick's eardrum is in direct contact with the molecules of vibrating air, it is also set into motion. This vibration of Nick's eardrum directly corresponds to the energy disruptions caused by Andrea's speech mechanism. Nick's eardrum begins vibrating with the timing, frequency, and force of the oscillating air molecules linking Andrea's speech mechanism to his ear. Vibrating air is the medium connecting the speaker and listener in the student union.

Attached to Nick's sensitive eardrum are three small bones called the **ossicles.** Because his eardrum is vibrating, they too vibrate, amplifying and transforming the acoustic energy into mechanical energy. Attached to the bones of his middle ear is a fluid-filled structure called the **cochlea.** Here, the vibrations that are Andrea's thoughts and ideas about Yellowstone are transformed into hydraulic energy. The fluid in his cochlea vibrates at a frequency and force that corresponds to the source of the vibrations. Within the cochlea are nerve fibers. When the fluid movement and pressure reach certain magnitudes or thresholds, electrochemical impulses travel up Nick's nervous system. Nick's brain allows certain auditory signals coming from the auditory nerve to be perceived while ignoring others such as the clink and clank of utensils, overhead music, and conversations of student union patrons.

Those neurological signals corresponding to the acoustic vibrations created in Andrea's throat and mouth now enter the receptive language center of Nick's brain. Here, Andrea's words about fishing, geysers, bears, and elk are decoded. Nick deciphers the grammar and syntax of the message. He automatically searches his memory for the meaning of her words. His experiences with fishing, geysers, bears, and elk are recalled as he listens to Andrea describe her adventure. Images and verbal associations come to mind. Of course, Nick's experiences with fishing, geysers, bears, and elk are not exactly the same as Andrea's. Thus, communication about them becomes the interpreting and sharing of associations. Andrea's thoughts, memories, experiences, and emotions about Yellowstone are not "placed" in Nick's mind. There is no direct neurological link between speaker and listener where thoughts are sent and received. In verbal communication, words carry the potential of meaning from speaker to listener.

Two college students sit in a restaurant on the first day of classes. To other patrons they simply appear to be enjoying good coffee and company. Yet, on a deeper level, what really is happening is the complex and intricate process of verbal communication. Andrea's thoughts are easily, rapidly, and automatically **encoded** into language. The grammar, syntax, and semantics of the English language are sent to the motor speech programming center of her brain where the program for the physical acts necessary to produce speech are created. There, her thoughts are programmed so that the muscles of her body can make them into speech sounds. In her lungs, air is compressed and, as it is expelled, her vocal cords, lower jaw, tongue, lips, and palates shape it into speech sounds. Acoustic energy radiates from her head and causes the molecules of air in the room to vibrate. Nick's eardrum vibrates in concert with the air molecules, as do the bones in his middle ear. The mechanical energy in the middle ear is transformed into hydraulic energy when the fluid-filled cochlea vibrates, setting off neurological impulses. Some impulses are ignored while others enter the receptive language center of Nick's brain. There, Andrea's messages are decoded and associations made with Nick's existing semantic references. The two people share thoughts and feelings about a summer's adventure in Yellowstone National Park. Through this marvelous process, they create a bridge to each other's consciousness and embark on a relationship that will be nurtured and maintained by communication.

Categories of Communication Disorders

Before discussing literature, media, and the social status of people with communication disorders, understanding the multiple ways communication disorders are classified is necessary. This section is an overview of major communication disorders (Table 1.1) and the way that they are typically referred to in literature and media. Three general classification methods are applicable to both children and adults.

The first method of classifying communication disorders is by listing them according to the *diseases* and *disorders* that can cause them. The list of diseases and disorders is extensive. For example, diseases such as Parkinsonism, multiple sclerosis, and muscular dystrophy can affect the brain and nervous system, resulting in problems making speech sounds and even the complete inability to speak. Cancers that affect the speech mechanism can result in slurred speech and loss of voice. When strokes and tumors affect the speech and language centers of the brain, they can result in difficulty remembering words or how to place them correctly into sentences. They can also impair the ability to understand the speech of others. When a head trauma damages a person's brain, the result can be impairments with thinking and memory, resulting in communication disorders. Birth defects such as cerebral palsy and cleft palate can also cause communication disorders. Virtually any disease or disorder that affects the brain, nervous system, and muscles of the speech mechanism can result in communication disorders. In the media, communication disorders are often referred to by the diseases and disorders that cause them.

The second method of classifying communication disorders is by the individual *processes of communication* that are affected. The individual processes of communication are the mental and physical aspects that comprise communication and were discussed in the Nick and Andrea example. Communication disorders can be categorized according to the aspect of communication that is disrupted. For example, some disorders involve the difficulty using and understanding language, and these disorders can be classified as primarily *receptive* or *expressive language impairments*. Communication disorders such as stuttering are disruptions in how smoothly or easily sounds, words, and phrases are spoken. These are called *fluency disorders*. When the vocal cords are impaired in their ability to vibrate normally, the result is a *voice disorder*. Some speech disorders involve how precisely sounds are made or whether one sound is substituted for another or omitted altogether; disorders in this category are called *articulation disorders*.

TABLE 1.1   *Categories of Communication Disorders*

Disorder	*Description*
Fluency disorders	Disruption in the rhythm and flow of speech (stuttering and cluttering)
Voice disorders	Disrupted vocal cord vibration and/or resonance characteristics of the neck and head
Articulation and phonology disorders	Disruption in production of speech sounds by the articulators; disruption of the sound system of a language
Language disorders in children	Impaired or absent communication abilities through the use of words or other symbols occurring during the developmental period
Hearing loss and deafness	Absent or partial hearing
Motor speech disorders and dysphagia	Impairments of respiration, phonation, articulation, resonance, and/or prosody (apraxia of speech and the dysarthrias); swallowing disorders
Aphasia in adults	Impaired or absent communication abilities through the use of words or other symbols occurring in adulthood
Communication disorders resulting from dementia	Disordered or absent communication abilities associated with generalized intellectual impairment
Communication disorders resulting from head and neck injuries	Disordered or absent communication abilities associated with traumatic brain or neck injuries

The third method of classifying communication disorders is by the *site of neurological or muscular damage* that occurs and the resulting type of paralysis or muscular impairment. This method of classification is often used by professionals for neurologically based communication disorders. For example, some communication disorders are a result of spastic muscles that occur when certain tracts in the brain and nervous system are damaged. Other communication disorders occur because of flaccid muscles of speech production. Damage to the parts of the brain responsible for coordination of speech movements results in certain types of communication disorders. Hearing loss and deafness can be classified by the site where the hearing mechanism is damaged.

Although each of the classification systems is used in different contexts to classify communication disorders, using a combination of them provides more detail and clarity. Combining the approaches is more descriptive and presents a realistic basis with which to understand them. The general public typically uses all three classification methods. A person might refer to someone as having the speech characteristics of Parkinsonism or multiple sclerosis, defining the communication disorder by the disease that caused it. A person could also refer to the process of communication that is impaired by commenting that a singer has a voice disorder. The colloquial phrase of calling someone's behavior "spastic" is an instance where the disorder is defined by the effects of damage to the brain, nervous systems, and muscles. The following classification is a combination of the systems and reflects the way communication disorders are discussed in this text.

Fluency Disorders

Fluency refers to the rhythm and flow of connected speech. It is the ease with which sounds, syllables, words, and phrases are made during connected speech. Most speech is occasionally produced with hesitations, repetitions, and other disruptions in its smooth flow. These are normal and typical of most speakers. All speakers have these normal **nonfluencies,** especially when they are hurried or excited. A fluency disorder is when the rhythm and flow of speech deviates significantly from the norm. Stuttering is the primary fluency disorder. In **stuttering,** excessive and/or abnormal **repetitions, prolongations,** and **hesitations** interrupt the person's speech. Besides the excessive **dysfluencies,** many people who stutter struggle with their speech, and they often grimace and show other body indications that they are forcing speech. Another type of fluency disorder is **cluttering,** whereby the person has trouble organizing thoughts into rhythmic utterances. It is a verbal thought-organization disorder. People who clutter often have short attention spans and stop and start over abruptly during speech. They typically talk rapidly, frequently revising their utterances, and appear to be impeded in their ability to easily and sequentially express their ideas. Whereas most people who stutter are aware of their dysfluencies, people who clutter typically appear unaware of their speech disorder. At present, the cause or causes of fluency disorders are controversial issues in communication sciences and disorders.

Voice Disorders

The term **voice** refers to sound produced by the vibration of the vocal cords, which are sometimes called vocal folds. The vocal cords are the source of sound produced in the voice box (larynx) when they vibrate. The frequency and force of their vibrations result in **pitch** and **loudness** characteristics of a person's voice. The **quality** of a person's voice is determined by the relationship between vocal cord vibration and the resulting resonance characteristics of the neck and head. This relationship between vocal cord vibration and head and neck resonance gives people their distinctive voice qualities. Voice disorders are caused by diseases, growths and blisters on the vocal cords, trauma, paralysis and weakness of the muscles responsible for vocal cord movement, and/or psychologically based problems affecting vocal cord vibration. A person has a voice disorder when his or her voice deviates significantly from the norm, with regard to pitch, loudness, or quality. Because of the relationship of resonance to voice quality, this category of communication disorders can also include disorders in which a person talks with too much or too little nasality. Cleft palate is an example of a birth defect that can affect resonance and voice quality.

Articulation and Phonology Disorders

Articulation refers to the production of speech sounds by the articulators: tongue, teeth, lower jaw, lips, and palate. The articulators are sometimes called the organs of speech. They are structures in the mouth that shape the compressed air coming from the lungs into meaningful sounds of a language. **Phonology** is one aspect of language and includes the rules by which the sounds are combined and articulated. A person with an articulation disorder may have difficulty producing one or several speech sounds. She might omit, substitute, or distort speech sounds. For example, an **omission** of a sound would occur when a person says "abbit" for "rabbit." She has omitted the /r/ sound beginning. A **substitution** of the /w/ sound for the /r/ sound occurs when the person says "wabbit" for "rabbit." A **distortion** occurs when a sound is produced indistinctly and inaccurately or it is clouded by too much nasality. Sometimes, articulation is impaired when there is a problem with the phonological rules relating to the combination and structure of the sounds of speech. When a person has difficulty producing many sounds, his speech might be so disordered as to render it unintelligible. Intelligibility is clinically defined in the field of speech–language pathology as the ability of a speaker to make himself understood by a listener; unintelligibility is usually measured in percent.

Language Disorders in Children

Language refers to communication through the use of words or other symbols. Language is also an important part of verbal thought, also known as *inner speech.* Language has multiple **modalities,** meaning that there are several avenues of language expression and understanding. The modalities are speaking, auditory comprehension, reading, writing, and gestures. A child with a language disorder may have difficulty with all or part of language including grammar, syntax, vocabulary, the social use of language, and using communication effectively. Children with language disorders often have difficulty sequencing ideas, describing events, following directions, understanding the speech of others, and socializing. There are many causes of language disorders in children, including birth defects, learning disabilities, diseases, mental deficiency, head traumas, environmental deprivation, and isolation from others during the speech and language development period.

Hearing Loss and Deafness

Hearing loss can range from a mild impairment in which the person's hearing is slightly less acute to **deafness** in which the person's hearing is nonfunctional. Hearing loss ranges from slight to profound, depending on how much residual hearing exists. A **hard-of-hearing** person has some hearing, usually with the help of hearing aids. A person may be born without some or all of the sense of hearing, or she may lose it later in life. The effect that hearing loss has on a person's speech and language abilities is in great part determined by when the hearing loss occurred. When hearing loss occurs in children during the speech and language development period, it can have dramatic effects on their ability to communicate. The effects of hearing loss on speech and language development also depend on what caused it, the severity of the hearing loss, and whether it involves high, middle, or low frequencies in the range of human hearing.

Motor Speech Disorders and Dysphagia

There are two categories of **motor speech disorders:** apraxia of speech and the dysarthrias. Motor speech refers to the motor aspects of the brain and nervous system that cause movements. Apraxia of speech is difficulty in programming the speech mechanism. Mild apraxia of speech is usually a nuisance in which the person has problems getting his mouth to make sounds or words; the person struggles with the correct programming of the utterances but is usually successful in verbally expressing himself. Severe apraxia of speech can render the person unable to communicate verbally because of the lack of the ability to program speech utterances. The **dysarthrias** are a group of neuromuscular disorders and are the result of damage to the brain, the nervous system, or the muscles of speech production. The speech patterns of patients with dysarthria depend on type of paralysis or movement problems affecting speech muscles.

Dysphagia is an impairment with the ability to chew and swallow food. Although it is not a communication disorder, the diagnosis and treatment of it have become a major part of the responsibilities of speech–language pathologists who are employed in medical settings. Dysphagia is a serious medical disorder and can be life threatening. Strokes, head traumas, and diseases are common causes of motor speech disorders and dysphagia.

Aphasia in Adults

Aphasia is a language disorder occurring primarily in adults. It can result from strokes, head injuries, and diseases that can damage the brain. Mild aphasia can result in occasional difficulties remembering the names of people and things and difficulty understanding complex expressions of other people. Severe aphasia can render a person unable to talk, read, write, and understand the speech of others. The ability to do math also involves language (some consider math the "universal language"). Aphasia can also eliminate a person's ability to perform and understand simple arithmetic. It can devastate relationships with family, friends, and business associates.

Communication Disorders Resulting from Dementia

The communication problems resulting from **dementia** include difficulty making speech sounds; problems with reading, writing, and arithmetic; impairments constructing sentences; and problems understanding the speech of others. These communication problems are associated with a generalized intellectual deterioration, and they often come on slowly. People with communication disorders resulting from dementia often have major problems with memory, judgment, and orientation. In severe cases, the person may be unable to communicate with loved ones and requires constant supervision.

Communication Disorders Resulting from Head and Neck Injuries

The communication disorders resulting from head injuries often result from memory deficits and disorientation. They are part of several symptoms of brain damage classified as **traumatic brain injuries** (TBIs). The communication disorders associated with TBI are sometimes called the language of confusion. Patients with severe head traumas often have major problems with memory, and their communication reflects their confusion. There are often behavior problems, too. Sometimes, when the speech and language centers of the brain are also damaged, aphasia and motor speech disorders are present, besides the confusion and memory deficits. Neck injuries sometimes result in communication disorders because the person cannot use and control her speech mechanism due to paralysis.

Incidence and Prevalence of Communication Disorders

Although communication disorders have been studied extensively, exact data about the number of people afflicted by them are difficult to obtain. The **incidence** of a communication disorder gives an idea of how many people have had it at some point in their lives, and the **prevalence** shows how many people currently have it (Guitar, 1998). With certain communication disorders, such as stuttering and childhood language disorders, these figures are highly variable for several reasons. First, many children outgrow their communication disorders. For example, both stuttering and lisping occur in some children, but either because of treatment or maturation, when they grow older, they do not present with the communication disorders. Second, in some instances, pinpointing exactly when a child has the disorder is difficult. Some disorders develop slowly. Particularly with stuttering, a child's self-report of when he started to stutter and when his parents noted its presence can differ greatly. Some parents misdiagnose normal nonfluencies as stuttering and thus believe the child is stuttering before the child feels that she is a stutterer. The third reason for widely differing incidence and prevalence figures in communication disorders concerns research methodology. Researchers who study communication disorders come from a variety of backgrounds. Speech and hearing scientists, linguists, psychologists, educators, physicians, and others study communication disorders, and they may have different standards for what constitutes a communication disorder. Because definitions differ so greatly, incidence and prevalence figures are highly variable.

The occurrences of communication disorders are skewed at both the younger and older ends of the human age continuum. Although most children easily learn sounds, words, grammar, and syntax, some youngsters do not acquire these abilities easily or completely. Many of these children are in special education programs. Some children may be in these programs only because of their communication disorder. Other children may have multiple special education needs including the communication disorder. Older adults are also susceptible to communication disorders because many diseases and disorders occurring in the elderly population also disrupt the ability to communicate. For example, strokes are more common in the later decades of life, and they often result in aphasia and motor speech disorders.

Although communication disorders are found more frequently in the young and elderly populations, some speech and hearing disorders occur in the middle years. People who experience automobile accidents, falls, or violent events sometimes suffer communication disorders. Additionally, certain diseases, such as multiple sclerosis, which can result in a speech pathology, frequently occur in people between the ages of 20 and 40.

In the United States and other industrialized countries, the prevalence of all communication disorders ranges between 5% and 10% (Ruben, 2000). There is a higher prevalence of communication disorders in children. The National Institute of Neurological and Communicative Disorders and Stroke (1988) reports that childhood speech and language disorders affect about 10–15% of school-age children. In the United States, hearing loss and deafness are the most common communication disorders (Public Health Service, 1994). In the elderly population, about 33% of people over the age of 65 years experience a hearing problem (National Center for Health Statistics [NCHS], 1988). According to Spahr and Malone (1998), approximately 15 million Americans have a swallowing disorder, which often occurs with major neurological disorders. Evaluation and treatment of swallowing disorders are part of the scope of practice for speech–language pathologists and they often occur with dysarthria, a neuromuscular speech disorder. Roughly 1 in 6 Americans have a communication disorder (Bello, 1995). Spahr and Malone (1998) report that "It is a rare family that does not have at least one close relative with a speech, language, or hearing problem."

Communication disorders are a significant economic loss to the United States, costing between $154 and $186 billion annually (Ruben, 2000). There are three aspects to be considered when discussing the economics of communication disorders. First, when a communication disorder prevents a person from entering the workforce or requires that an individual must leave it, a direct economic loss is associated with the goods or services that cannot be contributed to the gross national product. That person's contribution to society, business, and industry will never be fully realized. Sadly, that individual could have potentially discovered a medical cure for an illness, found a more efficient way of conducting business, or invented something to make life better for millions of people. Second, the cost to society in diagnosing and treating the communication disorder must be considered. Although these direct medical, psychological, and educational services create jobs, contribute to the goods and services of a country, and increase the tax base, they are expensive services and require a large financial commitment from individuals and their families. For many individuals and families, dealing with a communication disorder is a major financial burden. Third, many costs for the services provided to individuals with communication disorders are provided directly or indirectly by governmental programs and financially supported by taxes. There is a limit to the amount of taxes a society will bear, and services for people with communication disorders must compete with other tax-supported programs. The economics of communication disorders is likely to become more important in the future because the prevalence of communication disorders in the United States is likely to increase.

Particularly in the next 10 or 20 years, there will be more people with communication disorders. Spahr and Malone (1998) believe that the prevalence of communication disorders in the United States will increase for four reasons. First, because the population is increasing, there will be a growth in the number of people with communication disorders. Second, the population is also aging, and consequently, more elderly people will be susceptible to communication disorders resulting from age-related diseases and strokes. Third, more at-risk babies survive, often with a communication disorder. Compared to the past, fewer children and adults succumb to catastrophic accidents, and the survivors often have communication disorders. Finally, the scope of practice for speech–language pathologists has increased to encompass the evaluation and treatment of more disorders and disabilities. This increases the number of people in the population identified with communication disorders. Also, because of increased visibility (largely as a result of literature and media coverage), more people are aware of the services available to people with communication disorders and are motivated to seek out those services.

Since some 42 million Americans have communication disorders, it is not surprising that such disorders appear frequently in literature and the media. With the projected increase in the number of communication-disordered people, in the future there will likely be even more visibility in literature and media. Literature and media are powerful forces that shape society's attitudes. Explorations of how communication-disordered individuals are portrayed can provide insight into society's perceptions and treatment of people afflicted by them. It can cast light on attitudes and prejudices about these individuals. It can also provide a foundation for understanding their etiology, diagnosis, and treatment. Most important, the study of literature, media, and communication disorders provides an opportunity to dispel myths about these disorders and the people who have them.

History of the Perception and Treatment of People with Communication Disorders

Communication disorders have existed presumably since humans began to talk. References to communication disorders are found in early Egyptian, Greek, and Roman writing. Hippocrates described one speech disorder, probably aphasia, as "aphonos" and "anaudos" (Benton, 1981). Valerus Maximus (ca. A.D. 30) described a case of **alexia,** a reading disorder, that was of traumatic origin (Benton & Joynt, 1960). It is likely that Moses was afflicted with a speech disorder. In Exodus 4:10, there is a reference to Moses' communication problem: "And Moses said unto the Lord, O my Lord, I am not eloquent, neither heretofore, nor since thou hast spoken unto thy servant; but I am slow of speech and slow of tongue. And the Lord said unto him, Who hath made man's mouth? or who maketh the dumb, or deaf, or the seeing, or the blind? have not I the lord?"

Van Riper and Erickson (1996) note that disabled persons throughout history have been treated as intolerable nuisances, objects of mirth, pitiful beggars, and challenging problems and, more recently, as individuals who are challenged. Today, the tendency is to concentrate on what people with disabilities can do rather than emphasize their disabilities, but this has not always been the case.

As noted previously, communication disorders can occur alone, but they also frequently occur with other disabilities. In addition, many communication disorders occurring independently of other physical and mental disabilities place significant limitations on a person's ability to function in society. Thus, society's treatment of people with disabilities can also be generalized to those having communication disorders. Primitive societies tolerated no weakness in their numbers as they struggled for survival. The value of individual members was directly related to how well they could contribute to the safety and survival of the tribe or community.

Consequently, the treatment of people with disabilities has often been brutal. According to Van Riper and Erickson (1996), the inhabitants of ancient India cast the disabled into the Ganges, the Spartans hurled them from precipices, the Aztecs sacrificed them to the gods, and the Melanesians buried them alive. In ancient times, to be physically or mentally disabled was a major life-limiting event that cut dramatically into the person's quality of life and could result in survival obstacles. Many disabled were relegated to the life of beggars. In fact, some believe the word *handicapped* originated from the practice of disabled people "begging with a cap in hand" on street corners (Van Riper & Erickson, 1996). Their lives literally depended on the generosity of people who put money and food in their caps.

During the Middle Ages, disabled individuals were often thought to be possessed by supernatural forces. Their disabilities were believed to be caused by possession of evil forces or to be a manifestation of being out of harmony with nature. As a result, many people with disabilities were feared. Shamans, and other practitioners of magic, were called upon to treat the disorders by casting out the evil spirits and demons. Even today, some Native American religious ceremonies treat people with aphasia as having deviated from a path of harmony with nature (Huttlinger & Tanner, 1994). According to Van Riper and Erickson (1996), during the Middle Ages, people with disabilities did not dare to walk to the marketplace lest they be stoned. This fear and disdain of people with disabilities has persisted into modern times. During the 1940s the Nazis engaged in systematic extermination of people with disabilities as part of their misguided program of genetic cleansing. Large numbers of disabled were "euthanized" to rid their defects from the gene pool. Even recently in the United States, the sterilization of mentally impaired people was sometimes practiced (Van Riper & Erickson, 1996). These sterilization and mandatory birth control regulations were practiced officially as state laws or regulations of social service departments, or unofficially by coercing family members to comply.

People whose only impairment was a communication disorder have also been rejected by society. However, because communication disorders do not necessarily impose physical limitations, thus enabling the person to toil to the benefit of society, the rejection was less profound. As Ruben (2000) reports, "During most of human history a person with a communication disorder was not thought of being 'disabled.' The shepherds, seamstresses, plowmen and spinners of the past did not require optimal communication skills to be productive members of their society, as they primarily depended on their manual abilities" (p. 245). However, some people with communication disorders were also thought to be possessed by demons or simply looked upon as medical oddities. They, too, were objects of ridicule, relegated to a beggar's life, and often the butt of jokes. For food and shelter, some also depended on the kindness of strangers. As recently as the 1970s, some deaf individuals solicited money in public places, such as malls and supermarkets, by offering pencils or cards showing sign language and finger spelling. To the ire of many in the deaf community, some of these individuals were con artists using deafness as a means of solicitation. Ruben (2000) writes that "In the United Kingdom men with a hearing or a speech handicap were found more frequently in the lowest classes. They were also more likely to be out of the labor force—three times more likely for the hearing impaired and eight times more likely for the speech impaired than non-disabled persons" (p. 243). These sorts of employment trends occur in the United States as well.

Throughout history and even today, many people view people with communication disorders as being less intelligent, even retarded. Because communication disorders and mental deficiency sometimes occur together, some people view speech- and hearing-disabled individuals as being mentally deficient. According to this stereotype, because speech and language are mastered by young children, an adult with a communication disorder must be mentally deficient. The widespread myth that most people with communication disorders are retarded even applies to communication impairments that are not necessarily associated with mental deficiency, such as voice disorders, stuttering, cleft lip and palate, and articulation disorders.

This often unfounded assumption by the general public that people with communication disorders have low intelligence involves negative reactions to such words as *retarded*, *mentally disabled*, *challenged*, *alternately abled*, and *differently abled*. Today, many people object to those words because of their negative connotations. There is no consensus on a term or terms that are acceptable to denote people with low intelligence. For example, during the acquisition and developmental reviews for this book, reviewers took issue with the words used to indicate people with low intelligence. Unfortunately, this lack of a consensus for a politically correct word for people with low intelligence results in many words being offensive to someone or some group of activists. The names given to people with low intelligence do not negate their many and varied positive mental, physical, and personality attributes. These types of semantic issues have been around since the sixteenth century and earlier, and as Shakespeare remarked, "What's in a name? That which we call a rose/By any other name would smell as sweet."

Recent advances in science, education, and medicine have brought about more accurate perceptions and ethical treatment of people with disabilities. Unfortunately, scientific research conducted in the nineteenth century and the early twentieth century often viewed people who had communication disorders as medical or psychological oddities. Early scientific papers on communication disorders addressed the subjects' unusual symptoms, and theories were advanced about the neurological basis to them. Rehabilitation, quality-of-life issues, and adaptation of the patient to the disorder was largely ignored in these early scientific writings. The history of aphasia is replete with studies concentrating only on its neurology and ignoring the psychological and social implications of this major and potentially devastating communication disorder (Tanner, 2003). Early learning theories of communication disorders, those advanced in the early to middle twentieth century, sometimes portrayed these individuals as being lazy, having weak wills, and simply needing discipline. For example, during the late 1800s and early 1900s, stuttering was viewed as a bad habit, akin to biting fingernails. It was seen as a nervous reflex, a result of poor learning or a weak constitution, and was considered treatable with verbal punishment or a good flogging.

In the early part of the twentieth century, medical treatments of communication disorders sometimes made the cure worse than the disorder. For a time, some surgeons routinely cut the tongue muscles to cure stuttering (Van Riper, 1973). In addition, lisping and other articulation disorders were surgically treated by cutting the lingual frenulum, a tissue running from the bottom of the tongue to the lower jaw. Similar misguided and unsuccessful surgical remedies for communication disorders have persisted. As recently as the 1990s, some surgeons severed the laryngeal nerves of patients in an attempt to cure spastic voice disorders. Throughout history, dangerous and even lethal potions have been used to treat everything from stuttering to Tourette syndrome. *Tourette syndrome* is a neurological disorder resulting in tics, grunts, barks, and, in some patients, uncontrolled swearing. (Tourette syndrome is discussed in Chapter 7.) Even today, some individuals with anxiety and tension-based communication disorders use over-the-counter herbs that claim to help achieve relaxation and confidence. These medicinal herbs do *not* have the quality control of prescription medications and can have serious side effects.

Scientific approaches to the treatment of people with communication disorders began in the 1930s and 1940s with the development of university programs to educate and train "speech correctionists." The first major program was at the University of Iowa, and many other colleges and universities in the Midwest soon developed similar academic and clinical programs. Today, most major U.S. colleges and universities have undergraduate and graduate training programs in communication sciences and disorders. These departments go by several names including Speech–Language Pathology and Audiology, Speech and Hearing

Sciences, Communication Sciences and Disorders, and Communication Disorders. They are housed in colleges of health professions, arts and sciences, education, communications, or medicine.

Training programs in speech–language pathology and audiology often evolved from existing speech and drama, speech communication, or education programs. This was a natural academic evolution. Regardless of the names the departments go by or the colleges in which they are housed, all these programs have one thing in common: They rely on the scientific method to advance diagnostic and treatment methods for people with communication disorders. In the United States, the national association that represents speech–language pathologists and audiologists is the American Speech-Language-Hearing Association (ASHA). One of the purposes of ASHA is to advocate for the rights and interests of persons with communication disorders.

The American Speech-Language-Hearing Association

The American Speech-Language-Hearing Association has been in the forefront in representing and advocating for people with communication disorders. Founded in 1925, ASHA is a nonprofit organization and has approximately 100,000 members. For more than 75 years, ASHA has encouraged the scientific study of the process of human communication and has championed the rights and interests of people with communication disorders. ASHA advocates for the rights of the communication disordered by strong and effective lobbying efforts at the national level and assists many state speech and hearing associations with their advocacy issues. In addition, ASHA publishes brochures and pamphlets that present people with communication disorders in a positive light. ASHA also sets and enforces ethical standards for practicing speech–language pathologists and audiologists and has established high standards for training programs. One of its main functions is to certify practitioners who treat people with communication disorders. Currently, ASHA provides two certifications: (1) speech–language pathology and (2) audiology (these are discussed in detail in Chapter 11).

The propagation of scientific research into communication disorders is one of the major activities of ASHA. The association funds research, publishes several journals and magazines, and sponsors an annual national convention. By setting high clinical standards, advocating for the rights of the communication-disordered population, propagating scientific research, and lobbying, ASHA has been in the vanguard of the ethical treatment of people with communication disorders. The National Student Speech-Language-Hearing Association (NSSLHA) is affiliated with ASHA, and most colleges and universities have chapters of this organization, providing students an avenue for addressing on-campus issues and concerns regarding communication disorders.

Social Characteristics of Those with Communication Disorders

What is the current social status of people with communication disorders, and what factors affect it? Like millions of Americans who share a common religion, race, ethnicity, or sexual preference, people with communication disorders form a large social group with whom its members identify. They are a diverse group of people whose commonalities include delayed language, misarticulated speech, loss of voice, stroke-related amnesia for words, hearing impairment, cleft palate, and a host of other specific communication disorders. With few exceptions, members of this group are considered inferior to the mainstream population with regard to communication. Many people with communication disorders have been socialized into a belief that their communication is substandard rather than nonstandard. *Substandard* means that their communication abilities are below the norm, and *nonstandard* means that their communication abilities are simply different. Substandard connotes "inferior" and "less than," whereas nonstandard connotes "unconventional" and/or "atypical." Many people with communication disorders have had a disability all their lives and have spent years in remediation and rehabilitation programs trying to improve their communication abilities. Some have adopted the label "communication challenged" to refer to themselves; the assumption inherent in that label is that they should simply "try harder" to be like the mainstream population with regard to communication. Professionals have spent years helping them overcome their disorder and little if any time helping them to accept or even revel in their differences. Particularly with children, they have spent most of their lives in special education programs playing "catch-up" with their peers.

Many communication disorders in this social group involve fundamental disruptions in essential abilities to communicate. Because of mental deficiency, autism, strokes, learning disabilities, laryngeal cancers, head traumas, and the like, people in this group are significantly communication impaired or even incapable of communicating. Their communication disorders are obstacles to happy, productive lives and the richness to living that only functional unimpaired communication can bring. However, many people in this social group simply have obtrusive or cosmetic communication disorders; their communication stands out from the norm. For example, some people lisp, distort sounds, or stutter, and although their speech is perfectly intelligible to their listeners, they strive for "normal" communication. Because of standards set by professionals, literature and media stereotypes, society's prejudices, or their parents' or spouses' wishes, they endeavor to be just like others in articulation, motor speech, and fluency. Even though they have functional communication, they have accepted the belief that their communication differences are laughable, intellectually inferior, and indications of lower socioeconomic status. Many feel embarrassment and shame at their different speech patterns, even though they are functionally able to communicate; in this sense, their beliefs and feelings are products of society.

Why has society continued to consider these conspicuous patterns of speech substandard, rather than another example of human diversity and communication that is simply different? Why are these beliefs thoroughly entrenched in society? Part of the answer lies in the power of speech to communicate **intelligence** and social status. Recently, members of the deaf community have addressed this issue. Some people in the deaf community feel abnormal and isolated from society, although they can communicate through sign language, which is a rich language unto itself. Others take pride in their deafness and have formed a strong community. (See Chapter 6 for a discussion of the social implications of deafness.) In a society striving to recognize and accept diversity among its members, many people with obtrusive communication disorders are relegated to inferior positions, negatively stereotyped, and feel the brunt of social and vocational discrimination because of their atypical communication.

Many have been relegated to a substandard social position simply because their speech is different. This group of people with communication disorders has not participated in many of the gains in social equality made by other social groups over the past four decades. Perhaps the reason why people with obtrusive communication disorders have not become socially and politically active in changing societal views about their differences is because of the nature of their nonconformity. Political and social activism are fundamentally acts of communication, and this social group is limited in this basic requisite.

Group Size, Power, and Status

The number of people with communication disorders is large enough to constitute a social group and, as already noted, one that has an inferior position. With around 42 million communication-disordered individuals in the United States, it is one of the largest groups of people with disabilities. The largest number of people within this group are those with a hearing loss or deafness, and most of them are adults. People with speech, voice, and language disorders is the second largest subgroup, with most of them being children. The fact that the subgroup of people with hearing loss and deafness is made up primarily of older Americans gives them more power and status within society than the other groups. This group is mostly made up of people who previously had normal hearing and were able to establish power and status before their hearing became impaired; they are not likely to have had a communication disorder until their later years. Those with speech, voice, and language disorders, as a group, tend to be children, dependent adolescents, and adults with disabilities. Often this group has a low earning potential, a low socioeconomic status, and less economic power than other groups. Even smaller subgroups, such as those individuals with orofacial anomalies, stuttering, aphasia, or articulation disorders, have large enough numbers to constitute a viable social group with formal and informal structures. Formal structures include organized support groups for individuals with communication disorders and their families. There are support groups for almost any type of communication disorder, from people who have stuttering or aphasia to people with Tourette syndrome or multiple sclerosis. The formal structures of these groups also include national, state, and local associations, which lobby and advocate for their interests. Informal structures include loosely knit groups of people with communication disorders and their families, who socialize with each other. Primarily because they share the common thread of a communication disorder, these individuals and their families often interact with one another at sports events, school-related activities, and social gatherings and in Internet chat rooms.

Social Visibility and Cohesiveness

One factor that characterizes the social group of people with communication disorders is the visibility of the disorders. Unlike many other disabilities, communication disorders are not always readily apparent. Except for people with orofacial anomalies, Down syndrome, and other obvious disorders, most people with communication disorders appear normal until they engage in the act of communication. This lack of continuous visibility causes identification with other people with communication disorders to be irregular and communication dependent. Therefore, the cohesiveness of the group is reduced because of the lack of continuity of identification. The bonds of the group are not as strong because the members are separated from group identification during nonspeech activities. Many people with communication disorders only identify with other people with communication disorders during verbal activities. Unlike disabilities such as amputation and blindness, where the disability is easily identifiable as a physical or sight impairment, many people with speech and hearing disorders show their disorders only when attempting to communicate. A person with a stutter or lisp appears different from others only when she stutters or lisps. Consequently, there is only part of her **self-concept** related to stuttering and lisping. The severity of the types of communication disorders also influences the lack of cohesiveness. Communication disorders range from those that render a person mute to those that are barely perceptible differences in the way sounds are made. This causes some people to identify with the social group of people with communication disorders more than others.

Economic Disadvantage

As a rule, people with hearing or speech impairments tend to have lower incomes than people with normal communication abilities (Ruben, 2000). Effective communication has become a prerequisite for many present-day jobs. The best jobs, and those commanding the highest salaries, are those that require excellent communication abilities. The higher one goes up the corporate ladder, the more exclusively the job becomes one of communication. As a group, people with communication disorders are at an economic disadvantage.

In the twentieth century, a revolutionary change in the way people make a living came about. At the beginning of the 1900s, at least 80% of the U.S. labor force was primarily employed in tasks that depended on manual skills (Ruben, 2000). Their productivity was based on how much physical labor they could perform. Now, 62% of the U.S. labor force makes their living using skills based on their communication abilities. People in even the remaining farming and blue collar jobs depend on communication abilities to function effectively (Ruben, 2000). More and more jobs require good communication skills. As Ruben (2000) writes,

> The fitness of the person of the 21st century will be defined, for the most part, in terms of his or her ability to communicate effectively. Societal self-interest will drive an increased allocation of resources to optimize the communication ability of its population, for this is how society prospers. Communication disorders will be a major public health concern for the 21st century because, untreated they adversely affect the economic well-being of a communication-age society. (p. 245)

Social Inclusion through Accommodation

Political and technological accommodation brings people with communication disorders into mainstream social interaction. Political inclusion is a relatively recent event and largely the result of the 1990 Americans with Disabilities Act (ADA). From access to telecommunication systems to educational and vocational accommodations, this congressional act opened many aspects of society to the communication disabled. The Department of Justice's ADA Internet home page (see Appendix A) notes that census data, national polls, and other studies have documented that people with disabilities have inferior status in society and are severely disadvantaged educationally, economically, and vocationally. The ADA was created to prevent discrimination against individuals with disabilities in employment, housing, public accommodations, education, transportation, communication, recreation, institutionalization, health services, voting, and access to public services. The ADA has improved and will continue to improve the productivity and ultimately the social status and power of people with communication disorders.

Major advances in technology have also resulted in significant gains in accommodation. Most technological advances use silicon chips. Speech synthesizers, voice recognition devices, scanning instruments, digital hearing aids, communication boards, cochlear implants, and personal computers have increased social interaction and vocational opportunities for those with communication disorders. As a result, the productivity of people with communication disorders has improved, and this trend is expected to continue. It will result in greater socioeconomic gains, status, and power for the population of communication-disordered people. As Ruben (2000) comments,

> Today a fine high-school athlete—a great "physical specimen"—who has no job and suffers from poor communication skills is not unemployed, but, for the most part, unemployable. On the other hand, a paraplegic in a wheelchair with good communication skills can earn a good living and add to the wealth of society. For now and into the 21st century, the paraplegic is more "fit" than the athlete with communication deficits. (p. 245)

It follows, then, that as we enter the twenty-first century an able-bodied person with a communication disorder will be at a greater economic disadvantage than a paraplegic with good communication skills.

Social Perceptions and Stereotypes

How are people with communication disorders perceived? Social perceptions are based on judgments of fact and truth or on misinformation based on presumed traits. People's judgments may result from personal interaction and individual experiences with communication-disordered individuals; however, the greatest exposure many people have to the wide spectrum of communication disorders comes from literature and media. Beyond the experiences a person may have with an acquaintance, friend, or family member's particular communication disorder, the only exposure she may have to other disorders is through seeing their portrayal on television and in the movies or by reading novels containing characters who have such disorders.

Sometimes considerable difference exists between the portrayal of people with communication disorders in literature and media and what a person observes through personal and individual contacts. For example, rarely do movies about people with profound mental deficiencies or advanced dementia show the problems with toileting, grooming, and other aspects of personal hygiene. Apparently, television networks believe it is inappropriate to depict these aspects of disabilities in "afternoon specials" or during prime-time television.

However, many people with profound mental deficiency and advanced dementia do have problems with toileting, grooming, and personal hygiene. When there is a difference between actual and presumed traits, the observer experiences cognitive dissonance. *Cognitive dissonance* is defined here as the discrepancy between a person's perception of a stereotype and the actualization of a person who is labeled by the stereotype but does not fit the stereotyped perception. A person with a communication disorder can have many reactions and responses when confronted with public perceptions that are in conflict with the reality of her communication disorder. The most apparent reaction is an identity conflict. An *identity conflict* can occur when the person's concept of self with regard to the communication disorder is in conflict with society's beliefs about people with communication disorders. For example, if society falsely assumes that all individuals who stutter are dimwitted due to the way they are portrayed in movies and when a person who stutters knows that he does not fit that stereotype, the stutterer may feel uncomfortable and unable to express his intelligence purely as a function of societal repression. Stereotypes of communication-disabled people are usually broad and encompass all subgroups, and the result can be a general misconception of abilities and capabilities. When many examples of these conflicting views abound, and particularly when they occur during early self-concept development, they can have major effects on the identity of a person with communication disorders.

Impatience, ridicule, overt and covert rejection, and pity are common negative reactions to people with communication disorders. Because communication-disordered people often take longer to express themselves and/or understand others, they are frequently met with impatience, an increasingly common fact in our fast-paced society. Impatience can lead people to walk away midsentence or interrupt the speaker. Too often, people with communication disorders are subject to ridicule, or mockery, because of their speech impediment. Children are subjected to ridicule from their peers because of mild or severe communication disorders and the stigmas associated with them. An insensitive child will imitate a stutter or lisp to obtain laughter and approval from classmates. Speech disorders in adults violate societal norms. When an adult cannot easily or clearly give her address or telephone number, it is viewed as a lack of attention to societal expectations or a blatant disregarding of them. People ridicule and poke fun at things they do not understand. Televised situation comedies frequently use ridicule at the expense of a person with a hearing loss, lisp, stutter, or reduced intelligence, to make a joke. For example, during a situation comedy, when a character stutteringly tries to say something, another cast member may announce, "That's easy for you to say!" followed by a laugh track. This sort of ridicule is pervasive in our society and adds to the negative feelings that too many people with communication disorders are forced to live with. Communication-disordered people experience overt and covert rejection by family members, coworkers, and friends. Overt rejection is done openly, whereas covert rejection is subtle and disguised. An example of overt rejection is when a father interrupts a child and reminds him to stop being lazy with speech. Overt rejection specifically directed at stuttering was seen in the film *A Fish Called Wanda*. Covert rejection occurs when a hurried boss ignores what a stuttering employee is saying. Often, covert rejection is more detrimental and hurtful because it hides the intent and action of the person doing the rejecting. Consequently, there is no avenue for the person with the disability to confront it. Pity is a negative act for people with communication disorders. It solidifies feelings of inferiority in the disabled and creates a false sense of superiority in the mind of the pitying person. People with communication disorders usually just want acceptance of their disorder; they neither ask for nor want pity. Pity injures the recipient's self-esteem, albeit with good intentions. The role pity plays in people's perception of communication disorders was illustrated in the best-selling book and blockbuster movie, *Harry Potter and the Sorcerer's Stone*. The statement "Next to him, who would suspect p-p-poor, st-stuttering P-Professor Quirrell?" suggests that, because a person stutters, he could not be capable of bad deeds. Table 1.2 shows the negative reactions to communication disorders.

Literature, Media, and People with Communication Disorders

Literature and media have three functions in society: inform, entertain, and educate. Each function can affect the social status of communication-disabled people and society's **perception** of them. Literature and media have large audiences consisting of people from all strata of society. The audience is diverse, in that people from all walks of life read best sellers, watch television, and see movies. The role of literature and media in determining the social status of communication-disordered people is extremely important, especially in this age of information. Literature and media do a commendable job in educating and informing people about the various types of communication disorders. They inform their audiences about public figures who have communication disorders. They also educate their audiences to the nature, course, and symptoms of these disorders. They keep society knowledgeable about the causes, treatment, and cures for many disorders and diseases that plague humankind.

The print and electronic media are primarily involved in providing information. Newspapers and magazines have traditionally provided more in-depth coverage, although television news magazines now also provide detailed newscasts. For example, the Sunday newspaper insert *Parade* of January 6, 2002, had a cover article on actor Kirk Douglas and his stroke-related communication disorder. It has a huge circulation and examined Douglas's communication disorder and the way he and his family have coped with it (see Chapter 7).

TABLE 1.2 *Negative Reactions to People with Communication Disorders*

Reaction	Description
Impatience	Discourteous actions and comments to slow, labored, and impaired communication
Ridicule	Derision and mockery of impaired communication
Overt rejection	Explicit and open negative reactions to impaired communication
Covert rejection	Hidden and subtle negative reactions to impaired communication
Pity	Debasing and demeaning reactions to impaired communication, albeit with good intentions

The announcers and personalities in the electronic media usually have excellent communication abilities, speak standard American dialect, and thus set standards for unobtrusive speech. Not only do they inform, but they also provide examples of desirable communication abilities. Their credibility often depends on their communication abilities. For example, Walter Cronkite, a television news anchor, was once considered the "Most Trusted Man in America." This was due, in no small part, to his clear, concise articulation and strong, authoritative voice. Certainly other aspects contributed to his success as a newscaster, such as physical appearance, but his speech and voice were major factors in his credibility. It is doubtful that he would have had as successful of a career if he had a whiny voice or a lisp.

Books, films, television, and the Internet are powerful forces in educating a society. Books, from the Bible to college textbooks, are the oldest forms of educational material. Communication disorders are directly referred to in medical or educational books, to teach students about these disorders. They are also indirectly used to emphasize salient points about many disorders and diseases that have communication disorders as part of their symptoms. Films have used communication disorders for plot and character development since the arrival of movies with sound tracks, and frequently there has been an educational aspect to them. Audiences have learned about hearing amplification, speech synthesizers, sign language, mental deficiency, and other aspects of communication disorders by viewing these films. Television's widespread ability to educate society is well accepted. From The Learning Channel to the major networks, television functions to educate society. Television has indeed made the world a global village. The Internet is the most recent invention to serve an educational function for society. Home pages of people with communication disorders; Web sites for local, state, national, and international associations; and chat rooms—all provide an educational function in today's society.

When communication disorders are used to entertain people, literature and media get mixed reviews. Literature and media propagate stereotypes and also dispel myths about communication disorders. In movies and on television, speech pathologies, hearing loss, and deafness are frequently used as entertainment vehicles, primarily for their humor value. From situation comedies to novels, characters with communication disorders are often used for comic relief, whether it is an episode revolving around misinformation acted on by a hard-of-hearing person or a supporting character with an articulation disorder in a murder novel. Communication disorders are also used to add interest and humanity to a character. A deaf, mentally deficient, autistic, or lisping person in a major role of a film might be used to give dimension, depth, and uniqueness to personalities and plots. Part of the entertainment value of a film can be an actor's use of sign language and lip reading, as was seen in *Children of a Lesser God*. Mental deficiency and autism gave interest to the characters in *Forrest Gump* and *Rain Man*, and Leon Phelps, in *The Ladies Man*, lisps on virtually every word with an /s/ in it. His lisping in this movie gives him an unusual and unique persona. In a novel an author can develop a character around mental deficiency, as did John Steinbeck in *Of Mice and Men*. Communication disorders are frequently used in literature and media in an attempt to better entertain the audience.

Some have criticized Hollywood for portraying communication disorders in a humorous manner. Individuals and activist groups have condemned films where stuttering, mental deficiency, and other communication disorders were dealt with humorously. They have demanded that Hollywood either make certain communication disorders off-limits or portray them in a more positive way. This issue was recently addressed in *The ASHA Leader*, a publication of the American Speech-Language-Hearing Association:

> Hollywood sometimes portrays communication disorders in a humorous way, but this should not detract from its positive influences. Occasionally, Hollywood satirizes and pokes fun at all aspects of society: men, women, politicians, intellectuals, homosexuals, heterosexuals, saints, sinners and people who are overweight, underweight, bald, hairy, powerful, weak. With this in mind, is it correct to respond with outrage and demand that people with communication disorders be off limits to the sharp wit and witticisms of Hollywood? Would that not make us self-important and humorless? Would that response not further isolate people with communication disorders from mainstream society and provide fodder for even more extreme depictions? (Tanner, 2001a, p. 29)

Summary

Verbal communication is a complex cognitive, neurological, muscular, and acoustic process. The cognitive abilities include verbal thinking and putting thoughts into a language code that can be heard, decoded, and understood by other people. The neurological and muscular abilities include programming speech utterances and using the muscles of the body to make speech sounds. Speech is also sound waves that radiate outwardly from the speaker's body.

In industrialized countries as much as 10% of the population has a communication disorder, and these people form a large but diverse social group. Communication disorders range from those that are only a minor nuisance to debilitating ones that render a person mute and without the ability to understand the expressions of others. They can be caused by virtually any disease or disorder that can affect the brain, nervous system, and speech mechanism. Some communication disorders, like mild stuttering or a voice disorder, are only obtrusive or cosmetic, as opposed to disorders like multiple sclerosis, which can debilitate victims' speech mechanisms until their words are unintelligible. With cosmetic disorders, although speakers can effectively communicate, their speech stands out in a negative way. Historically, people with disabilities, including people who have communication disorders, have been misunderstood and treated poorly. Recently, there have been gains in the understanding and treatment of communication-disordered people. ASHA has been in the forefront in advocating for the rights and ethical treatment of people with communication disorders. Additionally, there has been more social inclusion due to technological and political advances.

Literature and media are powerful forces in informing, entertaining, and educating society. Their uses of and references to people with communication disorders have the power to create, eliminate, or reinforce stereotypes about this large population of people. Studying literature and media can provide a window into the lives of people with communication disorders and society's perception and treatment of them.

Study Questions

1. Besides those listed at the beginning of this chapter, give current examples of films, books, and public figures who have communication disorders.

2. What are the cognitive abilities involved in the process of communication?

3. Describe the speech programming activities that occur during verbal communication.

4. What function does respiration perform during the act of verbal communication?

5. Describe how humans produce voice.

6. Describe how humans articulate sounds.

7. List and briefly describe the categories of communication disorders used in this chapter.

8. Historically, how have people with communication disorders been treated?

9. What is the American Speech-Language-Hearing Association, and what functions does it perform?

10. In what ways are people with communication disorders at an economic disadvantage?

11. What role does communication play in the twenty-first century? How is this different from previous centuries?

12. In what two major ways have people with communication disorders been brought into society's mainstream?

13. What are some social perceptions, stereotypes, and reactions of people to communication disorders?

14. What are the three functions of literature and media in society and how do they relate to communication disorders?

15. What are your thoughts about the motion picture industry's portrayal of communication disorders? Do you think communication disorders should be used for humorous purposes?

Suggested Reading

Owens, R., Metz, D., & Haas, A. (2000). *Introduction to communication disorders: A life span perspective* (pp. 24–25). Boston: Allyn & Bacon. The authors provide a table showing major provisions of important federal legislation affecting people with communication disabilities.

Ruben, R. J. (2000). Redefining the survival of the fittest: Communication disorders in the 21st century. *Laryngoscope, 110:* 241–245. This article shows how most jobs now require effective communication. It also describes the economic impact of communication disorders.

Tanner, D. (2001). Hooray for Hollywood: Communication disorders and the motion picture industry. *ASHA Leader, 6*(6): 10. This article discusses several films that have characters with communication disorders.

Tanner, D. (2003). *The psychology of neurogenic communication disorders: A primer for health care professionals.* Boston: Allyn & Bacon. Read the short stories "Murder Challenged" and "Alternately-Abled" to learn about social stereotypes and people with communication disorders. Also, Chapter 1 provides a historical review of the social and psychological treatment of people with aphasia and related disorders.

Van Riper, C., & Erickson, R. (1996). *Speech correction* (9th ed., pp. 5–11). Boston: Allyn & Bacon. The authors give a brief summary of the history of the disabled.

2

Stuttering and Cluttering

Chapter Preview

Stuttering has existed since the beginning of recorded history. It is universal; it occurs in all languages and cultures. The cause or causes of stuttering have yet to be discovered. Some authorities believe that psychological problems cause or perpetuate stuttering. Other experts believe stuttering is simply a learned behavior. Currently, many scientists believe that stuttering is a physical irregularity and that genetics predispose a person to stuttering. There are many interesting aspects about this speech disorder, including the fact that most individuals who stutter can sing normally and that they seldom stutter when talking to nonthreatening audiences. Fortunately, stuttering can be prevented in most children who start to develop it. In this chapter suggestions are provided for parents and teachers to help prevent at-risk children from starting to stutter. Treatment strategies for stuttering are also presented. There is also a discussion of the portrayal of people who stutter in media and literature and the implications of this on society as a whole.

"An awkward tongue has molded my life," remarked Wendell Johnson, an early speech and hearing scientist, and someone who stuttered his whole life. Indeed, for many individuals, this speech disorder involves more than just occasional difficulties saying sounds and words. Stuttering affects their self-concept, personality, relationships with family and friends, and vocation. For other people, especially those with a mild problem, stuttering is just a nuisance.

Although some stuttering has a late onset, beginning in the teenage years or adulthood, in most cases stuttering begins in childhood. Stuttering can occur in children as young as 18 months but most often begins between the ages of 2 and 5 years (Guitar, 1998). The young child who finds herself unable to talk fluently has a strange feeling of verbal impotence. This panicky feeling of being out of control gradually builds as months and years of stuttered speech go by. At first, a few sounds or words are repeated or get blocked in the throat or mouth. As the disorder progresses, more and more sounds and words are stuttered, and the child begins to fear words themselves. And it seems, the harder that she tries to talk, the more difficult it becomes. The more the stuttering child tries to repair defective speech, the more frustrating speaking becomes. And worst of all, the more emotional or important the utterance, its propositionality, the more disrupted is the speech. **Propositionality** is the meaningfulness and amount of content in an utterance. Seeing peers talk easily, enjoying the act of communication without an impediment, only increases frustration. Sometimes, frustration turns to anger directed outward, other times, it is turned inward. Communication becomes not the easy enjoyable banter between friends but something dreaded and feared.

Rejection also fuels the fires of stuttering. The child watches cartoon characters that stutter and evoke laughter. All too soon, that same laughter is directed at him. Even loyal friends may laugh when he stutters to a clerk, teacher, or police officer. Children can be cruel, and it seems anyone who stutters is fair game for their demeaning jokes and hurtful remarks. A creative 9-year-old boy with a moderately severe stuttering problem put his feelings about rejection in a song (Tanner & Lafferty, 2001).

People Say Stupid Things
by Garrison Fawcett

People say stupid things,
I know why but they stink,
Makes me sad,
When they're bad,
I wish they would,
Be nice to me,
I wish they would,
Just go away,
Then I would have a better day

Chorus: Na na na na na

This is why people say,
Stupid things,
When they're mad,
They say stupid things.

This song is a clear picture of the difficulties that a stuttering child faces from peers. But other children are not the only source of frustration for a young stutterer. With the best of intentions, the child's parents often demand that she "try harder" to speak perfectly, but this only exacerbates the problem. Repeatedly, they remind her not to stutter, as though the stuttered words are due to nothing more than a lack of attention.

As the child grows into young adulthood, stuttering becomes a bigger part of his life. Stuttering amplifies the pangs of adolescence. He has the usual tortured angst of awkward teenage years, but with stuttering as an unwanted companion. Not only is there the stress of asking someone out on a date, but the stuttered words also add yet another dimension to this age-old ritual. Sometimes a prospective date's tolerance for stuttering becomes a major part of the romantic equation.

Stuttering contaminates the complexities of marriage and career. It can turn a sincere comment into something laughable. People, words, and situations are avoided because of the fear of stuttering. Navigating through a verbal society is complicated by stuttering. Feelings about stuttering can be as much a part of the disorder as the stuttering behaviors (Guitar, 1998). For millions of people who stutter, an awkward tongue is much more than a speech disorder.

Literature, Media, and Personality Profiles

Pearl Harbor

The film *Pearl Harbor* was released during Memorial Day weekend, 2001. Written by Dick Clement, Ian La Frenals, and Randal Wallace and directed by Michael Bay, it recounts the events immediately before and after the destruction of the U.S. Navy's Pacific Fleet while docked at the Pearl Harbor Naval Station in Hawaii. This film is noted for its special effects depicting the early morning sneak attack by the empire of Japan's air force on December 7, 1941.

One of the supporting characters is Red Winkle, a pilot who stutters. He is played by Ewen Bremner. Red is involved in a love affair with one of the nurses who is stationed at a hospital in Pearl Harbor. In this movie Red's stuttering is tied to anxiety. When asked if he stutters all the time, he reports, "Only when I'm nervous." Throughout the movie his stuttering appears during anxious periods but is conspicuously absent during most of the actual attack. One of the characteristics of his stutter is a nasal snort. A *nasal snort* is the substitution of the /n/ sound for another one during the moment of stuttering. There is an audible snorting noise during speech. Red displays this nasal snort while struggling to talk. Stuttering gives the character a likeble, vulnerable personality and provides comic relief from the tension associated with the events that prompted the United States to enter World War II.

The Howard Stern Show: *Stuttering John*

The Howard Stern Show is one of the country's most popular syndicated radio programs. It consists of a typical talk-radio format, with Robin Quivers providing support and backup for the outrageous Howard Stern. Celebrities and other guests are interviewed, and Stern is considered to be one of the most entertaining interviewers in media. Many of his guests reveal bizarre sexual behaviors or encounters. *The Howard Stern Show* is famous for its controversial content.

One of the personalities on *The Howard Stern Show* is John Melendez. "Stuttering John" is responsible for answering phones, screening calls, and doing errands. Stern and other members of the staff castigate and criticize him. They are not shy about taunting him because of his stuttering problem. Stuttering John is notorious for his celebrity interviews, which consist of brash, personal, and offensive questions asked with his stuttered speech. Stuttering John has recorded an album entitled *Everybody's Normal But Me*.

One Flew Over the Cuckoo's Nest

This classic film, an adaption of Ken Kesey's novel by the same name, won five Academy Awards in 1976. The film is a treatise on personal freedom and mental institutionalization. Jack Nicholson plays Randle Patrick McMurphy, an inmate of a psychiatric hospital. Louise Fletcher plays the role of Nurse Ratched, a cold, arrogant, and indifferent nurse. Billy Babbitt (Brad Douriff) is a young, awkward inmate with a severe stuttering problem. Toward the end of the movie, the inmates have an all-night party. After a sexual encounter, Babbitt's speech is remarkably fluent. However, the next day, as Babbitt begs Nurse Ratched not to tell his mother about the sexual encounter, his stuttering gets progressively worse. The film associates sexual frustration with stuttering.

My Cousin Vinny

This comedy-drama is about New York City lawyer Vinny Gambini, played by Joe Pesci. He and his brazen girl friend (Marisa Tomei) travel to the rural South to defend his cousin, Bill Gambini (Ralph Macchio), and his friend, Stan Rothenstein (Mitchell Whitfield). They are falsely accused of murdering a convenience-store clerk. Rothenstein hires a lawyer, Pendleton, who stutters. In one humorous scene, Austin Pendleton stutters in the courtroom, barely able to complete a sentence, let alone keep Rothenstein from a death sentence.

Warner Bros. Cartoon Character: Porky Pig

Porky Pig is perhaps the best-known stutterer among the baby boom generation. Also, he is many present-day children's first experience with the humorous portrayal of stuttering because Warner Bros. cartoons are widely available on tapes and on cartoon television networks. Most people are familiar with the popular portly pig concluding a cartoon episode by uttering the famous broken words "Th, th, th, th, that's all folks!" One of the most notable characteristics of his stuttering pattern is **circumlocution,** which is the substitution of an alternative word for a stuttered one. For example, Porky might substitute the more easily produced "bye" for the stuttered one, "night," when bidding farewell: "Good ni, ni, ni, uh . . . Goodbye." In the cartoons, much of the humor revolves around Porky's inept efforts to accomplish household tasks and to interact with other cartoon characters, especially his girlfriend, Petunia Pig.

The Cowboys

This classic 1972 film is about a rancher, Will Anderson, played by legendary actor John Wayne, who takes 11 boys on a cattle drive. During the drive, Anderson is killed by the antagonist Asa Watts (Bruce Dern). The youngsters are required to finish the cattle drive without benefit of their adult leader. It is a coming-of-age film about young men in the 1800s. One of the young cowboys is "Stuttering Bob," played by Sean Kelly. In the film, the screenwriter associates repressed anger and hostility with stuttering. Freely expressing anger and frustration at the intimidating John Wayne cures Stuttering Bob's speech disorder. The film attempts to make a serious statement about the cause and treatment of stuttering.

Mel Tillis

Country singer, television personality, and actor Mel Tillis is well known for his stutter, which has become his trademark. To the public, one of the most interesting aspects of Tillis's speech disorder is that he can sing without stuttering. He comments about it on his home page:

> The word began to circulate around Nashville about this young singer from Florida who could write songs and sing, but stuttered like hell when he tried to talk. The next thing I knew I was being asked to be on every major television show in America. To name a few: The Johnny Carson Show, The Merv Griffin Show, The Mike Douglas Show, The Dinah Shore Show, The David Letterman Show and The Phil Donahue Show. You name it, and I was on it. From there, I went on to make thirteen movies. Some of the more familiar ones are: "Smokey and the Bandit," "Every Which Way But Loose," "The Villain," and "Uphill All the Way."

The Sixth Sense

The Sixth Sense, released in 1999, stars Haley Joel Osment as Cole Sear and Bruce Willis as Dr. Malcolm Crowe. It is a thriller about a child psychologist trying to reach and help a fearful young boy. The source of Cole's fear is that he "sees dead people." During one scene where Cole is in school, a teacher lectures about the history of the school building. Cole remarks, "They used to hang people here." When the teacher repeatedly indicates that the building was just a courthouse, Cole angrily exclaims, "You're Stuttering Stanley. You

(continued)

Literature, Media, and Personality Profiles (continued)

talked funny when you went to school here." The teacher reverts to severe stuttering. He finally musters the ability to tell Cole, "Shut up you freak!" The teacher's regression to stuttering shows that Cole has psychic abilities: He can see clearly into the past. *The Sixth Sense* was nominated for six Academy Awards and was written and directed by M. Night Shyamalan.

Understanding Stuttering

Definition of Stuttering

Some authorities have defined stuttering in a narrow sense that only includes speech patterns that are frequent and obvious disruptions in speech fluency. **Fluency** is the act of speaking easily and smoothly with effortlessly produced speech, without hesitations, interjections, or repetitions. Others have used broader definitions of stuttering that include mild speech fluency disruptions such as occasional word revisions and hesitations. Unfortunately, both narrow and broad definitions of stuttering have been used throughout history, making it difficult to know what speech patterns were considered stuttering. Van Riper (1973, 1992) simply defines **stuttering** as *a word improperly patterned in time and the speaker's reaction thereto.* A word that is improperly patterned in time is one that may be blocked, repeated, or prolonged. The speaker's "reaction thereto" involves the speaker's struggle in the attempt to speak fluently and includes negative feelings associated with the speech disorder. Many clinicians consider the fluency disruptions the core aspect of stuttering and the speaker's feelings and reactions to stuttering as secondary behaviors. The following is an operational definition of stuttering applicable to the way this fluency disorder is discussed in this chapter. Here the thoughts, feelings, and behaviors of a person who stutters are included in the definition:

> An individual who improperly patterns phonemes, syllables, words and/or phrases in time; who experiences classically-conditioned negative emotional reactions to disfluent speech and associated stimuli and who may engage in visible avoidance and escape behaviors when confronted with disfluent speech or associated stimuli. (Tanner, Belliveau, & Seibert, 1995, p. 6)

Stuttering is a fluency problem. It is a speech planning, patterning, and coordination irregularity. The speaker's reaction to the irregularities is an important facet to stuttering. The various aspects of the preceding definition are discussed in detail in this chapter.

The History of Stuttering

Stuttering has existed since the beginning of recorded history; even the ancient Greeks referred to it. They may even have treated stuttering by having individuals so afflicted talk while lifting or holding heavy objects, speak with pebbles in the mouth, or shout above the noise of the sea (Van Riper, 1973). As noted in Chapter 1, there is even a reference in the Bible about Moses having a speech problem, which may have been stuttering. Famous stutterers include King George VI, Charles Darwin, and Winston Churchill. Entertainers with a stuttering problem include George Burns, Marilyn Monroe, Bob Newhart, James Earl Jones, and Bruce Willis.

Early researchers wondered if stuttering was found in all cultures and languages. They examined most of the languages of the world for words for stuttering. If there is no word for stuttering, then it is likely that the disorder does not exist in the culture speaking the language. Early observers thought that certain Native Americans in the West, especially the Bannock, Shoshone, and Ute tribes, did not have stuttering because they could not find words for it in these languages. This theory was disproved, and later researchers found that stuttering is universal: There is indeed a word for it in every language (Van Riper, 1973). The percentage of people who stutter is relatively low, about 1% of American adults, but 3–4 are male to every 1 female stutterer (Bloodstein, 1995; Lawrence & Barclay, 1998). Depending on the definition of stuttering used by researchers, the male-to-female ratio may be more evenly distributed in younger children.

Throughout history many different stuttering treatments have been attempted, from speech drills to punishment to folk remedies. The idea behind such treatments was that the stuttering person needed more control and coordination of the speech mechanism. Folk remedies were common treatments for many human maladies of the past and included jumping in cold lakes, drinking teas made from tree roots or the bulbs of plants, eating disgusting substances, and weathering cold temperatures. Many of these radical treatments were based on the idea that the stuttering person needed more stamina. The saddest period in the history of stuttering treatment was when it was believed that stuttering could be cured surgically (Van Riper, 1973). These surgical procedures likely began in the latter part of the 1800s and persisted into the early 1900s. During this period, a surgeon would cut the root of a patient's tongue in the belief that this would cause smooth speech. These painful surgeries were done at a time when anesthetics were often weak or ineffective. After the surgery, the speaker would have an extremely sore mouth and do little talking. Due to the pain, when she would talk, the speech sounds would be made slowly and carefully, giving the impression that the surgery was a successful stuttering cure. Of course, when the pain subsided, the stuttering frequently returned. As recently as the 1970s, some physicians would "clip" the lingual frenulum, which is a thin tissue running from the lower jaw to the base of the tongue, supposedly to cure stuttering. The idea was that the stuttering person was "tongue-tied" and that clipping the frenulum would cause fluent speech. In addition, stuttering has been treated with many drugs throughout history, including benzodiazepines, phenothiazines, calcium channel blockers, beta blockers, and anticonvulsants (Lawrence & Barclay, 1998). Some drugs are addictive, and most have serious negative side effects. Fortunately, present-day treatments of stuttering are more enlightened and ethical.

Stuttering Behaviors

In stuttering there are three ways words may be improperly patterned in time: repetitions, prolongations, and blocks. Repetitions are common stuttering behaviors and the usual way stuttering is portrayed in literature and media. Characters in novels and films who stutter often show only repetitions. These audible stuttering behaviors can include sound, syllable, word, and phrase repetitions. For example, sound repetitions occur in this example: "P . . , p . . , p . . , Please direct me to the student union." A person who is stuttering may say, "Wha, wha, wha, what time does the student union close?" thus repeating a syllable. When words are repeated, it may sound like this: "I want, want, want, want to go to the student union." Entire phases can be repeated: "Would you please, would you please, would you please direct me to the student union?"

Prolongations occur on continuant sounds. A **continuant** is a sound where the articulators constrict the airstream, but there is no complete cessation of airflow. (Continuants are discussed in Chapter 4.) When a person who stutters prolongs a sound, he stretches it out longer than what is considered normal. An example of a prolongation is when a person who stutters asks for directions: "Would you please direct me to the sssssstudent union?" Here the /s/ sound is prolonged. Sometimes a pitch rise accompanies a prolongation. This is due to increased tension in the vocal tract.

A **block** is the inability to get speech started. When a person who stutters blocks, there appears to be an obstruction of airflow in the speech tract. For example: "Would you please direct me to the student . . . , . . . , . . . union?" There is an unusually long delay between the words *student* and *union*. Blocks also occur within word boundaries such as "un . . . . . . ion." When a person who stutters blocks on a word, it often appears that the blockage is occurring on the lips, but it is also likely there is a blockage in the larynx and where the back of the tongue contacts the roof of the mouth. During a block, the obstructions may be at multiple sites along the speech tract. Sometimes during a block, extraneous sounds such as a nasal snort or a click made by the tongue can be heard. (Nasal snorts were prominent stuttering behaviors made by the stuttering character in the movie *Pearl Harbor*.)

There are also visible features to stuttering. Besides the audible ones just listed, many people who stutter try to force speech production, resulting in visible difficulties. Forcing speech results in obvious physical signs of struggle. A few common signs are an eye squint, tension in the jaw, or a hand slapped against the side of the body. Sometimes, particularly with advanced stuttering, there is a jaw or tongue tremor. These are sometimes called associated stuttering behaviors. As will be discussed later, they are attempts on the part of the speaker to avoid or escape from the stuttering moment.

Incidence and Prevalence of Stuttering

As was discussed in Chapter 1, the **incidence** of a communication disorder is the number of new cases that occur, and **prevalence** refers to the total number of people in a population who have it at a particular time. After reviewing the literature, Bloodstein (1995) reports that the incidence of stuttering, how many people have had it at some point in their lives, is about 5%. This number represents people who have stuttered for a period of 6 months or longer. The prevalence of stuttering shows that approximately 1% of the population currently stutters. There are approximately 300 million Americans. Thus, there are about 3 million Americans who currently stutter, and about 15 million people in the United States who have stuttered for 6 months or longer at some point in their lives.

Types of Dysfluent Speech

The specific type of dysfluent speech determines how stuttering is prevented, diagnosed, and treated. The three categories are *normal nonfluencies, confirmed stuttering*, and *developmental stuttering* (Table 2.1).

Normal Nonfluencies.   People are rarely completely fluent, and children, when they are first learning to talk, are often very dysfluent. Speech fluency can be likened to riding a bicycle: When first learning, the rider is clumsy and awkward, and the bicycle tips and wobbles. After a while, the rider learns to control the bicycle, and soon it becomes an unconscious, smooth activity. When children are first learning speech, they are awkward and clumsy. After a while, they learn to talk more fluently. They gain control of their "speech bicycle."

Both children and adults rarely produce perfectly **fluent speech.** Most of us repeat sounds, syllables, words, and phrases. We often prolong consonants or vowels. Sometimes, speech is broken up with hesitations, especially when we are thinking of what to say. Speech is said to be **normally dysfluent** when it contains a normal number and type of repetitions, prolongations, and hesitations (see Sidebar 2.1). In studies of large numbers of children and

TABLE 2.1   *Categories of Dysfluent Speech in Children*

Normal Nonfluency	Developmental Stuttering	Confirmed Stuttering
Few sound, word, and phrase repetitions	More than normal nonfluency but fewer than confirmed stuttering	Many sound, word, and phrase repetitions
Infrequent and short prolongations of consonants and vowels	More than normal nonfluency but fewer than confirmed stuttering	Frequent and longer prolongations of consonants and vowels
Infrequent hesitations, usually while trying to remember words	More than normal nonfluency but fewer than confirmed stuttering	Frequent blocks between and within word boundaries
Lack of awareness and concern about dysfluencies	May be aware and concerned on some level about dysfluencies	Awareness and concern about dysfluencies
No struggle to produce speech	Initial signs of struggle to produce speech	Struggle present to produce speech
Few occurrences of the vowel "uh" during dysfluencies	More than normal nonfluency but fewer than confirmed stuttering	Vowel "uh" often present during dysfluencies
Little muscular tension present during dysfluencies	Initial signs of muscular tension to produce speech	Excessive muscular tension present during dysfluencies

adults, speech and hearing scientists have identified aspects of speech fluency that is considered normal. Drawing from those studies, Van Riper (1992) has differentiated normal from abnormal dysfluency. For example, having more than two syllable repetitions per word and having prolongations that last longer than 1 second are indications that speech dysfluency is abnormal. Other aspects involve pitch, eye contact, frustration, breath support, struggle, tension, and awareness of the dysfluencies.

Punishing or making the child self-conscious about her normal dysfluencies can actually cause some children to develop a stuttering problem. According to Hall, Oyer, and Haas (2001): "Some preschoolers and school-age children show speech disruptions that are labeled 'stuttering' when really parents and others who apply this label are observing normal nonfluencies. To be sure, some of these youngsters might one day be stutterers. Most will not" (p. 85).

Confirmed Stuttering.   **Confirmed stuttering,** sometimes called true stuttering, affects children as young as 18 months and elderly adults as well. To determine the presence of the disorder, a speech–language pathologist needs to evaluate the problem because delay in diagnosing stuttering can make it more difficult to treat. When the disorder is confirmed (i.e., it is not simply a stage that the person is going through), treatment should be initiated. Stuttering is likely to get worse the longer that treatment is delayed because, without it, the person naturally forces speech in an attempt to stop stuttering; this is self-defeating behavior. With an early start, the person's thoughts, feeling, attitudes, and behaviors can be changed more easily.

Typically, confirmed stuttering is treated on a one-to-one basis three or four times a week but may also include group therapy. In group therapy, two or more people who stutter receive therapy at the same time. A comprehensive therapy program also involves parents, friends, and teachers because they play important roles in the person's life. "The aim of treatment is to increase the child's confidence and to reduce the fear of stuttering" (Lawrence & Barclay, 1998, p. 2177). The types of therapy are discussed in later sections.

Developmental Stuttering.   When are speech patterns of a child considered to be within the range of normal, and when do they indicate stuttering? Some children, particularly when they are excited, have many repetitions, prolongations, and hesitations. As with children with normal nonfluencies, these characteristics are common when these children are under stress. For some children, this is just a passing phase—one they easily outgrow. Unfortunately, for

SIDEBAR 2.1 • *Normal Dysfluencies and Professional Speakers*

Everyone has normal dysfluencies, even professional speakers. To show how common normal dysfluencies are, do this exercise. Set aside 3 minutes for analyzing your professor's speech. On a sheet of paper, list three columns: repetitions, prolongations, and hesitations. Listen to your professor speak and note each time there is a sound, syllable, word, or phrase repetition and make a mark in that column. Do the same for prolongations and hesitations. It may surprise you how normally dysfluent even professional speakers are.

other children, the dysfluencies continue to grow in frequency and severity; unless a prevention or treatment program is initiated, many of these children are on the road to a lifetime of stuttering. The category of **developmental stuttering,** also called incipient stuttering, includes atypical dysfluencies. Children with atypical dysfluencies may not have more dysfluencies than other children, but the ones they have are more significant. For example, a child with more normal dysfluencies than usual may have three or four repetitions of sounds when trying to say a word. A child with an atypical dysfluency, however, may gasp for air in the middle of a word; this child is at risk for stuttering. The problems with the rhythm and flow of speech are more than occasional hesitations, prolongations, and repetitions of speech.

Children with developmental stuttering require extensive evaluation, and early intervention is important. Thus, the child who appears to be stuttering should get a comprehensive evaluation. Parents are important in identifying the number and type of dysfluencies (Tanner, 1990a). Figure 2.1 shows a questionnaire that can be given to parents of children who stutter as part of the evaluation. Therapy for the developmental stutterer can be direct or indirect. In *direct therapy*, the clinician works individually with the child. In *indirect therapy*, parents, friends, and teachers are counseled to help reduce the child's stress and self-consciousness about speaking. With proper therapy and counseling, stuttering can be prevented.

Causes of Stuttering: Theories

Readers, television audiences, and movie-goers are understandably curious about what causes a person or character to stutter. Authors and playwrights sometimes allude to the cause of stuttering as they develop a plot and subplots. For example, in *One Flew Over the Cuckoo's Nest*, Billy's stuttering problem existed only until he has sex, probably for the first time, after which his speech becomes normal. In this film, stuttering is erroneously related to sexual repression. In *The Cowboys*, pent-up anger is assumed to cause Stuttering Bob's communication disorder. His speech becomes normal when he freely expresses his anger and frustration. Will Anderson treats Bob's stuttering by allowing expressions of anger. Also, while Stuttering Bob curses, Anderson has him repeat the words. Soon, the repetitions are done fluently, and the stuttering is apparently cured. In *The Sixth Sense*, Stuttering Stanley reverts to dysfluent speech when he is taunted by Cole Sear. In this case, the teacher's return to stuttering is triggered by ridicule and taunting and perhaps supernatural forces. In *Pearl Harbor*, stuttering is tied to nervousness.

In reality, determining the cause of stuttering has proven to be a difficult but necessary task. Determining the **etiology**—that is, the cause of a pathology—of stuttering is important because, when the cause is identified, developing a cure is easier. Researchers in speech and hearing sciences, psychology, psychiatry, genetics, medicine, and education have sought the cause or causes of this disorder for decades. To date, no single study or series of research projects have identified why some people develop stuttering and others do not. The path to discovering what causes stuttering is uphill and slippery at best. Three general categories of plausible causes or perpetuating factors of stuttering are psychological, learning, or organic theories (Box 2.1). A fourth category, multiple-cause theory, combines the psychological, learning, and organic theories.

Instructions: Circle the number that most accurately represents your child's speech behavior.

	Never		Sometimes		Always
1. My child struggles to get the words out.	1	2	3	4	5
2. When my child repeats syllables, he/she appears to be struggling.	1	2	3	4	5
3. When my child starts to talk, his/her lips appear to tremble.	1	2	3	4	5
4. There is a tremor (trembling) in my child's jaw when he/she starts to talk.	1	2	3	4	5
5. When my child repeats syllables, he/she repeats more than two syllables per word.	1	2	3	4	5
6. When my child repeats syllables, the time interval between those syllables is not regular.	1	2	3	4	5
7. My child repeats, prolongs, or hesitates on the schwa vowel "uh."	1	2	3	4	5
8. My child makes word substitutions when he/she talks.	1	2	3	4	5
9. When my child talks, he/she appears to avoid eye contact with others.	1	2	3	4	5
10. My child's voice changes pitch inappropriately when he/she is talking.	1	2	3	4	5
11. My child complains of a tense or strained feeling in his/her throat.	1	2	3	4	5
12. When my child repeats syllables, his/her airflow is interrupted with gasping.	1	2	3	4	5
13. When my child talks, the last part of the word ends suddenly.	1	2	3	4	5
14. There are gaps–silent pauses–that occur within the word my child speaks.	1	2	3	4	5
15. There are long pauses between the words in my child's speech.	1	2	3	4	5
16. There are unusually long silences or gaps before my child begins talking.	1	2	3	4	5
17. My child appears to be afraid to talk.	1	2	3	4	5
18. My child becomes frustrated because he/she cannot talk properly.	1	2	3	4	5
19. My child appears to be afraid to talk to people he/she does not know because of repetitions, prolongations, or hesitations.	1	2	3	4	5
20. My child is uneasy and strained when he/she is talking.	1	2	3	4	5

FIGURE 2.1   *Parental Diagnostic Questionnaire (PDQ)*

(Courtesy Academic Communication Associates)

BOX 2.1 • *Etiology of Stuttering*

Psychological
- Repressed needs
- Psychological shock
- Expectancy neurosis

Learning
- Rewards for stuttering
- Fluency-disrupting arousal

Organic
- Genetic predisposition
- Altered auditory feedback
- Neuromotor disorder

Psychological Theories

The idea that psychological factors cause stuttering has been around since the 1930s. They were most popular during the 1940s and 1950s and continue today. These theories of stuttering suggest that a person who stutters has some kind of psychological problem that causes his speech to be spoken in a struggled manner. Many of these theories view stuttering as a logophobia, an unrealistic fear of words. Most of these theories about stuttering deal with anxiety. Anxiety is either a causal factor or one that perpetuates stuttering. According to some of these theories, stuttering is a type of expectancy neurosis in which anxiety causes the person to be unable to perform tasks that were previously done automatically and with little forethought. In most literature and media examples, stuttering increases with anxiety.

As recently as the 1960s, some authorities believed that (1) stuttering was a "safe" manifestation of a deep-rooted psychological disorder and (2) no attempt should be made to cure people who stuttered until the stutterer first went through intensive psychotherapy. It was thought that if the stuttering was eliminated without the benefit of psychotherapy, the person who stuttered could become dangerous to herself and to others. The supposition was that when stuttering—the safe manifestation of the deep-rooted psychological disorder—was removed without a psychotherapist providing another alternative, the person who stuttered would resort to a dangerous alternative expression of her psychological distress. This belief has proven to be false. The scientific literature has never reported a case where eliminating stuttering resulted, directly or indirectly, in injury to anyone. No incident has been reported in which a person was cured of stuttering and replaced it with a destructive or harmful psychological substitute. The worst part of this false belief was that it portrayed people who stuttered as dangerously mentally ill.

No clear evidence proves that a psychological problem causes stuttering. Research on people who stutter has not found major differences in their psychological makeup. Stuttering people, as a group, do not have "repressed needs," "oral fixations," "sexual problems," or "major personality disturbances" any more than do people who do not stutter. Stuttering, in most cases, does not appear to be a symptom of a major underlying psychological disturbance. Van Riper (1992) believes that when maladaptive symptoms appear, they stem from communicative frustration and social penalties.

Learning Theories

The idea that stuttering is a learned behavior has been around since the late 1700s. This theory, prominent during the 1960s and 1970s, states that stuttering is a learned behavior that can therefore be stopped by drills, rewards, punishments, **desensitization,** or by sheer willpower. According to learning theory, stuttering is like the habit of biting one's fingernails. Initially, a person bites his fingernails out of boredom or because it satisfies a need. Apparently, to some people, it feels good or provides relief when they bite the tips of fingernails off, and this good feeling or relief rewards the behavior. Because it feels good, the person continues to do it.

According to learning theory, stuttering develops because speech dysfluency is rewarded, in some way, by family, peers, or teachers, and the disorder continues because of those rewards. There can be many types of rewards. Although stuttering may begin as a child's normal nonfluencies, under learning theory the child comes to enjoy the subtle rewards of accidental speech errors, until what was once a comforting way of seeking attention becomes a habit too hard to break. One of the most important unconscious rewards of stuttering is that the stutterer is not interrupted. There is also the reward of being "special." Every child wants to be special, and according to this learning theory, some children stutter because their parents and teachers then give them more attention. Reduction in tension and anxiety also perpetuates stuttering. Often, during the moment of stuttering, the person feels tense and anxious. However, when the stuttering stops, there is an immediate relief that rewards the behavior of stuttering. This kind of *behavior-reward* is seen in many types of maladaptive behaviors. For some people, stuttering becomes a cycle. It begins with the attempt to speak, followed by stuttering, and ending with the relief of overcoming the impediment. An example: "Do you wa-wa-wa-want (relief and loss of anxiety at finally speaking the word) to go the student union with me?" By learning theory, this relief at successfully speaking becomes a reward in itself; stuttering becomes a cycle, a ritualistic behavior. Some people engage in ritualistic behaviors, at least partially, because they are self-rewarded by doing them. Although there are several variations of learning theories, they can be summarized as follows: Stuttering is caused and perpetuated by the rewards provided by listeners and by the reduction in anxiety that occurs after the stuttering stops (Figure 2.2).

Learning does play a role in stuttering. All speech is learned, and consequently, learning must play an important part in its disorders, including stuttering. Learning to stop or control stuttering is the basis to many stuttering therapies, regardless of the cause or causes of it. Speech-language pathologists do not perform surgeries, do genetic engineering, or prescribe medications to treat stuttering; they provide therapies that are based on modern learning theories and counseling approaches. As is discussed later, many people who stutter can stop or reduce it by learning to think and act differently when speaking. After a while they learn to talk normally with only a minimum amount of attention given to the physical aspects of the speech act.

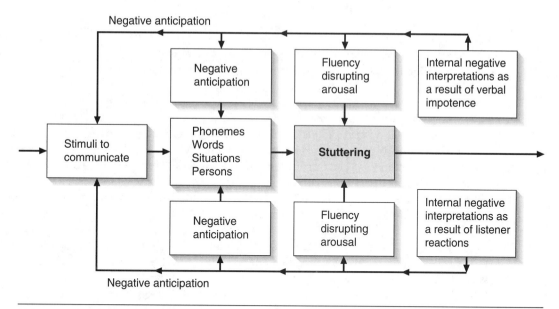

FIGURE 2.2   *Stuttering and Learning Theory.* Model of negative learning and stuttering.

Organic Theories

Organic, as used in speech pathology, refers to body structures or organs, such as the "organs of speech." When the term is used in reference to the *cause* of a communication disorder, it includes any impairment resulting from muscle weakness, biochemical irregularity, illness and disease, injury, physical structural deviation, or a genetic basis. As noted previously, organic theories have been popular throughout the history of the study and treatment of stuttering:

> In the 19th century, stuttering was widely believed to be caused by an anatomic defect in the oral cavity. Consequently, surgical procedures, often quite mutilating, were popular treatments. By the 20th century, the prevailing belief was that stuttering was a psychogenic disorder. Thus operant conditioning and psychoanalysis became the treatments of choice. (Lawrence & Barclay, 1998, pp. 2175–2176)

The organic theory suggests that stuttering is caused by physical irregularities. People stutter because their brains, nervous systems, or muscles are different or damaged. Today, the prevailing theory is that a verifiable neurophysical dysfunction disrupts speech timing (Lawrence & Barclay, 1998). Some organic theories suggest that stuttering is caused by brain chemistry deficiencies or by problems with auditory feedback.

A common question asked by parents concerns thought and speech: Is stuttering caused by the child simply talking faster than she thinks? Some people who stutter tend to have slight delays in language or articulation development (Guitar, 1998). Is the child's mind going too fast to allow speech to occur normally? Actually, everyone has thoughts that occur much more rapidly than their speech. We think in words much faster than we can utter them. So, the cause of stuttering is not that a person is thinking too fast for words, or we would all stutter.

Stuttering runs in families: "Fifty percent of people who stutter report that they have a relative who stuttered at some time in his or her life" (Owens, Metz, & Haas, 2000, p. 252). The hereditary aspect of stuttering is one of the most consistent facts emerging from decades of research. A child who has a father, mother, aunt, uncle, or cousin who stutters has a greater risk of developing stuttering. The question scientists are trying to answer about this observation concerns genetics: Is there a genetic basis to stuttering? There is a genetic basis to many illnesses, but some things run in families that are not necessarily related to genes. For example, a tendency to be overweight runs in some families, too. This might be because family members share a genetic basis for being overweight, but it also might be related to the way meals are prepared or the parents do not discourage eating junk food. Perhaps the family does not get enough exercise. Such environmental factors may also account for weight problems in several generations of family members. The reason stuttering runs in families might be related to genetics, but it also could be related to child-rearing practices. Currently, much research is being done on this aspect of stuttering.

One of the most perplexing statistics about stuttering involves gender differences. As reported previously, stuttering is more common among boys than girls. Although the ratio of stuttering between boys and girls varies among different studies, most find more boys than girls stutter. "The results from studies of people who stutter at many ages and in may cultures put the ratio at about three male stutterers to every one female stutterer" (Guitar, 1998, p. 17). For every girl that develops stuttering, three boys will have the problem. When trying to account for gender differences, again the question arises: Is it because of nature or environment?

Why boys stutter more than girls is not known (Lawrence & Barclay, 1998). Scientists who believe that the boy–girl difference is because of nature, that there is a genetic basis to stuttering, point out that many human maladies involve sex-linked genetic traits. Like male-pattern baldness, in which hair loss is directly attributed to genetics, the tendency to stutter may be passed on to generations of males. Stuttering may also be linked to other brain-related syndromes that occur more in males, such as attention deficit hyperactivity disorder (ADHD) and learning disabilities (Yeoman, 1998). On the other hand, scientists who argue that environmental factors cause children to stutter point to child-rearing differences between boys and girls and the different expectations of parents for boys and girls. Boys and girls also differ in their rate of speech and language acquisition: Girls are stronger at language acquisition, and boys tend to excel at motor skills.

Stuttering in twins has also fueled the nature-versus-nurture argument. When one twin stutters, the other one is likely to stutter, too. Although there are methodological problems with twin studies, the concordance rate is highest when the twins are identical (Booth, 1999; Van Riper, 1992). To scientists who believe in the genetic argument, this clearly points to a genetic basis for stuttering—after all, identical twins have identical genes. However, authorities who believe the disorder has to do with child-rearing practices and the environment point out that twins not only spend a lot of time together but also are often treated similarly by parents. This nature-versus-nurture controversy about the cause of stuttering could be easily resolved if a study could be conducted with groups of identical twins who were raised apart and one or both developed stuttering. If only one stuttered, this would support the nurture argument. If both children stuttered, this would support the genetic basis to stuttering. Unfortunately, there are no such cases available to conduct this type of a study.

Multiple-Cause Theory

As noted earlier, the kind of research currently being conducted about the cause(s) of stuttering often revolves around the age-old scientific question about human behavior: Is it because of biology and nature, or is it because of psychology, learning, environment, and nurturing? A third possibility would be a combination of all factors. Adopting a multiple-cause philosophy may be necessary. It is likely that there is more than one cause of stuttering. Some people develop stuttering because of psychological reasons. A psychological shock or trauma may cause a person to stutter. For example, soldiers in combat sometimes develop stuttering, as do civilians who undergo extreme bouts of stress. Other people may have learned to stutter; for them it is a learned behavior that is difficult to break. Evidence points to a genetic basis to stuttering as well. Most likely, it is a combination of genetics, learning, and psychology that work together to cause stuttering in a particular person.

Characteristics of Stuttering

Of all the communication disorders, stuttering has been studied the longest by researchers from a variety of disciplines. Yet, this disorder is still baffling to scientists even after decades of intensive research. Although much has been learned about stuttering, its cause, nature, and treatment remain controversial and challenging. It is a highly variable disorder in that it can be mild or severe. People who stutter vary greatly in their reactions to it and their resolve and ability to overcome the disorder. For some, stuttering is an inconvenience; for others, it is debilitating. Stuttering can come on suddenly or gradually. Sometimes, stuttering is consistently present, and at other times, it can disappear for weeks, even months. Certain sounds and words can set it off, as can speaking situations or a particular person. Most people stutter more when under stress, but some stutter when they are relaxed.

Stuttering and Singing

One of the most interesting facts about people who stutter is that most of them can sing without stuttering. As noted earlier, Mel Tillis has been interviewed on several television talk shows and stuttered when answering the hosts' questions. Then, when he performed, he sang without stuttering. Most people who stutter can sing without showing the disorder. There are several theories for this speaking–singing dichotomy. One hypothesis is that when a person sings, he is using a different part of the brain than what is used when speaking, thus controlling the rhythmic patterns differently. Singing without stuttering may also result from the rhythm of the tune. With a drum beat and guitar rhythm, words can be said more easily and smoothly. This phenomenon may also occur because when a person sings, he adopts a different role, the role of entertainer, and does not feel insecure or fearful while in that role. Finally, the fact that the person frequently rehearses the songs may also contribute to the normal fluency during singing.

Stuttering and Nonthreatening Audiences

Speaking is threatening for many people who stutter (Linn & Caruso, 1998). However, people who stutter tend to speak normally when they talk to babies, children, and animals. They also rarely stutter when talking aloud to themselves. This observation has baffled researchers, particularly those who believe that stuttering is the result of a brain irregularity or brain damage. Why would the fluency centers of the brain operate differently depending on whether the listener is an adult or a child? The stuttering person's audience plays an important role in how easily and smoothly speech is produced. According to Guitar (1998), one possible explanation for this phenomenon is that the speech production mechanism of a person who stutters is more vulnerable than that of normal speakers to the effects of arousal. Just as some people become obviously flustered and agitated when anxious, people who stutter may have more dysfluencies when they are under stress.

Stuttering, Speech Cues, and Self-Consciousness

People who stutter can often fluently repeat what someone else has spoken. They can also talk normally in unison with someone else. In both cases, normal speech may result from greater self-confidence. The person who stutters feels less pressure to talk in such situations. Another hypothesis involves the cues provided for the rhythm of speech. When repeating or talking in unison, the person who stutters gets cues about how to talk normally from the other speaker.

Stuttering and Noise

Noise, which blocks auditory feedback, leads to better speech in some people who stutter. For example, some people who stutter talk better when at parties where there is loud background noise. As well, when a therapist puts earphones on a person who stutters and creates masking noise, the stuttering is reduced. Masking feedback, whether resulting from therapy or with loud background noise, often causes a reduction in stuttering. This phenomenon is also related to the stuttering person's self-consciousness. Because of the noise, the stuttering is less prominent, and the speaker feels less self-conscious.

Stuttering and Delayed Auditory Feedback

One technique commonly used by speech–language pathologists to help people who stutter is **delayed auditory feedback** (DAF). Delayed auditory feedback is when there is a time lapse between what is spoken and when the speaker hears it. It has long been known that when normal speakers experience a delay between what they say and when they hear it, they tend to be very dysfluent. The longer the delay between what they say and when they hear it, the more they struggle. But an interesting thing happens to people who stutter when they experience DAF: Many of them speak more easily and smoothly. This phenomenon is thought to be a result of the increased concentration necessary to communicate while experiencing DAF. Some people who stutter are so focused on hearing themselves speak with a delay that they lose the self-consciousness that inhibits their speech.

Stuttering and Other Variables

Stuttering affects people differently. What is true for one person who stutters is not necessarily true for another. For example, some people who stutter report that they speak better when they are ill; others do better when they are feeling well. Some people stutter less when they have been drinking alcoholic beverages, whereas others stumble more with their speech under the influence of alcohol. Some people believe that their stuttering problem was caused when they tried to pitch or bat left-handed. It was common during the 1950s for teachers to force left-handed children to write with their right hands, and some believed this was a cause of stuttering. Even the weather can affect stuttering. Some people who stutter believe that the sun, wind, temperature, and rain affect their stuttering. Fatigue causes some people who stutter to talk better, whereas others are more dysfluent when they are exhausted. The complexities of stuttering, which are interesting to scientists, make it difficult for clinicians to treat it. Table 2.2 shows the variability of stuttering.

Key Aspects of Stuttering

What Is Heard

As was discussed previously, people who stutter have three types of struggled speech: repetitions, prolongations, and blocks. Some individuals have primarily repetitions. They stop and

TABLE 2.2 *Variability of Stuttering*

Factors	Effects on Some People Who Stutter
Singing and rhythm	Melody and rhythm improve fluency.
Audience	Nonthreatening audiences improve fluency.
Speech cues	Fluency improves when speaking in unison or repeating what has been spoken.
Noise	Masking noise improves fluency.
Delayed auditory feedback	DAF affects fluency.
Other	Illness, alcoholic beverages, handedness shift, weather, and fatigue may affect fluency.

start over when trying to get sounds, syllables, words, and phrases to come out. Sometimes, these repetitions happen two, three, or more times in rapid succession. An example of repetitions is seen in Billy Babbitt in the film *One Flew Over the Cuckoos's Nest.* His primary stuttering problem is repeating the first sounds of words.

Other people who stutter may prolong, or stretch out, vowels and consonants. Some people have abrupt stops in the flow of speech; they block at the beginning of an utterance or somewhere in the middle of it. Many people who stutter have all three types of dysfluencies. Sometimes, stuttering is so severe that an individual cannot functionally communicate through speech, but for others, stuttering is just an occasional nuisance. People with severe stuttering may stutter on more than 50% of their words, whereas those with a mild problem do so on less than 5% of them (Guitar, 1998).

What Is Seen

Struggled speech is often reflected in the bodies of people with confirmed stuttering, especially their faces. Eye squints, lip and jaw tremors, head jerks and nods, and hands slapped on the side of the face or on the hip accompany the stuttering person's struggled attempts to speak. Similar to what you can see on the face of a person lifting a huge weight, the visible aspects of forcing speech are apparent to those listening to persons who stutter. They often result from avoidance and escape behaviors.

Lack of eye contact, or closing the eyes in midsentence, are forms of *avoidance.* The person may be avoiding the expressions of the listener. *Escape behaviors* occur when the person who stutters tries to remove herself from the stuttering moment. A child may run from the room or an adult may turn away to escape the negative expressions of the listener. A disguise behavior occurs when the person who stutters tries to make stuttering look and sound like something else (Van Riper, 1992). Turning stuttered speech into a laugh is a way of trying to disguise the disorder. Some people with confirmed stuttering engage in all these behaviors, whereas others only occasionally have visible features of stuttering. Children often pick up more of these behaviors as they grow older and suffer more pangs of rejection from parents, teachers, and other children. Struggle, avoidance, escape, and disguises occur more frequently as they try harder to sound normal during speech.

What Is Felt

Not every person who stutters necessarily feels anxious and fearful. Sometimes, people who stutter have no negative feelings about stuttering. In addition, people who stutter have normal nonfluencies just like people who do not stutter. However, most people who stutter have negative feelings and anxiety during the stuttering moment. As Guitar (1998) writes, "Feelings may precipitate stutters; conversely, stutters may create feelings" (p. 13). This is particularly true when the stuttering is severe or lasts a long time. Increased anxiety leads to increased dysfluencies in individuals who stutter (Tanner, 1991; Weber & Smith, 1990). Adam Sandler, an actor and comedian, uses anxiety and stuttering for its humor value on several tracks of his comedy album *What the Hell Happened to Me?* The Excited Southerner, a character that Sandler plays, is a man who stutteringly tries to engage in several verbal activities. Some of the skits, where stuttering is used for its humor value, include trying to order in a restaurant, being pulled over by a police officer, interviewing for a job, and proposing marriage to a woman. One way to understand the negative feelings that some people who stutter have during a moment of stuttering is by comparing it to public speaking (Tanner, 1980).

Public speaking and stuttering are similar in that both cause anxiety and fear. High on the list of people's fears is speaking in public. Most people experience apprehension about speaking in front of groups, especially large ones. The reasons people give for fear of public speaking include fear of making mistakes, embarrassment, fear of forgetting the speech, or losing audience interest. The commonality among these reasons is the potential of rejection. The fearful speaker realizes that speaking to an audience carries a greater risk of rejection than when conversing with someone one-to-one. And to many people, rejection of what they are saying feels like total rejection. Most of us feel anxiety about the potential for rejection. The rejection may not actually be real; some speakers feel they failed when in fact they presented a good speech.

People who stutter often feel anxiety before they attempt to speak. This anxiety often continues through the stuttering moment and gets worse as the stuttering continues. They have feelings of embarrassment, fear, and being "out of control." Brutten and Shoemaker (1967) designed a therapy based on the belief that anxiety and negative emotions associated with speech cause stuttering. Their treatment plan minimizes or eliminates these fears to help stutterers achieve fluent speech. The association between stuttered speech and anxiety occurs through a psychological process called classical conditioning. Classical conditioning is the basis to many emotional responses and was first formally described by the Russian psychologist Ivan Pavlov. Pavlov conducted experiments with dogs: A bell would be rung, and immediately after hearing the bell, the dog would be given meat. Soon, the dog responded to the sound of the bell by salivating in expectation of meat to come. Pavlov proved that a previously learned neutral stimulus, when paired with a conditioned stimulus, can evoke the same emotional response; that is, two stimuli are paired to cause the same emotional response. The process is also called **Pavlovian conditioning.** Most stuttering therapies acknowledge the role that anxiety and negative emotions play in stuttering and try to alleviate them.

Effects on Personality

As noted earlier, research has shown that stuttering does not necessarily alter a person's personality. Although it is true that the disorder psychologically devastates some people, most individuals who stutter adjust well to it. However, stuttering, particularly severe stuttering, often results in the individual experiencing negative social interaction. Subtle rejection occurs when listeners turn to another activity while the stutterer is still struggling to speak. Not-so-subtle rejection occurs when jokes are made about the stuttering person resembling Porky Pig or another television or movie character with a stuttering problem. These obvious types of rejections often occur in the lives of people who stutter. They also start at an early age. The young person who stutters may also feel rejection when his mother remarks that the child's speech is substandard or when a child's father turns away from a stuttered conversation with a disapproving look on his face. Covert types of rejection go beyond words.

Occasional rejection is a part of life for all of us, but for an individual with a stuttering problem, rejection is more frequent and severe. According to Linn and Caruso (1998), stuttering can negatively affect the chances of an individual forming an intimate relationship, due to shame and guilt associated with the speech disorder.

People who stutter also often have confidence problems. The confidence problems usually revolve around social, school, and business activities. Standing in front of classmates and presenting an assignment is a fearful and anxiety-provoking situation for many children. They experience all of the usual fears of not having done the assignment well or not presenting the information clearly. Children may have concerns that their attire is not acceptable or fashionable, or they may fear that they will be the brunt of jokes. Children with a stuttering problem have these fears, too, but they also must be concerned about how they speak, even if they will be able to speak at all. As they grow older, the struggle to make friends becomes the struggle to find a partner, and as Linn and Caruso (1998) note, "Stuttering affects a person in many ways, but one of the most critical social activities an adult individual undertakes is that of finding a partner and maintaining an intimate relationship" (p. 12). Some people who stutter see their speech disorder as yet another obstacle in the task of finding a life partner. Some people who stutter develop the belief that speech is hard work and something to be avoided (Linn & Caruso, 1998).

The Prevention of Stuttering in Children

Clinicians, parents, friends, and teachers can do many things to reduce the likelihood of an at-risk child developing stuttering. The child who is at risk for developing stuttering is going through a period when she has more speech dysfluencies than usual, or having ones that are atypical, and is starting to be concerned about her speech. Some of them are obvious changes in child-rearing practices; others are more subtle. Understanding stuttering is an important part of the prevention program. Having information about stuttering can change attitudes and thus help the child who is struggling with speech fluency. Parents, friends, and teachers must work closely with the speech–language pathologist in the prevention program and follow directions carefully. Often, the speech clinician works directly with the at-risk child, but counseling parents, friends, and teachers is also an important part of the prevention program.

Strategies for Parents and Teachers

When it comes to stuttering, prevention is more successful than attempting to cure it after a confirmed-stuttering diagnosis. Some children become stutterers despite preventive measures. However, in the majority of cases, stuttering can be prevented. Adults can take several steps to prevent a child from beginning a lifetime of stuttering. These include changes in attitudes and commonsense activities that can help the child understand and cope with his speech dysfluencies. The goal of preventing stuttering is to make the child feel that his normal nonfluencies are natural, which of course they are. Because the most significant adults to the child are his parents and teachers, these suggestions focus on home and school activities. To help reduce speech self-consciousness in the at-risk child, Box 2.2 lists commonsense suggestions for parents and teachers.

BOX 2.2 • *Suggestions for Parents and Teachers to Reduce Self-Consciousness*

- Avoid using the words *stutter*, *stuttering*, or *stutterer*. Using these words around a child can make her hypersensitive to her own normal speech dysfluencies. Labeling a child a "stutterer" is a self-fulling prophecy, because the label can actually cause a child to become a stutterer. The theory that misdiagnosing normal nonfluencies as stuttering can actually cause stuttering is a well-accepted clinical concept and has been around for decades. First advanced by Johnson (1938; 1955), it is called the **diagnosogenic theory of stuttering.**
- Do not remind the child to "think before talking." Although this seems like a positive and constructive thing to do to reduce dysfluencies, it can cause the child to become self-conscious. Being too self-conscious about speech fluency can cause stuttering.
- Do not expect the child's speech to be perfectly fluent. As noted earlier, few, if any people ever have perfectly fluent speech.
- Do not let the child know that you are annoyed and frustrated about his speech. Do not say anything to show you are annoyed and frustrated. Watch your nonverbal communication, too. Your manners, gestures, and facial expressions should not indicate annoyance or frustration.
- Just as you do not let the child know that you are frustrated and annoyed by her speech, try not to reward her dysfluent speech. You can inadvertently reward dysfluent speech by paying more attention to the child when stuttering occurs.
- Do not make the child stop and start over when he is having trouble talking. This disrupts the normal flow of communication and makes the child self-conscious.
- Do not rush or hurry the child. Conversations should be as relaxed as possible. The child should know that the listener will take the time necessary to listen.
- Do not tell the child to slow her rate of speech. The child is talking as rapidly or slowly as is natural for her.

Professional Treatment of Stuttering

A person who has confirmed stuttering needs professional help to overcome the disorder. His speech patterns go beyond what are considered normal nonfluencies. A prevention program is not appropriate for a confirmed stutterer because it is too late to prevent the stuttering. A child with confirmed stuttering is usually aware, at some level, of his speech problem. Older children may talk about the problem with parents, teachers, and peers, whereas younger ones sometimes only express their awareness by crying or getting angry when they stutter. A person with confirmed stuttering struggles with speech, and he sometimes develops the identity of a "stutterer" and incorporates stuttering as part of his self-concept. Stuttering becomes more severe with age unless the child recovers with or without formal treatment (Guitar, 1998).

Most adult stutterers can benefit from therapy, no matter how long they have stuttered. However, with people who have stuttered for a long time, their response strength is usually higher. *Response strength* is the magnitude of reaction to a stimulus. The thoughts, feelings, emotions, and behaviors associated with stuttering are more established for adults than children. They have occurred more often and subsequently are harder to change or eliminate. Several types of therapies help reduce or eliminate stuttering in children and adults.

Types of Therapy

There are several types of therapies for confirmed stuttering. Some are specifically designed for children, whereas others are for adults. Some therapies are specific programs with detailed step-by-step instructions, drills, and exercises, whereas others are more flexible and focus on the therapeutic relationship between the clinician and the stutterer. All current treatments have two things in common. First, it usually takes at least 4–6 months of intensive therapy with periodic follow-up to cure or control stuttering. There is no quick, successful treatment that provides long-term gains. Second, stuttering therapies do not eliminate dysfluencies in all people who stutter. Some individuals do stop stuttering altogether, but many may only manage to control and reduce it. Unfortunately, some must learn to accept this speech pathology as a part of their lives.

Cure Versus Control

Can stuttering be cured? Some authorities on stuttering do not like to use the word *cure* to describe the effects of treatment. They believe that a person is never really cured of the disorder and the best a person who stutters can hope for is to control it. Stuttering can be likened to alcoholism. Like the alcoholic, a person who stutters may have the disorder under control, but she will always be a stutterer. Even authorities who believe that stuttering can be cured acknowledge that the memories of stuttering will persist. Certainly, a person who stuttered early in her life is not necessarily emotionally scarred because of it. However, the memory of rejection, ridicule, and taunting that occurred over speech dysfluencies must be acknowledged and integrated into her personality. We are products of our experiences, and in that sense, stuttering will always be a part of the person's life. All aspects of stuttering need to be addressed in therapy for a long-lasting cure.

Another problem with using the word *cure* to describe stuttering therapy concerns how much time should pass before treatment can be considered successful. In most people who stutter, becoming fluent is easy, for a short time. Sometimes, all that is necessary is to prolong each sound, such as by pretending to talk with a southern "drawl" or to concentrate on how the tongue feels inside the mouth. Others can talk fluently by tapping out a rhythm with their feet or by pretending that a hand puppet is doing the talking. Many people who stutter can use temporary tools to achieve near-normal speech . . . for a short period. When the novelty of the temporary tools wears off, most return to their typical stuttering speech patterns.

Some of the literature and media examples listed at the beginning of this chapter show quick "cures" for stuttering. Many people seeking stuttering therapy have been exposed to these ideas for a quick cure, either by seeing them in movies or by having friends and relatives recommend them. Unfortunately, this often creates unrealistic expectations about the goals and nature of stuttering therapy. In our fast-paced society, some people entering stuttering treatment look for a pill, hypnosis, surgery, device, gimmick, or miracle that will permanently eliminate the disorder. Most adults entering stuttering therapy have stuttered for years, perhaps decades, and it is unlikely that any therapy will result in an immediate elimination of the disorder. Movies propagate these myths. Although it is possible that Billy *(One Flew Over the Cuckoo's Nest)* was more fluent after having sex and that Stuttering Bob *(The Cowboys)* had improved fluency after expressing frustration and anger, these "cures" were probably short lived. For a true cure, it is necessary that the person maintain fluent speech for a long time. The length of time needed to evaluate the benefit from therapy depends on the age of the person, how long he stuttered, and the frequency of the treatment program. At least 2 years is required to determine whether the stuttering has been eliminated or controlled. Even after an extended period of fluency, some people who once stuttered have setbacks and need booster sessions to return to their best fluency levels.

Not all people who stutter accept the negative, inferior status portrayed in media and literature. Some people who stutter see the speech pattern as *different* rather than *disordered* and believe that it should be accepted by society. A radical and controversial notion gaining popularity is that stutterers are better off learning to accept stuttering rather than striving to overcome it (Yeoman, 1998). Many people who stutter, particularly those unsuccessful in improving their speech, believe that society should be more accepting and tolerant of them. They, and their speech patterns, should be viewed as simply "different." This issue was addressed in Chapter 1.

Treating Essential Aspects of Stuttering

As noted previously, there are four aspects to stuttering. Regardless of what the treatment philosophy or program is, for stuttering therapy to be successful, all aspects must, essentially, be addressed. The four aspects are (1) what is heard, (2) what is seen, (3) what is felt, and (4) what effects the disorder has had on the person's personality (Tanner, 1994; Tanner, Belliveau, & Seibert, 1995; Tanner, 1999b). Each aspect can be treated individually and sequentially. However, a combined approach where the clinician simultaneously addresses all aspects of stuttering can be used for older children and adults.

Treating Stuttering: What Is Heard.   The audible symptoms are the most prominent aspects of stuttering. The purpose of this aspect of stuttering therapy is to modify the audible symptoms so that the person who stutters reduces the number and severity of dysfluencies. The goal for the person who stutters is to speak easily and gently and to produce speech only with normal nonfluencies (Tanner, 1994; Tanner, Belliveau, & Seibert, 1995; Tanner, 1999b).

If a person who stutters is told to "stop stuttering," he often stutters even more. However, if the person who stutters is told to stutter easily and gently, he can learn to modify speech efficiently with training. When the person learns to stutter easily and gently, most of the time, he can become so effective that the stuttering is unnoticeable. By learning to stutter easily and gently, the stutterer has permission to stutter and does not appear to be stuttering. When people who stutter speak this way, or *stutter fluently*, most nonprofessionals do not know they are even stuttering. This type of therapy is also called symptom modification, or fluent stuttering, and was advanced by Van Riper in the 1970s. A popular stuttering therapy, it is used by many present-day clinicians.

For therapy purposes, stuttering can also be operantly conditioned. *Operant conditioning* is a type of behavior modification therapy: If normal speech is rewarded and stuttered speech discouraged, the amount of stuttering can be reduced or eliminated. In this therapy, the person who stutters is given some kind of reward by the clinician when speech is made without stuttering. Usually, the therapy starts with noncomplex, simple types of utterances and gradually increases to normal, rapid speech. The rewards can range from simple verbal praise to tokens, candy, toys, and school privileges. Stuttered speech is discouraged by reminding the person to monitor her speech and to use the tools of fluent speech to prevent or modify stuttering. The main tool of fluent speech is easy contact in which the articulators gently touch each other during stuttered speech. The use of other tools depend on the nature of the person's stuttering problem and may include slowing the rate of speech, maintaining adequate breath support, slightly prolonging sounds, and paying attention to vocal cord vibrations.

Clinicians have other ways of helping the stuttering person's speech sound as normal as possible. Some therapies involve helping rid the individual of negative emotions associated with speech, using DAF, and gradually reducing the delay—concentrating on breathing, the way the tongue feels inside the mouth, and talking to the timed click, click, click of a metronome.

Parents and teachers are often important parts of this aspect of therapy for children with confirmed stuttering. Changing the way a person talks requires a lot of cues, and parents and teachers are an integral part of this aspect of therapy. A *cue* is a verbal or nonverbal indication to monitor how speech is being produced. A teacher, for example, may need to remind a child to use his tools of fluent speech in the classroom several times during the day. At the dinner table, parents may also need to remind the child to relax his speech muscles and to say sounds gently. Sometimes these cues and reminders are suggestions whispered in the child's ear, or they may be given nonverbally. For example, when a teacher puts her fingers to the mouth, this can cue the child to use what he has learned in therapy. A speech–language pathologist may also want parents and teachers to help by providing rewards for fluent speech.

Treating Stuttering: What Is Seen.   The visible aspects of stuttering include excessive eye blinking, head jerking, trunk twisting, lack of eye contact, and facial grimaces. The goal of this aspect of stuttering therapy is to eliminate the abnormal visible features of stuttering during speech. Because the visible features of stuttering are obvious and observable, clinicians and others can work to eliminate them by rewarding normal facial expressions and body movements and discouraging abnormal ones. Often, simply bringing visible features to the attention of the person who stutters is enough to cause her to stop doing them. Videotapes can be used for this purpose. Teenagers and adults who see their own visible aspects of stuttering either on videotape or in a mirror often stop them on their own. They learn to maintain eye contact or to stop squinting their eyes during stuttering. Young children with confirmed stuttering may have rewards given to them, such as tokens, which can purchase toys, candy, or privileges. Praise from parents and teachers also helps children learn to stop the visible features. Rewarding normal facial features and body movements during speech is usually successful in helping a speaker appear more natural during speaking. This is true of all the visible features except tremors of the lips, tongue, and jaw. Excessive muscular tension is necessary for stuttering tremors (Van Riper, 1992), and these can be eliminated through relaxation therapy. *Relaxation therapy* for stuttering is a systematic method of achieving muscular relaxation that includes progressively tensing and relaxing muscle groups, autosuggestion, and meditation (Tanner, 1991). The elimination of abnormal visible features, combined with helping the person who stutters learn to talk easily and fluently, does away with two of the most apparent aspects of stuttering: What is heard and what is seen. Many confirmed stutterers, however, often continue to feel tense and anxious when they speak.

Treating Stuttering: What Is Felt.   Clinicians have many ways of reducing anxiety and negative emotions. Certain medications cause a reduction in anxiety but may be habit forming and have other negative side effects. Biofeedback devices can be used to monitor and reduce anxiety. With biofeedback, the person is taught to reduce tension by attending to tones of differing pitches or loudness. By responding to the tones, people can learn to relax their muscles. Counseling and support groups can also help people learn to relax in speaking situations. All these strategies can be used to help people reduce high levels of speech-related anxiety and tension.

One particularly useful way of managing the anxiety and negative emotions associated with stuttering is called systematic desensitization. Systematic desensitization is a method of reducing negative emotions that have been associated (classically conditioned) with certain stimuli. Positive or neutral emotions are created to counter the negative ones previously associated with the stimuli. In **psychology,** systematic desensitization is used to treat anxiety disorders and phobias. Systematic desensitization works well for most individuals to reduce the anxiety and associated negative emotions that occur during stuttering. This is done primarily with relaxation training, but may also include counseling, role playing, and using positive suggestions. Relaxation training is a natural way to reduce anxiety and negative emotions. People who stutter can use audiotapes for training in these techniques (Tanner, 1991). For example, a person who stutters may be desensitized to a frequently stuttered word by saying it repeatedly in a variety of contexts while experiencing neutral or positive emotions. Gradually, the person is desensitized to anxiety and associated negative emotions previously associated with the word. The aspects desensitized are *sounds, words, situations,* and certain *people* or types of people (Brutten & Shoemaker, 1967).

People who stutter often experience negative emotions when they must say certain sounds or words. This happens because in the past they have stuttered on them. They may have been the objects of ridicule and felt out of control. Soon, the thought of having to say these words causes negativity that in turn worsens the problem. Besides certain sounds and words, certain situations can cause negative emotions. Talking in front of a classroom, asking for directions, arguing with someone, or asking a person out for a date are examples of situations that may cause more stuttering negativity. Certain people may also cause anxiety and associated negative emotions in some stutterers. A particular teacher or the school principal may evoke negative feelings when the child must talk to them. People in a hurry, authority figures, professors, relatives, doctors, and the police may also elicit negative emotions in a person who is struggling with speech fluency.

The goal of systematic desensitization and other forms of counseling and instruction is not to eliminate all negative feelings during speech, which would be unattainable, but to break the link between broken speech and negative feelings. Replacing negative feelings and anxiety with positive ones desensitizes the person to certain sounds, words, situations, and people. Figure 2.3 shows how anxiety and associated negative emotions are deconditioned over time.

Treating Stuttering: Effects on Personality.   In stuttering therapy the whole person is treated, not just his speech disorder. Stuttering therapy includes improving the person's speech-related **self-esteem,** or ego strength. Speech-related self-esteem and ego strength are the feelings of confidence and well-being experienced by a speaker during verbal communication:

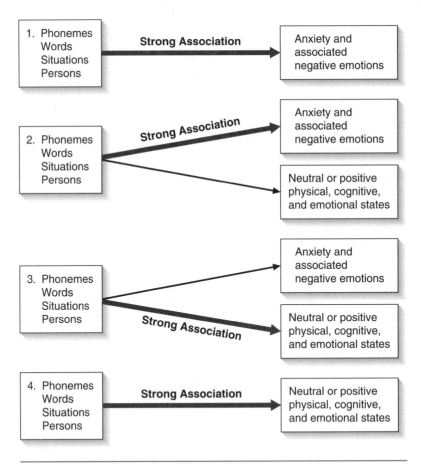

FIGURE 2.3 *Deconditioning Stuttering Responses.* Deconditioning and counterconditioning of anxiety and associated negative emotions to phonemes, words, situations, and/or people.

Ego strength is difficult to define, but we know when it's low and we know when it's high. It rises and falls in all of us depending upon our success–failure ratio, but its basic ingredients are love, faith, and opportunity. Some of our stuttering children are denied all three. (Van Riper & Erickson, 1996, pp. 275–276)

Improved speech-related self-esteem is an important aspect of successful therapy. Group therapy helps with speech-related self-esteem because discussing stuttering with other people who stutter helps individuals learn that they are not alone with their fears. They can learn others' strategies and methods of coping with rejection. Sometimes, it is comforting and therapeutic simply to talk about these issues to others. Speech clinicians also are trained to counsel people who stutter about how to deal with their feelings associated with stuttering. Using speech-related self-esteem exercises, the clinician encourages and rewards what is communicated, as opposed to how fluently it is said. Parents and teachers are involved in this aspect of stuttering therapy. They learn ways of ignoring broken speech without rejecting the child.

One of the most important ways of building self-esteem is the unconditional expression of love and approval. Teachers can do this by remarking to the child that she is valued in the classroom, not for good grades or behavior, but for being herself. Parents can improve their child's self-esteem by regularly expressing their love and acceptance. It is important that parents express these things when the child is doing something neither good nor bad. If love and praise are only given when the child is succeeding at something, she may learn to have these feelings only when she is doing well. Obviously, a child should never be praised for doing things that are wrong or undesirable. One of the best times for parents to express their love and acceptance of the child is before bedtime or just upon awakening. During these times, the child is not succeeding or failing at anything, and statements such as "You are a wonderful child," "We are very proud of you," and "We think the world of you" said repeatedly can help create a strong foundation of self-esteem and confidence. When the child hears these statements regularly, the child feels good about herself, and these good feelings can help deflect the inevitable blows to her self-esteem caused by stuttering.

Effectiveness of Treatment

As noted previously, the number of people who have stuttered for 6 months or longer (5% of the population) is 5 times larger than the number of people who currently stutter (1% of the population). A large number of people who have a stuttering problem recover with or without treatment. Actually, this assumption may not be as simple as it appears because of research methodology problems. Many people who report stuttering only to have it go away may in fact never have actually had a stuttering disorder. They may have only had excessive normal nonfluencies and not truly have developed the self-sustaining patterns of stuttering. The definitions of stuttering used by researchers create problems when comparing several studies.

Stuttering is easier to prevent than to cure. The incidence of stuttering is declining (Van Riper, 1992). This decline may be due to many factors including public information programs sponsored by the American Speech-Language-Hearing Association and early prevention and treatment programs provided by speech–language pathologists, particularly those in public schools. The decline in stuttering may also be a result of changes in parental and societal attitudes toward stuttering and more acceptance of dysfluencies as a normal part of human speech patterns. The majority of people who stutter can benefit from programs provided by speech–language pathologists, either to cure and eliminate the stuttering or to minimize and adjust to it.

Other Fluency Disorders

Cluttering

Many communication disorders have disrupted fluency as part of their symptoms. In particular, motor speech disorders, which are discussed in Chapter 7, often have as part of their symptoms disruptions in how fluently the patient can talk. Disorders of the brain, nervous system, and muscles can cause ill-coordinated, ill-timed speech production. However, besides stuttering, cluttering is *primarily* a fluency disorder.

Cluttering is a verbal thought-organization fluency disorder characterized by short attention span, excessive rate of speech, and omissions and substitutions of sounds and words. Clinically, the person who clutters often speaks rapidly, with sentence fragments, word repetitions, and many revisions. He appears to be unable to organize thoughts clearly and is persistently unsatisfied with the output. The following is an example of cluttering:

> I would like to go. What I want to do after class is to go to the, go to the, uh. Hey, why don't you and I go to the student union. The thing is that a cup of coffee would taste good at the student. . . . Would you like to go to the student union and have a cup . . . Espresso coffee is good at the student union. Hey, let's go to the student union and have a cup of espresso.

In movies and on television, people who have cluttering tend to be perceived as anxious, scatterbrained, disorganized, and flighty. Excited people often clutter their thoughts, but people who have the communication disorder of cluttering persistently talk with disturbed fluency. Clinically, cluttering is rarely diagnosed and treated independent of other communication disorders. Sometimes, it is evaluated and treated concurrently with stuttering. Table 2.3 compares the definitions of both fluency disorders.

Literature and Media Stereotypes

Books, films, and television often give a simplistic view of stuttering. This simplistic view portrays the person who stutters as a humorous, anxious, and befuddled character whose speech disorder can be easily eliminated. When literature and media do address the cause of the disorder, it usually has a psychological theme, related to anxiety, repressed anger, or sexual dysfunctions. Although people who stutter may experience anger at people's insensitive remarks and rude behaviors, stuttering is not caused by repressed anger. Neither is stuttering linked to any type of sexual dysfunction. It is not the manifestation of an oral or any

TABLE 2.3   *Differences Between Stuttering and Cluttering*

Stuttering	Cluttering
A fluency disorder	A fluency disorder involving verbal thought organization
Person is aware of the problem	Person is unaware of the problem
Usually a slow rate of delivery	Usually a rapid rate of delivery
Dysfluencies related to specific sounds, words, people, and situations	Dysfluencies not related to specific sounds, words, people, and situations
Person has normal concentration and attention span	Person may have poor concentration and reduced attention span

other type of fixation. Without exception, in literature and media, frustration is shown to increase the amount and severity of stuttering.

Literature and media stereotypes give lower status and power to stutterers. People who stutter are typically less valued by society than fluent speakers (Linn & Caruso, 1998). Porky Pig is consistently inept, whereas many other cartoon characters are wily and clever. This lower status and power are especially true of vocations and professions requiring extensive communication, such as the legal or teaching professions. The exception to this observation is the movie *Pearl Harbor*. The character Red Winkle is a fighter pilot despite his stutter. However, today it is unlikely that a person with a severe stuttering problem would pass the extensive flight training and tests to become a military pilot. Pilots are required to be able to communicate quickly and effectively with the control tower and other airplanes, often during anxiety-provoking events. In these situations, a stutter could be fatal. Stuttering problems are often used as an interesting aside to the general plot or theme development, as in *The Sixth Sense*. Sometimes, the rejection is covert with little overt ridicule or taunting. A look or glance at the stuttering person carries ridicule. Literature and media often place the person who stutters in an inferior role, one that negates his effectiveness, such as in the stuttering scene in *My Cousin Vinny*.

Not all portrayal of stuttering in literature and media is negative. Stuttering often gives the character a likable, vulnerable personality. For example, in the movie *Pearl Harbor*, the stuttering that occurs when Red asks the nurse for a date—and later in the movie, marriage—provides the audience with a way of identifying with the tension associated with those types of questions. The same type of likable personality characteristics are seen in Mel Tillis movies. In some instances, stuttering shows a vulnerability of character with which all of us can identify. Stuttering can give depth to a character.

It is remarkable that in *The Cowboys*, *The Sixth Sense*, *The Howard Stern Show*, and *One Flew Over the Cuckoo's Nest*, the stuttering characters are primarily labeled as "stutterers." The word *stutterer* in the films, credits, and reviews precedes their names. The characters are not simply Bob, Stanley, John, or Billy, they are Stuttering Bob, Stuttering Stanley, Stuttering John, and Stuttering Billy. This shows how the label of stuttering can be an overriding aspect of a person's identity.

Summary

Stuttering is an age-old communication disorder with many possible causes and treatments. Stuttering consists of what is heard and seen by the listener and what is felt by the person doing the stuttering. Stuttering also affects the person's personality, especially with regard to speaking self-esteem and ego strength. Aspects of stuttering make it both interesting to study and difficult to treat. A highly visible communication disorder, it is often used by authors and playwrights to provide comic relief.

Study Questions

1. How is verbal impotence and the propositionality of an utterance related in stuttering?

2. Provide three examples of circumlocution.

3. What problems are raised by the lack of a consistent definition of stuttering when comparing the results of research?

4. List and describe the three ways words may be improperly patterned in time.

5. What are the incidence and prevalence statistics for stuttering?

6. Compare and contrast *normal nonfluencies*, *confirmed stuttering*, and *developmental stuttering*.

7. Discuss the three theories of the causes of stuttering.

8. List and discuss the variables that can affect stuttering, such as speech cues, self-consciousness, noise, and the like.

9. What are the key aspects of stuttering, and how are they treated in stuttering therapy?

10. What is the *diagnosogenic theory of stuttering*, and how might it explain the cause of stuttering?

11. What are your thoughts about cure versus control of stuttering?

12. Compare and contrast *stuttering* and *cluttering*.

13. What are some myths about the cause and treatment of stuttering?

14. Overall, how does literature and media treat the subject of stuttering?

15. What steps could the media take to disprove myths about stuttering and improve the lives of stutterers?

Suggested Reading

Lawrence, M., & Barclay, D. M. (1998). Stuttering: A brief review. *The American Family Physician, 5*(9): 2175–2178. This article, written by physicians, reviews the etiology, diagnosis, and treatment of stuttering.

Linn, G. W., & Caruso, A. J. (1998). Perspectives on the effects of stuttering on the formation and maintenance of intimate relationships. *Journal of Rehabilitation, 64*(3): 12–14. In this interesting article, stuttering—and its effect on intimate relationships—is reviewed from the perspective of rehabilitation counselors.

Tanner, D. (1999). *Understand stuttering: A guide for parents.* Oceanside, CA: Academic Communication Associates. Written for parents, this guide describes stuttering and provides helpful suggestions to parent and teachers.

Yeoman, B. (1998). Wrestling with words. *Psychology Today, 31*(6): 42–47. This article provides an alternative view of stuttering as a disorder. It suggests that some people should learn to accept stuttering, rather than striving to overcome it.

3

The Voice and Its Disorders

Chapter Preview

The human voice is remarkable. It is necessary for the physical act of speaking, and there would be no song without it. In this chapter the interplay between head and neck resonance and vocal cord functioning is discussed, particularly as they contribute to individual voice characteristics. There is a discussion of the relationship between respiration and voice production. The muscles and cartilages of the larynx are described, particularly their roles in adjusting pitch and loudness, along with the aerodynamic and muscular forces that permit the vocal cords to vibrate rapidly. In addition, the perceptions people draw from differences in voice quality are analyzed. Voice and resonance disorders including those resulting from cleft lip and palate, vocal cord paralysis, diseases, and psychological factors are reviewed. The role vocal strain and abuse play in certain voice disorders is explained, as well as how society views people with voice disorders.

The study of the human voice and its disorders is a journey into the core of our ability to produce speech. Voice is the foundation of speech. It is a remarkable aspect of our evolution. From the birth cry of a newborn to the vocal stylings of Linda Ronstadt, Eminem, and Britney Spears, we delight in the human ability to create sound and song. Like most things human, the voice is complex, intricate, and dynamic. Although speech and hearing scientists have discovered much about this ability, there is still much to learn about the neurology, physiology, and acoustics of the human voice.

People in the public eye, such as politicians and entertainers, often benefit from a desirable voice quality. The voice can be a powerful window into the personality and can prompt the listener to draw conclusions about the speaker. Such perceptions can be accurate or inaccurate. Some people with weak characters have voices that accurately reflect their personalities. In other people, undesirable voice qualities can be misleading, and people may erroneously think they perceive something not actually there. A person's voice can be a friend or foe as one deals with the world.

Voice disorders can be minor nuisances or devastating disabilities. For people who do little talking, a voice disorder can be of minor consequence. For those who rely heavily on verbal communication, it can be devastating to job and career. Hundreds of diseases and disorders can impair, or even eliminate, this marvelous ability to produce voice and song. The treatment of a voice disorder can be as simple as reducing the amount of one's talking or it can be as all-encompassing as learning to talk without a larynx.

The Human Resonating System

The human voice is more than just the sound made by the vocal cords when they vibrate. Voice is the interplay between vocal cord vibration and the resonance in the air-filled cavities of the neck and head. **Vocal resonance** is the amplification and damping of the vibratory sound produced in the larynx by passage through the resonating chambers in the neck and head. The vocal cords are the source of voice, and the resonating chambers modify the energy coming from them. In this acoustic view of voice production, voiced speech sounds are produced through amplification and damping of the vibratory energy coming from the larynx.

This principle of speech production was advanced by Hermann von Helmholtz in the 1800s. Acoustically, the speech production mechanism is a double Helmholtz resonator. In this sense the human voice can be likened to brass and reed musical instruments. The sources of the sound for these instruments are the vibrations of the reed or the lips in the mouthpiece of the brass instrument. Then, the texture, shape, length, and cavities of the musical instruments give them their unique sound quality. The tones are an interplay between the vibratory source and the musical instrument's resonance characteristic. Acoustically, the voice is similar to a musical instrument in that a sound source interplays with resonating chambers in the neck and head. The vocal cords create vibratory energy, and certain aspects of that energy are amplified or damped in the neck and head. There is empty space in the cavities of the neck and head, and these cavities are filled with air and resonate when the vocal cords vibrate. This resonance gives people their individual voice qualities. For the most part, a person's voice sounds like her because of the way her head is shaped.

Respiration and Voice

When a person speaks, he creates sound waves by compressing the air in the lungs and sending it through the vocal tract where it is shaped into speech sounds. **Respiration** is the driving force for the voice. Although the respiratory system is essential for speech communication, its primary function is to allow the exchange of gases to and from the environment. For life-sustaining purposes, the respiratory mechanism is a chemical-processing system allowing for the exchange of oxygen for carbon dioxide. For speech purposes, respiration is an overlaid function. It is a mechanical act that compresses the air, enabling the production of speech sounds. The primary function of respiration is to sustain life, and speech communication is a secondary ability that evolved. The life-sustaining function of respiration always has the highest priority. Test this the next time you run a long distance or do something else that taxes your respiratory system. During strenuous activity, if you try to speak, you will see that

Literature, Media, and Personality Profiles

Julie Andrews

Actress and singer Julie Andrews was born on October 1, 1935, in Walton-on-Thames, England. When she was a young girl, her parents noted that she had a voice with a range of four octaves, and she began singing lessons at the age of 8. In the 1960s she became an international star with two musicals: *The Sound of Music* and *Mary Poppins*. She has received the title of Dame from Queen Elizabeth in a ceremony at Buckingham Palace. In 1999 Andrews filed a malpractice suit against a hospital and two physicians. She alleged that they ruined her ability to sing due to unnecessary surgery to remove noncancerous tumors on her vocal cords. She was starring in *Victor Victoria* on Broadway at the time of the surgery. According to the suit, she was not informed of the risk of permanent irreversible loss of voice quality. In November 2000, Andrews was awarded $20 million in damages for the loss of her singing voice.

William Jefferson Clinton

William Jefferson Clinton was elected the 42nd president of the United States on November 3, 1992. During the 1990s, President Clinton's chronic voice disorder received national attention during his first presidential election campaign. During the early primaries, he was forced to limit his oratories and was occasionally completely unable to speak in public. The news media reported that his voice disorder resulted from allergies and extensive public speaking. The voice disorder was described as *laryngitis*, which means inflammation or swelling of the vocal cords.

During both terms of office, Clinton suffered periodically from the voice disorder. The problem was so chronic that his public speaking voice was characteristically hoarse. His voice disorder often punctuated his speeches, interviews, depositions, and public statements. Some people judged the veracity of his statements based on the strength of his voice. Several comedians mimicked his voice quality in impersonations. Fervent critics of the president, such as Rush Limbaugh, also imitated Clinton's voice quality when ridiculing him or his political views.

Jack Klugman

In 1974 Jack Klugman won a Golden Globe award for Best Television Actor in a Musical or Comedy for his role as Oscar Madison in the long-running show *The Odd Couple*. *The Odd Couple* revolved around the lives of two men, Oscar, a messy slob, and Felix, played by Tony Randall, who was compulsive about neatness and cleanliness. The humor of the show evolved from their conflicts as roommates. They were longtime friends but constantly got on each other's nerves. Oscar Madison was typically seen playing poker, wearing a torn sweat shirt and baseball cap, and smoking an ever-present cigar. Reruns of *The Odd Couple* are widely syndicated.

Klugman was diagnosed with throat cancer in 1989 and underwent a partial laryngectomy, the surgical removal of the larynx. In Klugman's case one of his vocal cords was removed. For several months after the surgery, he was unable to speak. With therapy his voice returned, albeit with a forced, breathy quality. Since the surgery he has done several commercials and an episode of the science fiction television show *The Outer Limits*, and continues to perform on Broadway.

Kenny Rogers

Kenneth Ray Rogers was born on August 21, 1937. Considered one of today's best country–western and crossover singers, he is also an actor. Rogers began his singing career as a member of the New Christie Minstrels and then joined The First Edition; after they disbanded he began a highly successful solo career. His notable songs include "Ruby Don't Take Your Love to Town" and the Grammy Award–winning tune "Lucille."

Rogers's musical appeal is based in part on his low-pitched, sullen voice quality. Frequently during his songs, his voice drops into a mode of vibration known as vocal fry. *Vocal fry* is a low-pitched, pulsating voice quality sometimes described as "gravelly." The effect of Rogers's distinct voice quality depends on the theme of the song. In "Lucille" and "Ruby Don't Take Your Love to Town," the theme is rejection and infidelity. His **glottal fry** voice quality expresses a sense of desperation, hurt feelings, and seething anger. Vocal fry is a distinct voice quality, not necessarily the result of a pathology. However, Rogers developed a voice disorder and consequently received medical treatment for it.

Stacy Keach

Walter Stacy Keach was born in Savannah, Georgia. He has starred in several television shows, most recently *Titus*, and has made several guest appearances in others including *Maverick*; *Dr. Quinn, Medicine Woman*; and *Bonanza*. He usually wears a moustache to cover scarring that resulted from his cleft lip surgery. Keach, who is Honorary Chair of the Cleft Palate Foundation, has been active in attempts to reform insurance coverage for children born with birth defects. He was a speaker at a congressional briefing addressing denial of insurance coverage for congenital defects and pediatric deformities.

Randy Travis

Country singer and actor Randy Travis (born Randy Traywick) was born on May 4, 1959, in rural North Carolina. At an early age, Travis and his brother Ricky had their own duo and played at private parties, VFW halls, and fiddlers' conventions. At age 16 he won a solo competition on a talent show and subsequently began performing and recording. In 1981 Travis moved to Nashville. During his first decade as an internationally recognized country singer, he sold more than 20 million records. He is one of the country's top-grossing touring attractions. He has made several movies—including *The Rainmaker* and *Fire Down Below*—and has had guest appearances on television shows such as *Touched by an Angel* and *Matlock*. Travis is known for his strong resonant voice, which has a distinctive nasal quality. This type of voice quality typifies the country music genre; it is sometimes called a "country twang." Perceptually, Travis's voice helps carry an honest, sincere, and "down-home" message, which many people feel embodies country music.

The Godfather

The Godfather, released in 1972, stars Marlon Brando as Don Vito Corleone, a Mafia boss. Although Brando does not have a voice disorder, he has built his career on the distinctive quality of his voice. *The Godfather*, based on the novel by Mario Puzo, depicts the life and times of the Corleone family from the early 1900s to the mid-1950s. The film won the

(continued)

Literature, Media, and Personality Profiles (continued)

Academy Award for Best Picture, and Brando won for Best Actor. Two sequels followed it, both of which are considered remarkable and compelling films.

Brando's character, Don Vito Corleone, has been frequently imitated. The line "I'm gonna make him an offer he can't refuse" is delivered with a distinct breathy voice quality that helps give it the dual meanings. Technically, a breathy voice quality is not pathological but an example of the power of the voice to reflect and amplify a person's character. Rarely does Corleone raise the volume of his voice or show vocal indications of tension and stress. Throughout the film, Corleone's voice quality suggests a cold amorality about "the family business" and corruption. Corleone's soft, breathy voice quality embodies an unscrupulous sincerity to engage in criminal acts. While others may shout threats and have their voices carry their inflamed emotions, in *The Godfather*, when a Mafia boss decides to engage in criminal acts, he does so quietly, and his voice projects businesslike resolve.

the demands of the body for the exchange of gases will override your ability to talk. It is difficult, if not impossible, to carry on a conversation while breathing hard.

The Biological Pump

Viewing the respiratory system as a biological pump is a useful way to understand how air flows in and out of the lungs, both for gas exchange and for speech communication. The phase in which air flows into the lungs is called **inspiration. Expiration** is the phase in which the air flows from the lungs, during which voice can be produced. The human body pumps air in and out of the body by changing the size of the **thorax**—the upper part of the torso that contains the heart, lungs, and ribs. The lower part, the abdomen, contains the digestive organs and glands. More than a dozen muscles are involved in respiration. The *diaphragm*, a dome-shaped muscle separating the thorax from the abdomen, is one of the most important.

When the diaphragm contracts, moves downward, and compresses the contents of the abdomen, other muscles of respiration expand the size of the thorax, and the pressure inside the lungs decreases relative to the outside air. When this happens and there is an open pathway to the external atmosphere, air moves into the lungs. When these muscles relax and gradually return to their starting position, greater pressure is inside the lungs, and air moves outward to the external atmosphere. This is how the biological pump works. It works because of **Boyle's law:** Gas pressure and volume are inversely proportional to one another. The *kinetic theory of gases* helps explain this law as it relates to respiration: "Provided volume and temperature are held constant, the force exerted on the walls of the containing vessel is a function of the number of gas molecules within the vessel" (Zemlin, 1998, p. 34). As the size of the thorax changes, air moves from a region of higher pressure to one of lower pressure. This is done automatically for life-sustaining functions and for speech purposes. When we talk, expiration usually lasts longer, allowing more efficient use of the compressed air to create speech sounds.

The Larynx

In addition to structures in the mouth, one of the main sources for sound production is an anatomical structure called the larynx (lair-rinks), commonly called the "voice box." It is made up primarily of muscles and nine cartilages. *Cartilage* is firm connective tissue, which is softer than bone. Three cartilages of the larynx are paired: arytenoids, corniculates, and cuneiforms. The *arytenoids* are pyramid shaped, and the vocal cords attach to them. The *corniculates* are small cartilages attached to the upper part (apex) of the arytenoids. The *cuneiforms* are wedge shaped. The unpaired cartilages are the thyroid, cricoid, and epiglottis. The *thyroid cartilage* is the largest cartilage (the "Adam's Apple" is part of the thyroid cartilage and is more prominent in males). The *cricoid cartilage* is shaped like a signet ring and lies below the thyroid cartilage. The *epiglottis*, which has a free end projecting upward, closes over the larynx during swallowing to protect the lower air passageways.

Intrinsic laryngeal muscles are those that have both their origin and insertion within the larynx. They are important for pitch adjustment and loudness control. **Extrinsic laryngeal muscles** are those with their origin outside the larynx, and they help hold it in place. Sometimes called strap muscles, extrinsic laryngeal muscles have their attachment within the laryngeal system. The **vagus nerve,** also called cranial nerve X, has branches in the neck region, some directly serving the speech mechanism; damage to it may result in several voice disorders (Zemlin, 1998). The **hyoid bone** is U shaped, supports the tongue, and helps hold the larynx in place. Figure 3.1 shows anterior (front), posterior (back), and lateral (side) views of the larynx.

The larynx serves two important functions. Because food traveling to the stomach and air to the lungs both pass through the oral cavity, the larynx is important to speech and swallowing. In speech, when the vocal cords vibrate, phonation, or voicing, occurs. **Phonation** is the transformation of acoustic energy (vibration of air particles) within the larynx by means of vocal cord vibration—any vibratory sound produced at the level of the larynx. During swallowing the vocal cords close off and help protect the airway from getting food or liquid in it (see Chapter 7). Biologically, the larynx is a protective device for the lower respiratory tract (Zemlin, 1998). The lower respiratory tract includes the trachea, bronchial tubes, and lungs. The larynx also closes, capturing air in the lungs, to help stabilize the body during lifting and other strenuous tasks. The sound of grunting occurring during these activities is the controlled release of the compressed air and the accompanying vocal cord vibration.

When referring to the vocal cords, **fundamental frequency** is the rate at which they vibrate and is measured in cycles per second. The typical adult male's vocal cords vibrate, on average, about 130 cycles per second. The typical adult female's vocal cords vibrate more rapidly, on average, about 250 cycles per second. (See Box 3.1 for an example of how many times vocal cords vibrate during extensive speaking.) The higher rate of vibration in the female voice occurs because the larynx is typically smaller and shaped somewhat differently. This gives the typical female voice a higher pitch. **Pitch** is the psychological perception of frequency of vibration. **Loudness** is the psychological perception of the force, or strength, of vibration. Frequency and intensity are physical phenomena, functional properties of matter, whereas pitch and loudness are psychological perceptions. The physical properties of frequency and intensity and the psychological perceptions of pitch and loudness are not interchangeable. For example, frequency of vibration and pitch are not linearly proportional.

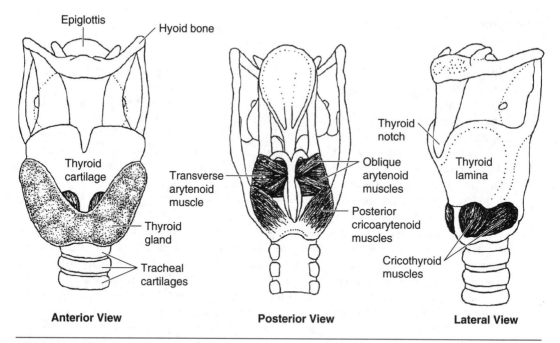

FIGURE 3.1   *Three Views of the Larynx*

Source: From W. Culbertson & D. Tanner, *Introductory Speech and Hearing Anatomy and Physiology Workbook.* Copyright 1997. Reprinted by permission by Allyn & Bacon.

Although a positive relationship exists between an increase (or decrease) in frequency of vibration and the consequent increase (or decrease) in the psychological perception of pitch, it is not a 1:1 relationship. A unit increase in frequency of vibration does not necessarily translate into a proportional unit increase in pitch. The same is true for amplitude of vibration and the psychological perception of loudness (see Chapter 6).

BOX 3.1 • *Continuous Vocal Cord Vibration*

The vocal cords of a professor giving an hour-long lecture might open and close thousands of times. Assuming that about three-quarters of the 44 sounds of English are voiced, all the vowels and more than half the consonants, the professor's vocal cords would vibrate, open, and close, about 9,000 times in 1 minute of continuous talking. This figure is obtained by multiplying an average frequency of vocal cord vibration of 200 cycles per second by 60 seconds and then multiplying the product by 75%. There are 60 minutes in an hour, so the professor's vocal folds would vibrate 540,000 times in one lecture of continuous talking. Of course, this is a gross estimate and does not account for pauses, pitch modulations, or other variables, but it does demonstrate how rapidly and continuously the vocal cords vibrate.

The Pitch-Changing Mechanism

A person makes both pitch and loudness adjustments by changes in respiratory support and by small movements of the muscles and cartilages of the larynx. To alter pitch, the frequency and manner of vocal cord vibrations are changed similar to the way a musician tunes a guitar. Tightening a guitar string raises the pitch; loosening it lowers the pitch. As well, all other things being equal, a thick guitar string has a lower pitch than a thinner string. The respiratory system and the larynx work together to make similar changes with the vocal cords. The arytenoid cartilages are important in changing pitch. Because they slide, rock, and rotate, they cause the vocal cords to become longer or shorter. Working with other muscles of the larynx, they cause the vocal cords to become thinner or thicker. Figure 3.2 shows the vocal cords and the way the arytenoid cartilages slide, rock, and rotate to help change pitch and loudness.

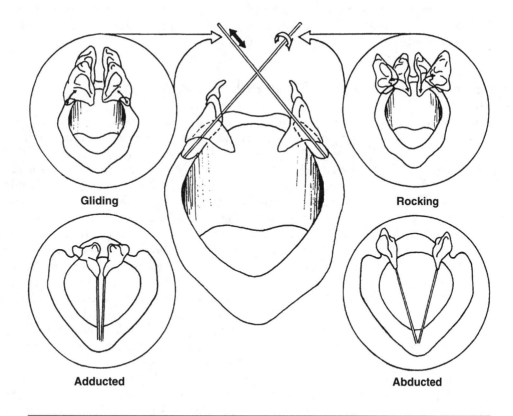

FIGURE 3.2 *The Arytenoid Cartilages Move to Help Change Pitch and Loudness*

Source: W. Perkins & R. Kent, *Functional Anatomy of Speech, Language, and Hearing.* Copyright 1986. Reprinted by permission by Allyn & Bacon.

Another way of looking at the pitch-changing process is by the relationship of the length to the thickness of the vocal cords, or their mass per unit length. Mass relates to the size or thickness of the vocal cords, and the length is how much they are stretched. When the mass per unit length of the vocal cords is increased, frequency of their vibrations decreases, with a consequent reduction in pitch. Decreasing the mass per unit length of the vocal cords results in more vibrations per second, thus increasing pitch. Several factors are involved in pitch adjustment, but primary is the amount the vocal cords are stretched in relation to their thickness. Pitch change is the result of the interplay between the sliding, rocking, and rotating of the arytenoid cartilages, intrinsic laryngeal muscles that move and adjust the cartilages of the larynx, and increase and decrease in air pressure below the vocal cords. The pressure below the vocal cords is the **subglottal air pressure** (Psub). The extrinsic laryngeal muscles, however, can play a minor role in pitch adjustment.

The amazing frequencies at which the vocal cords vibrate result from the physics of motion and laryngeal neurophysiology. How is it possible that the vocal cords can vibrate more than 500 times per second? This vibration cannot result from individual muscular contraction because human muscles cannot contract and relax that rapidly. People can talk for minutes, even hours, at a time with little effort. How is it possible that a professor, singer, debater, or student, having easy conversation with a friend over a cup of coffee, can move their vocal cords so rapidly and effortlessly?

Aerodynamic and Muscular Forces in Voice Production

Vocal cord vibrations result from finely coordinated air-pressure changes and muscular forces. Without these pressure changes and muscular forces, the vocal cords would not vibrate effectively; they would simply be blown apart rather than set into vibration. The main aerodynamic force that helps close the vocal cords results from the **Bernoulli principle,** named after a Swiss mathematician who discovered that the velocity of air flow through a tube is inversely related to its pressure against the side of the tube. When air flows through the *glottis* (the opening at the level of the vocal folds), negative pressure is created, and the vocal cords are sucked together. Once they contact each other, the suction is stopped, and they are blown apart again. The next cycle of vibration occurs when the subglottal air pressure builds to a sufficient extent to blow them apart, again permitting the flow of air, followed by contact with each other, and cessation of airflow, and another cycle begins. You can create the Bernoulli effect by holding two sheets of paper together and blowing through them. The curved parts of the sheet of paper create an airfoil and cause them to be sucked together, creating a vibration similar to what happens with the vocal cords. (See Sidebar 3.1.)

In addition to the airflow factors involved in vocal cord vibration, muscular forces are at work. Muscles have *elasticity*. Like a balloon or rubber band, a muscle tends to resist deformation and to recover its original shape once the force of deformation is removed. During phonation, the vocal folds and supporting muscles and tissues are stretched, and their elasticity causes them to regain their original shape. This tendency of muscles to return to their original shape and the force of their contractions help close the vocal cords and assist in vibration. Both aerodynamic and muscular forces are important in pitch and loudness adjustments. Together, these forces are the basis of the *aerodynamic myoelastic principle of voice production*, which describes the aerodynamic and muscular forces during phonation.

SIDEBAR 3.1

> The Bernoulli principle accounts for the lift that airplanes have when they reach certain speeds. The wing of an airplane is an airfoil. This means that the air going over the top of it has farther to travel than the air moving under the wing. The curved top of a wing gives it lift because a negative pressure, or suction, is created. The faster the wing travels through the air, the greater is the lift. The inside borders of the vocal cords are like airfoils.

Voice Quality

Humans have a marvelous ability to sense the mental and emotional status of a speaker. Much of the information about a speaker's frame of mind results from nonverbal communication. **Nonverbal communication** is the information expressed outside of word meanings that gives the listener information about the speaker's **affect,** or the temperament, mood, and feelings associated with a thought or statement. A person's voice—including quality, pitch, loudness, nasality, and modulation—provides a rich source of these nonverbal cues. These voice-quality cues can be normal differences found in people's voices and also the result of voice pathologies. To illustrate the power of the voice in nonverbal communication, suppose a student is chronically tardy to class. If the professor says, "It is okay that you come to class late each day" with a normal voice, the words clearly indicate that tardiness is not an issue. However, if the professor says the same words with a low pitch, stressing each sound, with a harsh voice quality and a frown on his face, the nonverbal message is different. These negative nonverbal cues suggest the message that tardiness is not acceptable. When there is a conflict between the verbal message and the nonverbal one, as in this case, the listener usually believes the latter. Greater weight is given to the nonverbal message and reflects the student's belief in the professor's intentions. Although the words say that being tardy is okay, the student knows that the professor would rather he be on time for class. This type of communication, also called the *nonverbal agenda*, plays an important role in human interaction.

Causes of Differences in Voice Quality

Although the frequency and intensity of vocal cord vibrations cause differences in pitch and loudness, voice quality involves the complexity of the tone. As noted previously, voice quality refers to both nasal resonance and vocal cord vibration. (See Box 3.2 for an experiment on how to change your voice quality.)

When a person's **velum,** or soft palate, is lowered during the making of a speech sound, air and acoustic energy is directed through the nasal cavity. In English, there are three nasal sounds: /m/, /n/, and "ng." During the production of all other sounds, the velum is elevated, effectively closing off the nasal cavity (Figure 3.3). When there is a defect, such as a hole in the palate or weakness of the velum, some speakers have too much nasality on nonnasal sounds; these speakers are said to be **hypernasal.** Nasal emission, where there is an audible escape of air through the nose, may also be present. Conversely, when the nasal passages are

BOX 3.2 • *The Helium Voice*

Many youngsters have breathed helium from a balloon and spoken with the "Munchkin" voice. Children delight in the voice change that results from breathing helium. Also, several movies and television situation comedy shows have used the helium voice for its humor value. Why does the voice change so dramatically when a person breathes helium? There are several principles at work, but the primary one is that helium changes the resonance of a person's voice.

The resonance characteristics of the voice result from the vibrations of the larynx and the effect of them on the neck and head's resonating chambers. When a person breathes helium, the vocal tract and resonating chambers are filled with gas of lower density. This changes the resonance and creates a different sound.

occluded and there is too little nasal resonance, the speaker is said to be **hyponasal.** They sound as if they have a "cold in the nose." There is much variability in normal nasal resonance; some people have more or less than others, especially while singing. Excessive nasal resonance is considered characteristic of many country singers. Popular actor and country singer Randy Travis is characteristically nasal in his speech and songs.

Descriptions of Voice Quality

Differences in a people's voice quality may be a result of genetics, learning, diseases, and disorders. People have a wide range of voice qualities. You can appreciate this by listening to the different voice qualities during a classroom discussion. Note the many different attributes, traits, and characteristics of the speakers' voices and try to describe them. Accurately describing voice quality is difficult because so many adjectives are commonly used. Some people characterize a voice as masculine, feminine, strong, weak, whiny, metallic, powerful, tinny, hard, sexy, raspy, and throaty, to name some descriptions. These words used to describe a particular person's voice are usually ill-defined and not valuable in the diagnosis or treatment of voice disorders. Three terms consistently used by the general public to describe voice quality are breathy, harsh, and hoarse. These voice qualities are easily distinguishable from one another and, at least in part, are related to too much or too little laryngeal muscle tension.

Breathy Quality.   A **breathy** voice quality is one in which the vocal cords do not close completely or the period of closure is very brief. "Besides having a higher fundamental frequency, women tend to have a breathier voice quality" (Kent, 1997, p. 133). A breathy voice quality in a woman is often considered sexy. The whispered quality gives the voice an intimate, bedroom effect. Marilyn Monroe spoke and sang with a breathy voice quality that accentuated her persona as a sex symbol. There is no better example of this sexy quality than when she sang "Happy Birthday, Mr. President" to John F. Kennedy. Actress Kathleen Turner also has a characteristically breathy voice quality. In a male a breathy voice quality is

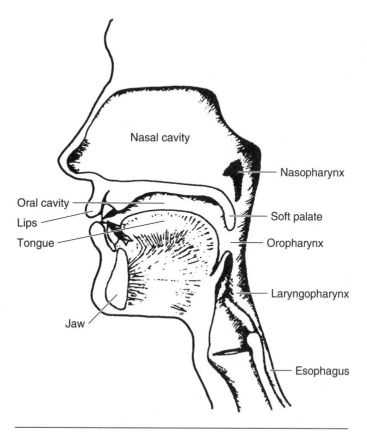

FIGURE 3.3 *Sagittal Section of the Head and Soft Palate (Velum)*

Source: W. Perkins & R. Kent, *Functional Anatomy of Speech, Language, and Hearing.* Copyright 1986. Reprinted by permission by Allyn & Bacon.

often used to signal a sinister or evil personality. Actor Vincent Price often used a breathy voice quality when playing evil characters or monsters. Marlon Brando, as the Mafia boss Don Vito Corleone in *The Godfather*, spoke with a breathy voice quality that helped develop and define his character.

A breathy voice quality may be learned in an attempt to project a particular image, be a natural voice quality due to genetics, or the result of a pathology that interferes with the complete closure of the vocal cords.

Harsh Quality. Harsh voice quality—sometimes called **strident**—is the opposite of a breathy one. A **harsh** voice quality results from the vocal cords closing with excessive force. Both males and females with a harsh voice quality appear tense, hurried, aggressive, and/or insensitive. Entertainers with a harsh voice quality include the late blues singer Janis Joplin, singer Rod Stewart, and actor Joe Pesci.

Hoarse Quality.   A hoarse voice combines breathy and harsh qualities, often with a high-pitched characteristic. Hoarseness often results from uneven closure of the vocal folds due to **edema,** or swelling. The edema can be caused by vocal abuse, diseases, and disorders, although some people constitutionally have a hoarse voice quality. Because of the uneven closure, areas along vocal folds do not close completely, allowing the air to escape and the breathy perception. When the speaker attempts to compensate for the breathiness by forcing closure, this gives hoarseness its harsh quality (Tanner, 1990b). Actor Demi Moore and soul singer James Brown sometimes have this hoarse voice quality.

Other Terms for Voice Quality

Other terms sometimes used by clinicians to describe voice include vocal fry, hard glottal attack, strangled, and wet-strangled voice qualities. As previously noted, a *vocal fry* is a low-pitched, pulsating, bubbling voice quality used in some songs by Kenny Rogers. The cartoon character Elmer Fudd, hunter of the wily rascally rabbit, "Bugs," also talks in vocal fry. **Hard glottal attack** is like the harsh voice, but the excessive force is primarily on the initial sounds of a word and the tension is reduced on the rest of the word. There is increased loudness, stress, and force on the initial part of the words. *Strangled* and *wet-strangled* voice occurs in progressive neuromuscular disorders such as multiple sclerosis and amyotrophic lateral sclerosis. The strangled sound occurs because the voice is being forced through tight muscles. It sounds much like it would if a person were physically being strangled. The wet component occurs in some patients because liquid can build up in the oral tract. You can make this type of voice quality by talking with a small amount of water in the back of your throat.

There are other entertainers whose voice quality, pitch, or loudness characteristics have become part of their persona. Robert "Bobcat" Goldthwait, a comedian and voice of the rabbit Mr. Fluffy on the television show *Unhappily Ever After*, sometimes has voice tremor, tension, and unusual pitch rises at the end of utterances. Tiny Tim was noted for his **falsetto** songs, as is vocalist Bonnie Tyler for her harsh, low-pitched 1980s hit tune "It's a Heartache." Tyler's voice is the result of surgery on her vocal cords. The following lists a few common terms, and Table 3.1 shows clinical terms and their definitions as used to describe voice quality.

Some Common Terms

feminine	metallic	strong
hard	powerful	throaty
husky	raspy	tinny
masculine	sexy	weak

Disorders of Resonance

Cleft Lip and Palate

A slang and demeaning term for a cleft lip is "harelip." Ancient myths about cleft lip and palate include mistaken beliefs that they are punishment for parents who are in disfavor with

TABLE 3.1   *Some Clinical Terms and Definitions for Voice Quality*

Term	Definition
Breathy	Vocal cords do not completely close or the period of closure is very brief.
Hard glottal attack	Harsh voice with excessive force primarily on initial sounds.
Harsh	Vocal cords close with excessive force.
Hoarse	Uneven closure of the vocal folds (breathy and harsh).
Hypernasal	Too much nasality on nonnasal sounds.
Strangled	Voice being forced through tight muscles.
Vocal/glottal fry	Pulsating low pitch.
Wet strangled	Harsh with liquid buildup in the oral tract.

God or that the child was not really wanted (Hall, Oyer, & Haas, 2001). **Cleft lip** and **cleft palate** are congenital birth defects. Part of a larger group of disorders called *craniofacial abnormalities*, these are disorders or defects of the cranium (head) and facial regions of the body. During the early weeks of pregnancy, the lips, dental arches, uvula, and hard and soft palates fuse. Sometimes this process is disrupted, and the result is a cleft, or hole, in the lip and/or roof of the mouth. Medical science has not isolated a single cause of this birth defect. In some cases craniofacial anomalies probably result from genetics; in other cases they occur because of irregularities during the early weeks of pregnancy. The incidence of cleft lip and palate is about 1 in 700 live births (Williams, Sandy, Thomas, Sell, & Sterne, 1999).

There are many types of clefts, and some are minor and barely noticeable. Others are severe birth defects requiring extensive corrective surgery and habilitation to correct. **Habilitation** is the development of an ability that is absent at birth or during the developmental period, whereas **rehabilitation** is the restoration of an ability that was once present but is now lost. Clefts are either bilateral or unilateral. A **bilateral** cleft is on both sides of the face; a **unilateral** cleft is limited to one side. A cleft palate occurring without a cleft lip is called an isolated cleft palate. Isolated clefts of the lip are rare, occurring in fewer than 5% of cases (Shprintzen, 1997).

Some people have **submucous cleft palates.** These are not visible because a mucous membrane in the mouth conceals the lack of fusion of the palate. Feeling the palatal region with a finger can detect submucous clefts, a diagnostic procedure called *digital palpation*. A bifid or deviated uvula sometimes accompanies a cleft. A **bifid uvula** is one that is divided into two parts. Technically, a bifid uvula is a cleft of that muscle. A deviated uvula is one that leans to one side, usually because of muscular weakness.

Several speech pathologies can result from clefts. There is often an overlap of the systems involved in communication disorders, and cleft lip and palate can also be categorized as articulation disorders. (See Chapter 4, Structural Defects of the Articulators.) Obviously, when there is a cleft lip, the ability to make sounds with the lips, such as /b/ and /p/, can be compromised. When the cleft includes the teeth and gums, production of sounds such as /t/ and /d/ can be impaired. A cleft can cause the teeth to be missing or jumbled. This can negatively affect the production of dental sounds such as /s/ and /z/.

Hypernasality is the primary resonance disorder associated with cleft palate. As discussed earlier, hypernasality is the presence of too much nasality during speech. In an unrepaired cleft palate, there is an opening into the nasal cavity. Hypernasality can also result from **velopharyngeal incompetence,** in which the soft palate does not adequately approximate the throat. A cleft palate can also cause nasal emission, which is the audible perception of air through the nose, a sniffing sound. This occurs primarily on pressure sounds like /t/ and /p/.

In addition to these speech pathologies, many children with clefts also have a hearing loss. Typically, it is a conductive hearing loss involving the middle ear (see Chapter 6). The hearing loss is related to the failure of the eustachian tube to equalize pressure in the middle ear. Children with clefts have also been found to be generally slower in their language development (Weiss, Gordon, & Lillywhite, 1987). Slower language development is probably related, at least in part, to the negativity and self-consciousness that they experience in social situations due to their speech disorder and possibly related to genetics or other disorders.

The Cleft Palate Team

Medical management of a child with a cleft lip and/or palate involves a team effort. The cleft palate team usually consists of a reconstructive surgeon, orthodontist, pediatrician, audiologist, and speech–language pathologist. A medical social worker also may be called upon to help the family navigate through the expensive and complicated medical procedures and therapies. Other cleft palate team members can include educators, psychologists, otolaryngologists, radiologists, genetic counselors, and dentists who specialize in treating children, depending on what is required in a particular case. (Table 3.2 lists the specialists on a cleft palate team.) The child's parents should be pivotal members of any cleft palate team.

The type and duration of therapy for cleft lip and palate depend on the severity of the birth defect. A prosthodontist is sometimes called upon to build **prostheses** to help with speech production and other functions. Prosthetic devices are appliances such as palatal lifts, dentures, and bulbs that help speech, chewing, sucking, and swallowing. The effectiveness of cleft lip and palate therapy to bring about normal speech often depends on the success of such appliances and surgeries. Reconstructive surgeries usually begin when the child is very young. Cleft lips are usually repaired surgically within the first 3 months of life, and cleft palates are typically repaired around 12 months of age (Dalston, 2000). The goal of cleft palate repair is to restore its continuity and to create an adequate velopharyngeal sphincter (Williams et al., 1999). It is effective in improving the child's speech production and appearance. "In the hands of a competent surgeon, approximately 80–90% of patients who undergo primary repair of the palate (primary palatoplasty) will have adequate velopharyngeal closure. The other 10–20% may need to undergo secondary physical management" (Dalston, 2000, pp. 273–274).

TABLE 3.2   *Specialists on a Cleft Palate Team*

Team Member	Responsibilities of Each Member
Audiologist	A specialist responsible for the identification and measurement of hearing disorders associated with cleft lip and palate
Medical social worker	A specialist responsible for counseling patients and their families regarding all aspects of cleft lip and palate habilitation
Orthodontist	A dental specialist responsible for correcting jaw and teeth irregularities associated with cleft lip and palate
Otologist	A specialist responsible for the medical management of hearing disorders associated with cleft lip and palate
Pediatrician	A physician responsible for the overall health and development of infants and children and treatment of their diseases
Prosthodontist	A dental specialist responsible for the construction of appliances that replace missing teeth or restore parts of the oral cavity
Reconstructive surgeon	A physician responsible for surgically repairing cleft lip and palate and reconstructing other facial deformities associated with them
Speech–language pathologist	A specialist responsible for the habilitation of speech, voice, and language disorders associated with cleft lip and palate

Voice Disorders

Evaluation of Voice Disorders

The evaluation of a voice disorder is a comprehensive process involving (1) review of medical records, (2) patient interview, (3) assessment of voice perceptual features, and (4) specialized laryngoscopic examination if warranted. Only after a comprehensive evaluation are therapies provided to treat the voice disorder.

Prior to seeing the patient for an evaluation, a speech–language pathologist reviews the medical records. Patients with voice disorders who first come to a speech–language pathologist are always referred to a physician for a medical examination, because some symptoms of a voice disorder can be the result of serious medical conditions. These can include tumors, paralysis, diseases, and structural or glandular problems. In addition, medications can affect the voice. The interview is conducted to determine the patient's perspective on the voice disorder and plausible causes of it. During the interview the speech–language pathologist reviews patterns of behavior that may be causing the voice disorder, such as the extent of talking, shouting, singing, preaching, or other factors that may be vocally abusive. The patient's motivation to engage in therapy and expectations for treatment are also determined. The assessment of voice perceptual features includes looking for pitch breaks, inappropriate pitch, loudness variability, hoarseness, breathiness, tremors, and strained or strangled phonation. The degree of the voice impairment is also noted and whether it occurs regularly. Several specialized instruments can be used in the voice evaluation, including a video **stroboscope,** which flashes light in such a way that the vocal cords appear to slow or stop vibrating. Other instruments include flexible or rigid scopes for viewing the larynx and for high-speed photography. There are also instruments for assessing pitch and looking at the complexity of the acoustic speech signals (time, frequency, and energy).

Vocal Cord Paralysis

Paralysis occurs when a muscle loses its ability to contract or move due to neuromuscular damage. **Paresis** means the muscle has the ability to partially contract or move. Paralysis or paresis of the laryngeal muscles can result in **aphonia,** the total loss of voice, or **dysphonia,** an impairment in the ability to produce phonation. Voice disorders due to paralysis usually impair the ability of the vocal cords to *approximate*, or contact, one another. Paralysis of the vocal cords can affect their ability to open, *abduct*, or to close, *adduct*. When the paralysis is limited to one side of the body, it is called unilateral paralysis. Bilateral vocal cord paralysis refers to both vocal cords being paralyzed.

Causes of Vocal Cord Paralysis.   Vocal cord paralysis can result from several factors. Often, damage to a nerve causes paralysis. Diseases (such as multiple sclerosis), tumors, and traumas can damage or sever a nerve, causing the muscle or muscles enervated by it to be paralyzed. The type of paralysis depends on where in the nervous system the nerve is damaged. (See Chapter 7 for a discussion of the types of paralysis.) Muscles can have reduced mobility, weakness, or slow, jerky movements, depending on where the damage occurs. Other causes of paralysis include muscle degeneration, wasting away, and problems at the myoneural junction. The *myoneural junction* is the site where the nerve and muscle come together, and several chemical reactions cause the muscle to contract and relax. These communication disorders can be caused by several diseases including muscular dystrophy, polio, multiple sclerosis, and cerebral palsy.

A common paralytic voice disorder is caused by **unilateral adductor paralysis.** This voice disorder results from paralysis, on one side of the larynx, of the muscles of phonation that are responsible for closing the vocal cords. This disorder can be caused by strokes, tumors, diseases, and trauma in which the nerve is damaged by a blunt blow or penetrating object. Unilateral adductor paralysis is usually characterized by breathiness. In patients with unilateral adductor paresis, the individual sometimes has hoarseness because she compensates for the breathiness by forcing the vocal cords closed. As was discussed previously, hoarseness is a combination of breathy and harsh voice qualities.

Treatment of Vocal Cord Paralysis.   The therapy for unilateral adductor paralysis involves straining and strengthening exercises. The goal of these therapies is to get the nonparalyzed vocal cord to cross the **midline** (the center part of the glottal opening) and approximate the impaired one, thus compensating for the reduced movement of the paralyzed cord. The vocal cords can be brought together by attempting phonation while doing strenuous activities, which include push-ups, lifting heaving objects, and isometric exercises. Also, in some patients, a physician can inject a solution into the paralyzed vocal cord to make it thicker and to help bring it closer to the midline. These therapies and medical treatments are often successful in helping the patient with unilateral adductor paralysis achieve phonation. (Medical treatments and straining and strengthening exercises are also used to treat the other kinds of vocal cord paralysis discussed earlier.)

Cancer and Other Diseases of the Larynx

Because normal voice is produced by fine adjustments of respiratory and laryngeal muscles, it is susceptible to many neurological and muscular diseases. In fact, minor changes in the voice may be one of the first symptoms of several diseases. Weak, slow, or tense muscle activity can cause pitch, loudness, and quality changes. Many degenerating and debilitating diseases result in voice pathologies. Multiple sclerosis and Parkinson's disease can impair or eliminate a person's voice. Other diseases that can affect the voice include muscular dystrophy, myasthenia gravis, and polio. These diseases, and the effects they have on the ability to phonate, are discussed in Chapter 7. Because these diseases often involve multiple motor speech systems, they are discussed in the section on dysarthria.

One of the most serious diseases of the larynx is cancer. Laryngeal tumors can be malignant or benign. Many noncancerous, or **benign,** tumors result from of vocal strain and abuse and are discussed later. However, some laryngeal tumors are **malignant** carcinomas, a specific type of cancer that develops on the tissue of the larynx. Smoking and other tobacco products cause cancer of the larynx.

Both malignant and benign tumors affect the voice in a similar manner, especially early on. They disrupt the way the vocal cords vibrate. A hoarse voice quality is often one of the earliest signs of a mass on the vocal cords. Another common indication of a laryngeal tumor is a sensation of having a foreign body on the vocal cords, resulting in attempts by a person to remove it by coughing or throat clearing. Everyone, especially smokers, who has a voice quality change or the sensation of a foreign body on the vocal cords for 2 weeks or longer should see a physician. If cancer is suspected as the cause of the voice quality change, a biopsy will be performed to determine whether the growth is benign or malignant. A *biopsy* is the process of removing tissue and examining it for diagnostic purposes. Most laryngeal cancers, if diagnosed and treated early, are curable. If left untreated, laryngeal cancers can **metastasize,** or spread to other parts of the body.

There are three conventional treatments for throat cancer: Radiation treatment, chemical therapy, and/or surgery are used to remove or destroy the tumor and to prevent it from returning. Recent advances and refinements in chemotherapy have reduced the need for surgery. New generations of medications can reduce or eliminate the tumor's genetic ability to grow, and antiangiogenesis drugs cut the blood supply to them. However, surgical removal of the larynx, a **laryngectomy,** is sometimes necessary for the treatment of cancer or laryngeal trauma. A partial laryngectomy is surgical removal of part of the larynx, such as one vocal cord, as was the case with Jack Klugman. A complete laryngectomy is removal of the entire larynx. Radical laryngectomy is the surgical removal of the larynx and adjacent parts of the body such as lymph glands, muscles, and tissues. A person who has undergone a laryngectomy is sometimes called a *laryngectomee.*

When all or part of the larynx is removed, so too is the ability to produce voice. A laryngectomee breathes through a hole in the neck called a **stoma.** There is no longer an air passage to the oral–nasal cavities and the lungs because the trachea now opens in the neck. Besides losing the ability to speak, the laryngectomee's abilities to smell, blow his nose, lift a heavy weight, and filter and warm the outside air are compromised. Because there is an open hole in the neck leading directly to the lungs, the laryngectomee must of course be careful around water, dust, and pollution.

Alaryngeal Speech

For people with laryngectomies, there are several options to regain speech. None of the options discussed next is clearly superior to the others, nor do any of them return a laryngectomee's speech to normal pitch, loudness, and quality. However, they do enable most patients to regain some ability to speak. The options for **alaryngeal** (without a larynx) speech are (1) surgery, (2) electronic devices, and (3) esophageal speech.

Surgery for alaryngeal speech involves creating a **pseudoglottis,** an artificially created pair of vocal cords. The air from the lungs is used for vibration. The vibrating source can be surgically created from existing tissue or by using an artificial device with a reed as a vibrating mechanism. These surgical procedures are evolving and improving, but not all patients are candidates for them. In addition, some patients prefer nonsurgical options.

Battery-powered vibrating sound sources have been used for decades to provide alaryngeal speech. The **electrolarynx,** a handheld vibrating device, projects its sound through the neck and head of the patient. The sound energy radiates upward into the head resonators, and the patient mouths the words. The advantages of the artificial larynx are that it is relatively easy to master and it creates speech that is understandable (intelligible) to most listeners. The disadvantages are that the patient must use one hand during communication to hold it in place, and the output is a metallic, buzzing sound. Some artificial devices are oral, in which a tube is placed in the side of the patient's mouth, providing a sound source. There is a buzzing in the cheek from which speech sounds are produced. In the cartoon series *South Park*, a cartoon character, Ned, uses an electrolarynx.

Many laryngectomees prefer to learn esophageal speech, also known as "belch talking." **Esophageal speech** consists of taking a small amount of air into the mouth and pushing it partially down the esophagus. It is not a true belch because the air usually does not come from the stomach. Several methods help get the air into the esophagus; the goal is to piston, or push, the air into the esophagus by the tongue, lips, and cheeks. The air is then gradually expelled while the person shapes the resulting sound into speech. Although esophageal speech is the most natural method of alaryngeal speech, some people cannot master either the injection method or intelligible output. For people proficient with esophageal speech, their speech can become so normal that listeners often only think they have a cold and a raspy voice.

For most people with a laryngectomy, these options can enable speech. For individuals who are unable or unwilling to use or master them, writing, gesturing, and mouthing words can provide avenues of expression. Box 3.3 shows how to produce esophageal speech. For some, belch talking is easy, whereas for others it is unnatural and difficult to learn.

BOX 3.3 • *Esophageal Speech: "I Want to Talk"*

You can experiment with esophageal speech. Find a secluded place and learn what it is like to speak without a larynx. First, open your mouth wide and capture as much air as possible and close your lips. Next, touch your tongue to the alveolar ridge, which is where the tongue and upper gums meet to make the sound /t/. With a piston motion, compress and move the air to the back of the throat and partially down the tube leading to the stomach. Swallow the air but do not allow it to go all of the way to your stomach. Now, relax and allow the air to return to your mouth. With the back of your tongue and throat, create a belching sound as the air escapes and shape it into the word *I*. Repeat the procedure and produce the word *want*. Again repeat the procedure and produce the word *to*. Finally, repeating the injection procedure, say the word *talk*. Now, do all four words as fast as possible. You may find that you can produce two or more words on one injection. You are now talking with esophageal speech. With instruction and practice, many people can be very efficient using esophageal speech.

Psychogenic Voice Disorders

A **psychogenic** disorder has a psychological cause rather than physical or organic causes. Voice disorders may also cause psychological reactions, and depression is a common reaction. Smith et al. (1996) investigated the social, psychological, vocational, physical, communicative, and quality-of-life effects of voice disorders on 174 patients. They found that 75% of the subjects believed the voice disorder negatively affected their social functioning.

Several psychogenic disorders can result in impairment or complete loss of the voice. The most common is a conversion reaction, sometimes called a hysterical disorder.

Conversion Reactions

A **conversion reaction** occurs when psychological conflict or trauma is transformed into a physical disorder. Aronson (1990) defines a conversion reaction as any loss of voluntary control over normal striated muscle movements, or over the senses, resulting from environmental stress or interpersonal conflict. These are serious psychological reactions sometimes causing institutionalization. As a rule, in this type of disorder, the patient's loss of voice symbolizes the nature of the emotional upheaval. Some psychiatrists believe there is a choice of symptoms in psychogenic disorders. The patient can manifest psychological distress in several ways. For example, an individual who sees a terrible act or event may lose her sight, which is symbolic of the psychological trauma. Psychogenic deafness can be symbolic of listening to traumatic or distressing sounds. When a person's loss of voice cannot be traced to physical causes and has a psychological cause, it can be symbolic of trauma or distress related to verbal communication. Also, psychogenic aphonia or dysphonia can represent the distress caused by a lack of meaningful relationships or an empty, dangerous, or unsatisfying one. Psychogenic voice disorders also often have an inner conflict at their core—the need to express a thought, feeling, or attitude and fear of doing so. Additionally, a person with a conversion voice disorder may act indifferent, even relieved, at having the disability. This is sometimes called *la belle indifference*, which, in French, means "the beautiful indifference." In some patients, having the voice disorder relieves them of overt psychological distress.

Hysterical Aphonia.   **Hysterical aphonia** occurs when a patient consistently whispers during speech and will not vibrate the vocal cords to achieve voiced speech. There is a loss of voice because anxiety becomes unbearable, and it is converted into physical symptoms—in this case, loss of voice. With these patients, testing whether the aphonia has a physical cause is easy. Most patients can usually laugh or hum a tune normally, which suggests no organic pathology. Often, these patients can gradually regain their speaking voice by humming and then shaping the sound into words and phrases. When the person experiences a gradual transition from humming to speech, a normal voice can be achieved.

Hysterical Dysphonia.   **Hysterical dysphonia** is a chronic impairment of the voice. It can include quality changes, pitch breaks, loudness reductions, and whispering. Sometimes the dysphonia occurs in regular cycles, periodically, such as in the morning or after lunch; in other patients the symptoms occur at irregular periods or aperiodically. In these patients, the impaired voice cannot be traced to any physical or organic cause. These patients are similar to the ones with hysterical aphonia, with anxiety playing a major role. The main difference between dysphonia and aphonia is the degree of voice impairment.

Treatment of Psychogenic Voice Disorders

The treatment of psychogenic voice disorders requires evaluation by a psychologist or psychiatrist. In these patients the defective or absent voice is a symptom of an underlying psychological disorder. Eliminating or reducing the voice disorder treats only the symptoms and does not address the underlying psychological cause(s). Psychologically, they should be viewed as a voiceless "cry for help." Experimental and clinical data support the effectiveness of therapy for the treatment of psychogenic voice disorders (Ramig & Verdolini, 1998).

Disorders Related to Vocal Strain and Abuse

Some people who strain and abuse their voices get vocal nodules, polyps, or contact ulcers. A vocal nodule is a small growth on the vocal cords, about the size of a peppercorn; it is sometimes called a singer, screamer, preacher, or teacher's node. They are more common in women, and teachers are particularly vulnerable to the detrimental effects of voice disorders. More than one-third of teachers with voice disorders report that the voice problems interfered with their ability to teach effectively (Sapir, Keidar, & Mathers-Schmidt, 1993). Cheerleaders chanting over screaming crowds are also vulnerable to nodules.

A **polyp** is a fluid-filled blister on the vocal cord. A sessile polyp is broad-based, whereas one hanging down from a stem is pedunculated. Vocal polyps may arise from a single episode of extensive strain and abuse such as cheering on a favorite sports team, engaging in a heated verbal argument, or shouting loudly in a noisy, crowded bar. Asthma and allergies may also be causative factors in the development of vocal polyps (Hall, Oyer, & Haas, 2001). **Contact ulcers** are abrasions or holes on the vocal cords, and they occur more often in men. Some vocal contact ulcers are granulated and have a rough ridge. Nodules, polyps, and contact ulcers can be unilateral or bilateral.

Causative Factors

Not everyone who strains and abuses their voices get vocal nodules, polyps, or contact ulcers. Just as some people are prone to migraine headaches or stomach ulcers, some people are more susceptible to nodules, polyps, and contact ulcers. The reason(s) why some people are prone to them is not known, but genetics, learning, and the environment may play important roles. In addition, some people might frequently strain and abuse their voices for years, even decades, without developing nodules, polyps, or contact ulcers, only to get them when they get older. This happens because aging reduces the strength and resiliency of the vocal muscles and tissues.

Singing can be vocally abusive, especially in people who have not been trained properly. The act of singing involves extreme variations of pitch and loudness, often done for long periods. Professional singers can sometimes strain their voices. For example, Leann Rimes, at age 17, was diagnosed with a strained right vocal cord and ordered to rest her voice for 60–90 days and to undergo therapy. Even singing teachers can have voice problems. According to Miller and Verdolini (1995), 64% of singing teachers reported past vocal problems.

Vocal strain and abuse can take many forms. Some people have chronic hard glottal attacks in which, during the initial production of words, their vocal cords close together too hard. Talking too loudly is abusive because it involves more forcibly closing the vocal cords. The louder the voice, the harder the vocal cords contact each other. Clearing one's throat is abusive, but some people form habits of doing it frequently. Throat clearing can irritate the vocal cords, causing the feeling that something foreign is on them. A cycle of having the sensation of a foreign body on the vocal cords followed by throat clearing can develop. Nicotine and alcohol use can also be abusive to the vocal cords. Both affect the vascular system: Alcohol dilates the blood vessels in the larynx, and nicotine constricts them. In addition, people who drink alcohol often talk too loudly and smoke more frequently and heavily. Strong chemical fumes are also causal agents, particularly causing contact ulcers.

Another cause of nodules, polyps, and contact ulcers is talking in a pitch that is either too high or low. Everyone has an **optimal pitch,** which is the easiest and most natural to produce. Given the size and shape of a particular person's larynx, there is an optimal frequency of vocal cord vibration. A person's optimal pitch is usually about one-quarter up from the bottom of his total range. **Habitual pitch** is the pitch most often used, the one that has become a habit. Sometimes, for a variety of reasons, a discrepancy exists between the optimal and habitual pitch in a particular person. For example, a male may want his usual pitch to be lower than what is natural for him; he may want to sound more masculine. A radio or television announcer may use an unnatural pitch to accentuate her broadcast personality. Generally, the more the discrepancy between a person's optimal and habitual pitches, the greater is the vocal abuse. Box 3.4 shows how to determine your optimal pitch.

BOX 3.4 • *Finding Your Optimal Pitch*

The following is a way of determining your optimal pitch. When doing this exercise, it may be helpful to use a piano, pitch pipe, or tape recorder. You may have to try this several times to get an accurate appraisal of your optimal pitch.

Sing "ah" beginning anywhere on the musical scale. Then sing down to the lowest note you can produce clearly. Then, sing "ah" on successive notes upward until reaching the highest note, including falsetto, while counting the number of notes between the lowest and highest pitch. Count the total number of notes, which is your range, and divide the total by 4. Now, do the above again and count from the lowest note to the one identified as one-quarter of your total range. This should be your optimum pitch. Prolong the sound and say a few words, using it to see if this is your typical, or habitual, voice. This exercise provides you with a way of knowing whether you typically speak in your optimal pitch. If you have a large discrepancy between optimal and habitual pitch and if your voice is frequently impaired or fatigues easily, you may want to see a speech–language pathologist for an evaluation.

Treatment of Disorders Related to Vocal Strain and Abuse

The goal of therapy for disorders related to vocal strain and abuse is to reduce laryngeal hyperfunction and muscular imbalance and to prevent the need for laryngeal surgery or maximize its long-term results (Ramig & Verdolini, 1998). Surgery involves removing or reducing the size of the growths on the vocal cords. Laser surgery is common, although some surgeons prefer to use a scalpel. Vocal cord surgery can sometimes dramatically alter a person's voice, as was the case with singer Bonnie Tyler. She states the nature of her husky voice on her home page (http://members.nbci.com/_XMCM/bonnietyler/bio.htm): "I had nodules on my throat, singers often have it. But unfortunately the doctor who operated on me cut off a little bit more and now I have such a husky voice." (For more information see www.bonnietyler.com/bio.html.)

There is a psychological component to the development of nodules, polyps, and contact ulcers, which is addressed in therapy. They are often anxiety- and tension-related disorders, which result from patients pushing themselves too hard. Stress often predisposes and precipitates these voice disorders. Excessive muscular tension in the voice production mechanism can perpetuate them. In some patients these growths or ulcerations on the vocal folds occur because they are hypersensitive to a deficient body function. They hear changes in their voices and feel an irritation in their throats. Because they have a low tolerance of temporary voice imperfections, they overcompensate by forcing voice. This results in increased laryngeal tension and irritation that eventually increases the severity of the voice pathology. A vicious cycle of impaired voice and overcompensation is the result, which further irritates the nodules, polyps, and contact ulcers.

Figure 3.4 shows how the cycle develops. First, in normal voice, there is an appropriate amount of muscular tension in the respiratory and laryngeal mechanisms. The self-concept evaluator, the part of the personality that monitors whether the voice is normal, does not detect abnormalities in the voice, so it is not activated. As used in this context, the self-concept evaluator receives information about the voice from the senses and makes judgments about its normalcy. Because of vocal strain and abuse, a nodule, polyp, or contact ulcer begins to develop. Vocal strain and abuse occur from frequent hard glottal attacks, excessively loud speech, frequent throat clearing, discrepancies between optimal and habitual pitch, excessive use of alcohol and nicotine, and others. Because the developing nodule, polyp, or contact ulcer impairs complete closure of the vocal cords during the closed phase of voice production, excess air escapes and is heard as breathiness. The voice sounds different from what the speaker is accustomed. The person may also feel foreign sensations including pain, tickle, and irritation. To compensate for these changes, the person forces the vocal cords together by using more muscular force. This creates a harsh quality and further irritates the developing nodule, polyp, or contact ulcer. Because of this pathology on the vocal cords, glottal closure is incomplete, causing the breathy quality. This is the cause of the hoarse voice quality, which is a combination of breathy and harsh voice qualities. Vocal nodules, polyps, and contact ulcers can be considered *reactive voice disorders* because of the person's reactions to changes in his voice; muscular relaxation training is an important part of therapy (Tanner, 1990b). Through muscular relaxation, patients learn to use their voices with less force. Initially, without overcompensation, there is a breathy voice quality, which gradually subsides as the growths become smaller and eventually are eliminated.

Regardless of the particular voice disorder, voice therapy has two goals: to optimize existing function and to minimize the disabling effects. "The goal of voice treatment is to maximize vocal effectiveness given the existing disorder and to reduce the handicapping effect of the voice problem" (Ramig & Verdolini, 1998, p. S101).

Voice production plays a critical role in self-expression, well-being, and functional daily living. (See Box 3.5 for vocal hygiene tips.) Disordered voice can negatively affect personal relationships, employment, and productivity. The effective treatment of voice disorders can positively affect quality of life (Ramig & Verdolini, 1998, p. S112).

Literature and Media Stereotypes

The voice brings speech and song to human existence. From the fine muscular changes involved in changing pitch to the enormous speed at which the vocal cords vibrate, voice is a highly evolved, dynamic function. Given the complexities of the respiratory structures, larynx, and resonating system, it is not surprising that many diseases and disorders can impair or even eliminate the voice.

Voice serves as the form for speech communication, and it is also involved in nonverbal communication. A person's voice on film, radio, television, or in song sends the audience several cues about character and frame of mind. These cues go beyond the objective meaning of the words. They provide information about how the speaker or singer feels about what is being spoken or sung. Whether the voice reinforces Don Vito Corelone's cold, detached Mafia ways or projects Kenny Rogers's desperation and pain, it helps define a character's intent and projects the singer's emotions.

Society has come to identify and stereotype aspects of voice with certain personality traits. Men with high voices are often thought of as having more feminine traits, and women with low voices as having more masculine ones. In film, men with breathy voice qualities are

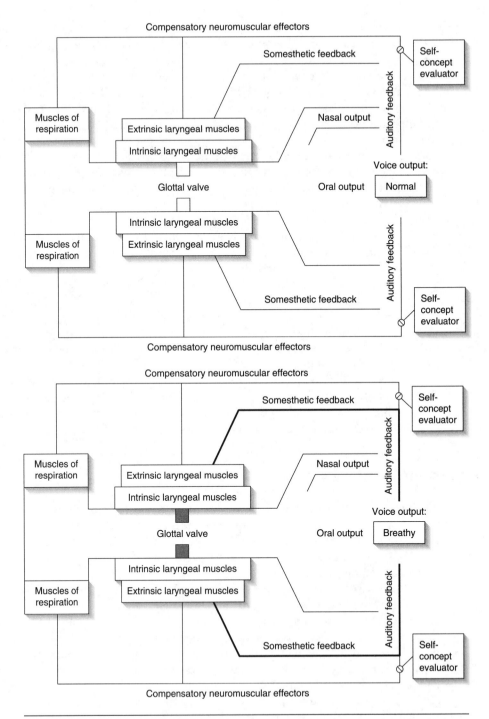

FIGURE 3.4 *Excessive Muscular Force Contributes to the Development of Nodules, Polyps, and Contact Ulcers*

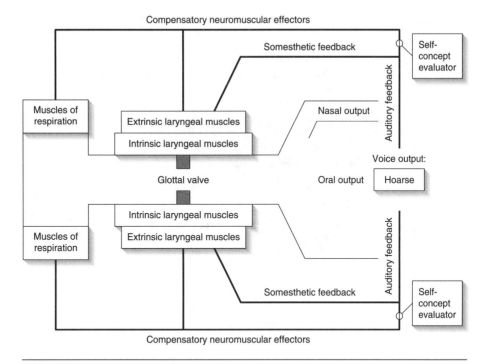

FIGURE 3.4   *Continued*

more cold and evil, whereas women with the same quality project an intimate, sexy personality. Too much or too little nasality also carries nonverbal information. The stereotypical hypernasal country tune brings to mind the image of a cowboy and reinforces the idea, to some people, that those types of songs are more simple, honest, and straightforward. The complete absence of voice can reduce or even eliminate an actor's ability to project feelings and attitudes with a particular line or an entire script. Even a "stage whisper," a loud whispered utterance, does not have the inflection, stress, and emphasis power of the voice. These stereotypes exist because people are judged by their nonverbal vocal cues. Successful actors, television announcers, radio personalities, and singers use them to create and amplify their persona. A distinctive voice can add power and authority to people and institutions, as with James Earl Jones's low-pitched declaration: "This is CNN."

Summary

A person's voice can be a window into his personality. For better or worse, people draw conclusions about an individual's character based on his voice. Voice is the essence of song, and a talented singer can communicate the range of human emotion through it. Many diseases and disorders can impair or even eliminate a person's voice. Fortunately, medical procedures and

BOX 3.5 • *Vocal Hygiene Tips*

1. Drink plenty of water.
2. Don't drink alcoholic beverages, smoke, or use other tobacco products.
3. Don't talk loudly or shout for long periods.
4. Don't whisper for long periods.
5. If you find a change in your voice quality, don't force it to sound normal.
6. Get professional singing instructions if you sing a lot.
7. Don't engage in excessive hard glottal attacks.
8. Talk and sing with relaxed throat muscles.
9. Talk in a pitch that is optimal for you.
10. Don't clear your throat or cough excessively; swallow and drink water to clear and soothe your throat.
11. If you are prone to voice problems, limit the amount of talking.
12. Check with a physician if you have a voice-quality change, pain, or a foreign-body sensation on the vocal cords that lasts longer than 2 weeks.

therapies are successful in treating most voice disorders and can minimize the disabilities caused by them.

Study Questions

1. How can the human voice be compared to a musical instrument?
2. Describe the processes involved in the biological pump of respiration.
3. Draw the larynx and identify the nine cartilages.
4. What are the factors associated with changing pitch?
5. Describe the aerodynamic myoelastic principle of voice production.
6. Provide an example of how voice can affect nonverbal communication.
7. Describe *breathy, harsh,* and *hoarse* voice quality.
8. What is *velopharyngeal incompetence*?
9. List and describe the responsibilities of the members of a cleft palate team.
10. What is *unilateral adductor paralysis*?
11. What are some options for people with laryngectomies to help them regain the ability to communicate?
12. Compare and contrast *hysterical dysphonia* and *hysterical aphonia*.
13. What are the disorders related to vocal strain and abuse? What causes them and how are they treated?
14. What are some stereotypes associated with different voice qualities?

Suggested Reading _____

Aronson, A. (1990). *Clinical voice disorders: An interdisciplinary approach* (3rd ed.). New York: Thieme. This graduate-level, interdisciplinary text provides comprehensive, detailed information about the voice and its disorders.

Ramig, L. O., & Verdolini, K. (1998). Treatment efficacy: Voice disorders. *Journal of Speech, Language, and Hearing Research*, *41*: S101–S116. American Speech-Language-Hearing Association. This article provides an extensive table summarizing selected studies on the effect of voice treatment. The table provides information about subjects, treatment(s), designs, measures, and results.

Tanner, D. (1990). *Tanner muscular relaxation program for voice disorders*. Oceanside, CA: Academic Communication Associates. This program provides information about reactive voice disorders and their treatment. It includes an instructional cassette tape that helps patients learn to relax respiratory and laryngeal muscles.

Articulation and Phonological Disorders

Chapter Preview

In this chapter you will learn how the structures of the oral cavity shape the compressed air coming from the lungs into speech sounds. The way consonants and vowels are categorized is explained, as are the acoustic and sequential units of speech. Ongoing speech production is an extremely sophisticated motor act, and you will learn about the many facets that go into it. Several causes of articulation disorders are discussed, and you will learn how articulation disorders are evaluated and treated. There is also an interesting discussion of dialects and accents. Finally, the way literature and media have typically portrayed people with articulation and phonological disorders is explored.

Most humans are omnivorous and eat a variety of vegetables, grains, fruits, eggs, nuts, and meats. The first stage of digestion occurs in the oral cavity, and we have the capability of biting, tearing, sucking, chewing, and swallowing many different types of food. Over millions of years, humans evolved the ability to sustain life by using the lips, teeth, tongue, and other structures of the oral cavity. During our evolution, we also learned to use those structures for an entirely different type of function: speech articulation, the end product of our ability to make sounds with the lips, teeth, tongue, and palate. No other creature on the planet can make as many sounds or make them so precisely. We are so proficient at making sounds that we can produce understandable speech in excess of 500 words per minute, or about 8 to 10 per second. And we talk on and on, most of our waking lives, seldom appreciating how sophisticated and intricate is this ability.

Hundreds of muscles and thousands of neurological impulses per second go into the act of talking. We move our articulators so rapidly that sounds become a stream of acoustic energy emanating from our bodies. Minor adjustments of the oral cavity affect this stream of energy. The lips open, close, and round, and the tip of the tongue bounces back and forth, up and down inside the mouth. The velum opens and closes to adjust the nasality of each sound.

The tongue rapidly moves from teeth, hard palate, and velum to affect the acoustic energy from which meaning will be derived.

Sometimes, what a person says is overshadowed by the way she makes the sounds of speech. The presence of a lisp, slur, or drawl in a person's speech can diminish the most eloquent of expressions. A statement is only as good as the speech that carries it. In many ways, clear, articulate speech is the flagship of our public selves. Good speech projects not only breeding and education but also suggests intelligence. When someone is described as "articulate," the implication is that he has the clarity of speech that comes from crisp thinking.

Articulation disorders range from mild impairments, such as substituting the /w/ for the /r/ sound (e.g., "wabbit" for "rabbit"), to the complete inability to produce speech that is understandable. The implications of not having understandable speech is apparent. For practical purposes speech falls on deaf ears: Needs go unmet, thoughts remain unexpressed, and emotions are not shared. There can even be unfortunate implications to a mild articulation disorder. Making speech errors that are typical of toddlers can diminish an opinion, business briefing, marriage proposal, or political oratory. A lisp can negate the potency of a statement. Although articulation disorders are not life threatening, they can have a profound impact on a person.

The Speech Articulators

As previously noted, speech is an overlaid function. The primary function of respiration is to replenish the cells of the body with oxygen; breath support for the production of speech is secondary. The primary function of the larynx is to protect the air passageways; phonation is secondary. The primary functions of the tongue, lips, teeth, and palates are biting, sucking and mastication (chewing); articulation, an overlaid function is secondary.

When people articulate they use the same oral structures that are used when eating. The oral structure used in making speech sounds are called **articulators.** The articulators can be divided into fixed and mobile structures. The primary *fixed articulators* are the **hard palate,** upper incisors, and **alveolar** ridge. The *mobile articulators* are the tongue, velum, **mandible,** and lips. Sometimes, articulators are classified by whether they are hard or soft. The main *hard articulators* are the teeth, mandible, hard palate, and alveolar ridge. The soft ones are the lips, tongue, and velum. Table 4.1 shows the articulators by their functional designation.

Speech is produced by alternating the shape of the vocal tract by these articulators. The lips form a sphincter at the opening of the oral cavity. They can completely *occlude* (close off) the oral cavity or articulate with the teeth to make sounds. The mandible and the tongue work synergistically during speech, particularly in the fine adjustments necessary for consonant production. The **velum** is a movable muscle that couples or uncouples the oral and nasal cavities. It is closed off during sucking so that negative air pressure in the oral cavity can be created. It also closes off during chewing to contain liquid and food. The tongue compresses and shapes food particles into a manageable ball (bolus) for swallowing (see Chapter 7).

The tongue is the most important speech articulator. Like the larynx (see Chapter 3), it has both extrinsic and intrinsic muscles. **Extrinsic tongue muscles** have their attachment outside the tongue. Intrinsic tongue muscles have both their origin and insertion within the

Literature, Media, and Personality Profiles

Barbara Walters

Barbara Walters was born on September 25, 1931, in Boston, Massachusetts. She received a Bachelor's of Arts degree from Sarah Lawrence College. Her first job was at an advertising agency in New York City. She became host of *The Today Show* in 1961. In 1976 Walters was employed by *ABC Evening News,* and in 1977 she went to work for the news magazine *20/20.* She is considered one of the best interviewers on network television and a role model for women aspiring to the telecommunication professions. She has won an Emmy and a Matrix Award.

Whether Walters's distinct articulation is the result of her Boston accent or a speech pathology known as a *w/r substitution,* several comedians have parodied her speech. The great comedian Gilda Radner, on the weekly television show *Saturday Night Live,* mocked Walters with her character "Barbara Waa Waa," which has become a comedy icon. Barbara Waa Waa would attempt a serious interview and ask the questions with the defective articulation. The comedic effect of asking serious questions with the exaggerated articulation error was one of Radner's most humorous skits. More recently, Cheri O'teri, on *Saturday Night Live,* has spoofed Barbara Walters's speech pattern.

Warner Bros. Cartoon Characters: Elmer Fudd, Tweety Bird, and Sylvester the Cat

Several Warner Bros. cartoon characters have articulation errors. The voice of these characters was Melvin Jerome Blanc, known as the "Man of 1000 Voices," who was born in San Francisco in 1908. Early in his career, he starred on the Jack Benny radio and television programs, and he created the Woody Woodpecker laugh. Blanc signed a contract with Warner Bros. in the 1940s to provide the voices of their cartoon characters. Some of the voices he provided include futuristic Cosmo G. Spacely on the *Jetsons,* bumbling Barney Rubble of the *Flintstones,* lovesick and odoriferous Pepe Le Pew, loud-beaked Foghorn Leghorn, and the elusive Roadrunner. Elmer Fudd, Tweety Bird, and Sylvester the Cat were all created using several types of articulation errors.

Elmer Fudd has a /w/ for /r/ substitution similar to the Gilda Radner character Barbara Waa Waa. Elmer is known for his ill-fated attempts to hunt the wily cartoon character Bugs Bunny (also the voice of Mel Blanc). "I'm going to shoot dat pesky wabbit" is typical of Elmer Fudd's speech.

Tweety Bird and Sylvester the Cat had separate cartoon careers before teaming up. Tweety Bird is noted for the statement "I tot I taw a putty-tat." Although Blanc gives Tweety Bird several articulation errors, the primary one is a /t/ for voiceless "th" substitution (tot for thought). Sylvester, a cat with a serious /s/ problem, teamed up with Tweety Bird in the 1940s. Blanc died in 1989, and on his tombstone is written "That's All Folks."

Sean Connery

Thomas Sean Connery was born on August 25, 1930, in Edinburgh, Scotland. He started playing James Bond in 1962 with the film *Dr. No.* A school dropout at age 13, Connery has won an Oscar and a Tony, and in 1999 he was awarded the Kennedy Center Honors Lifetime Achievement Award.

Many consider Connery to be the definitive James Bond. Connery's Bond is noted for fast, technologically advanced cars, a quick wit (especially with sexual double entendres), and his affinity for martinis. When ordering a martini, Bond is quick to tell the bartender it should be "shaken, not stirred." The words *shaken* and *stirred* are articulated with the airstream partially diverted to the sides of the tongue. This minor lateral lisp is as indelible as is the idea that his cultured palate can appreciate the difference between a stirred and shaken martini.

The World According to Garp

The writer John Irving is best known for *The World According to Garp*, which was first published in 1978 and reissued in 1994 by Ballantine Books. He studied at the University of Vienna and is the author of several best-sellers including *The Hotel New Hampshire*, *A Prayer for Owen Meany*, and *The Cider House Rules*.

The World According to Garp, considered by many to be a modern classic, is the story of T. S. Garp. It is filled with bizarre humor and sadness. There is an illustration of how a child's perception of speech can cause him to have defective articulation. Garp's son's confusion of "under toad," for the "undertow" of the ocean's current is typical of the type of confused auditory perception that leads to some types of childhood articulation disorders. Because the child has no reference for "undertow," he perceives the words *under toad* (a toad is a natural reference for a young boy). Another example of his auditory misperception is "gradual student" for "graduate student." Some articulation disorders in children are a result of similar misperceptions. Substituting one sound for another can be the result of not clearly perceiving differences in the words. When this auditory perceptual confusion persists, it can lead to several types of articulation errors.

My Fair Lady

The movie *My Fair Lady* was released in 1964 and received Academy, Directors Guild of America, and Golden Globe Awards. Starring Rex Harrison and Audrey Hepburn, it is about an upper-class English professor who attempts to transform a lower-class flower girl into a high-society lady. The difficult transformation is in no small part a result of changing speech patterns. Much of the perceptions of lower status is the result of a Cockney dialect. This film demonstrates the role accent and dialect play in perceptions of social class and status.

The Ladies Man

Released in 2000, this comedy is a spinoff from a character developed on *Saturday Night Live*. It is the goofy story of a radio personality, Leon Phelps, who gives disgusting sex advice to callers. Irate husbands of his vast number of sexual conquests meet on the Internet and form a gang intent on revenge. In this film, Leon Phelps lisps on virtually every /s/. The comedic effect of the severe lisp happens on three levels. First, the lisp helps create Phelp's character; it gives him and his hedonistic pursuits an innocent, almost childlike quality. Second, the lisp contrasts with the characteristics typically associated with a womanizer. He also appears oblivious to it, as are the women he pursues. Third, this type of speech disorder is not typically associated with a radio personality; it is unusual to have a lisp and work in radio. *The Ladies Man* stars Tim Meadows, as Leon Phelps, Will Ferrell, Tiffani-Amber Thiessen, Billy Dee Williams, and Lee Evans. Distributed by Paramount Pictures, it is directed by Reginald Hudlin.

That '70s Show

That '70s Show is a weekly television comedy about the trials and tribulations of growing up during the 1970s. One of the bell-bottomed characters is Fez, a foreign exchange student

(continued)

Literature, Media, and Personality Profiles *(continued)*

from an unidentified country. Always one step behind the rest of the high schoolers, Fez is forever trying to fit in and learn the subtleties of Wisconsin suburbia. Fez's attempts at cultural assimilation are complicated by a speech pattern called *fronting*, which is the tendency to substitute sounds produced in the front of the mouth for those occurring farther back in the oral cavity. It is a common phonological substitution found in preschoolers.

Fez is played by Wilmer Valderrama, who was born in Miami, Florida. His mother is Colombian and his father Venezuelan. He has appeared in several television shows including *Hollywood Squares*, *1999 Teen Choice Awards*, and *The Donny and Marie Show*. In real life he has a mild Venezuelan accent and does not have the speech pattern seen on *That '70s Show*.

Passions

Passions, an unusual daytime soap opera, is a story about the East Coast town of Harmony, witches, supernatural events, and a doll that has magically come to life. It is similar in nature to the popular *Harry Potter* stories. The doll, Witch Tabitha's "one-of-a-kind friend," is played by 18-year-old Josh Ryan Evans. The diminutive Evans is 3 feet, 2 inches tall and has appeared on *P. T. Barnum* (as Tom Thumb), *The Grinch*, *Ally McBeal*, and *Baby Geniuses*. He also has a prominent frontal lisp, which is consistently present and particularly noticeable when referring to Tabitha as "princess"; it is said as "printeth."

tongue. Both groups of muscles are important for making the fine adjustments necessary for the production of speech sounds. Both intrinsic and extrinsic tongue muscles help move liquid and food to the back of the throat for swallowing.

Phonetic Transcription

Phonetics is the science of speech sounds. Phonetic transcription is a method of representing one and only one sound, by one and only one letter. There are 44 sounds, or **phonemes,** in the English language. The English alphabet contains 26 letters **(graphemes).** Representing

TABLE 4.1   *Articulators by Their Functional Designation*

Soft	*Hard*	
Tongue Lips Velum	Mandible	**Movable**
	Teeth Hard palate Alveolar ridge	**Fixed**

the individual phonemes by traditional graphemes is confusing because one letter can be used to represent more than one sound and vice versa. For example, the "th" letters are used to represent both the voiced and voiceless "th" sounds. It is confusing to know whether the "th" letters refer to the voiceless sound in "think" or the voiced one in "that." They are different sounds represented by the same letters (see Box 4.1).

The International Phonetic Alphabet (IPA) eliminates transcription confusion. Several professions use the IPA, including radio and television announcers, linguists, and actors. Speech clinicians must be able to transcribe accurately and rapidly both normal and abnormal speech. All speech clinicians use the IPA because knowing the sounds and their symbols is important. Table 4.2 shows many of the IPA symbols and common pronunciation of sounds.

Place and Manner of Production

The muscles of articulation produce the consonants and vowels of speech. **Consonants** are speech sounds made by modifying the airstream in the oral and/or nasal tracts. **Vowels** are voiced speech sounds that are the result of relatively unrestricted acoustic energy through the speech tract. Unlike consonants, all vowel sounds begin as a single common sound produced by the vocal cords (Pickett, 1999). Consonants are divided into several categories, based on how they are made by the articulators. **Place of articulation** classifies sounds by the points in the oral cavity *where* they occur. For example, **bilabials** are sounds produced by both lips. (See Box 4.2.) Other places of articulation are **labio-dental** (lips and teeth), **lingua-dental** (tongue and teeth), **lingua-alveolar** (tongue and alveolar ridge), **lingua-palatal** (tongue and palate), **lingua-velar** (tongue and soft palate), and **glottal** (vocal cord) sites (Figure 4.1). Approximately 16 different places of consonant articulation are in the world's languages (Ladefoged & Maddieson, 1988).

Manner of articulation deals with the *type* of speech sound production (Figure 4.2). It classifies them by the manner of air stream modulation, or the process of shaping and valving the compressed air coming from the lungs. In this classification system, consonants are divided into two categories: stops and continuents. **Stops** are made by momentarily ceasing completely the airstream and subsequent acoustic energy in the speech tract. **Continuants** have continuous air flow rather than an abrupt release. **Plosives** result from explosions of air, and **affricates** are explosions of air shaped into continuents. **Fricatives** involve constriction of the airstream and are associated with higher frequencies of acoustic energy. **Glides** are

BOX 4.1 • *Cognates*

A **cognate** is a pair of consonants that differ only by voicing. They are produced motorically in the same way—that is, they have the same place and manner of articulation—but one of the pair is voiced and the other is unvoiced. To appreciate voicing difference, plug your ears with your fingers and produce the voiceless cognate. (By plugging the ears, you can better hear the effects of voicing.) Then, begin voicing and note how the phoneme changes. Do the following cognates: /s-z/ and /f-v/. You can also experiment with stops such as /k-g/ and /t-d/.

TABLE 4.2   *IPA Symbols and Common Pronunciation*

Consonant Pronunciation	Vowel Pronunciation
n as pronounced in now	I as pronounced in his
t as pronounced in tag	ɑ as pronounced in mop
d as pronounced in dog	æ as pronounced in cat
s as pronounced in soap	ɾ as pronounced in see
w as pronounced in water	ɛ as pronounced in head
r as pronounced in rabbit	o as pronounced in over
m as pronounced in milk	ʌ as pronounced in mother
ð as pronounced in that	ɔ as pronounced in all
k as pronounced in comb	u as pronounced in you
l as pronounced in lamb	U as pronounced in cook
g as pronounced in go	ɝ as pronounced in bird
z as pronounced in zipper	e as pronounced in ache
ŋ as pronounced in sing	
b as pronounced in button	
p as pronounced in pig	
h as pronounced in hurt	
v as pronounced in very	
f as pronounced in fine	
θ as pronounced in think	
ʃ as pronounced in shoot	
ʤ as pronounced in jump	
j as pronounced in yellow	
ʧ as pronounced in chicken	
ʒ as pronounced in beige	

produced by a gliding motion of the articulators from one position to another (see Box 4.3). Your articulators must move in the production of glides. **Nasals** involve the activation of the nasal resonance chambers in their production. They are produced by movements of the tongue or lips to completely occlude the oral tract and by the lowering of the velum (Pickett, 1999).

BOX 4.2 • *Ventriloquism*

Have you ever wanted to be a ventriloquist? Although many talents and skills are required to be a ventriloquist, you can practice this art by simply learning to speak *without* bilabials. Say this sentence with normal articulatory movements: "I can talk without moving my lips." Now, to practice ventriloquism, say them and keep you lips partially open and stationary. To produce the bilabials in the sentence, valve with your tongue rather than your lips. For example, say "noving" rather than "moving." Try to make the /n/ as much like an /m/ phoneme as possible and do not move your lips. While doing this, make your facial expressions as normal as possible and try to direct the audience's attention away from your face.

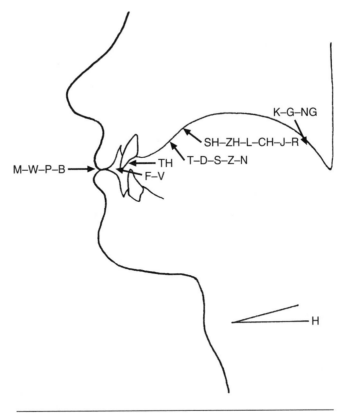

FIGURE 4.1   *English Consonants by Place of Articulation*

Source: W. Perkins & R. Kent, *Functional Anatomy of Speech, Language, and Hearing.* Copyright © 1986. Reprinted by permission by Allyn & Bacon.

Vowels are made by shaping acoustic energy into various patterns by altering the tongue and its position within the oral cavity. Vowel sounds depend on the height and front-to-back position of the tongue in the oral cavity (Figure 4.3). For example, some vowels are high-front sounds produced by the tongue high and prominent in the front of the oral cavity. Other vowels are classified as low-back, high-back, low-front sounds, etc.

Syllables

The **syllable** is the basic acoustic, perceptual, and motoric unit of speech. Phonemes, the basic sequential units of speech, are always embedded in syllables (Pickett, 1999). Syllables consist of a vowel that can stand alone or be surrounded by one or more consonants. The vowel nucleus is where the energy of the syllable is dissipated. There are several types or shapes of syllables, and they are designed with the letters C (consonant) or V (vowel).

Words can be described in terms of how many syllables they have. **Monosyllables** have one syllable, **bisyllables** have two syllables, and **polysyllables** have more than two syllables.

Continuants															Stops							
Nasals			Glides				Fricatives									Affri-cates		Plosives					
ŋ	n	m	j	r	l	w	ʒ	z	ð	v	ʃ	s	θ	f	h	dʒ	tʃ	g	d	b	k	t	p

FIGURE 4.2   *English Consonants by Manner of Articulation*

Some syllables are *open*, which have a vowel ending, and others are *closed*. Open syllables are rare in English, and their shapes can be CV ("high"), CCV ("sleigh"), or CCCV ("straw"). Closed syllables are the most common. Their shapes can be CVC ("man"), CCVC ("stone"), CCVCC ("spark"), CVCC ("heart"), CVCCC ("parked"), CCCVC ("strap"), and CCCVCC ("strange") (Culbertson, 2001).

The way a sound is produced in isolation, such as saying the sound /k/ alone, is called *static articulation*. Humans rarely produce sounds that way. Most speech is in the form of connected utterances, or dynamic articulation.

Dynamic Articulation

Motor speech production is a sophisticated act. Articulation is one of the most complicated aspects of motor speech. When you talk, your articulators must move rapidly from one position to the next, shaping the breath stream and acoustic energy into recognizable sounds. And to make the act even more complicated, the tongue movements must be made synergistically while atop a rapidly moving mandible. Vladimir Nabokov (1955) lustfully describes speech movements at the beginning of his erotic book, *Lolita*: "Lolita, light of my life, fire of my loins. My sin, my soul. Lo-lee-ta: the tip of the tongue taking a trip of three steps down the palate to tap, at three, on the teeth. Lo. Lee. Ta" (p. 9).

When minor movement errors or missed points of contact with the articulators occur, your speech becomes distorted. Greater movement and placement errors can cause your speech to be unintelligible. **Intelligibility** is the ability to be understood and is usually measured in percent. Reduced intelligibility is used for its humor value in the cartoon comedy *King of the Hill* and the film *Snatch*.

BOX 4.3 • *Gliding Sounds*

The glides are /w/, /r/, /l/, and /j/. They are called glides because the articulators must move from one point of contact to another in their production. Say each sound aloud and note the movement of the articulators. Try to say them without moving your articulators. You will see that they cannot be said clearly without articulatory movement.

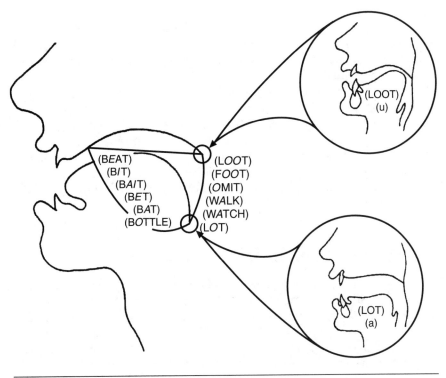

FIGURE 4.3 *English Vowels*

Source: W. Perkins and R. Kent, *Functional Anatomy of Speech, Language, and Hearing.* Copyright 1986. Reprinted by permission by Allyn & Bacon.

Articulation happens so rapidly that, in connected speech, many sounds are *approximated;* they only come close to being made by their precise, ideal points of contact. The stream of speech is so fast that rarely does a person make a "perfect" sound. Her articulators are moving so rapidly that they only come close to the points of contact necessary to produce an ideal sound. For example, if you say the word *literature*, the tip of your tongue must move to the alveolar ridge to make the /l/ sound. Then, in an instant, it must make the height and front-to-back adjustments necessary for the "ih" vowel. The /t/ consonant requires the tongue's return to the alveolar ridge, and then the "er" and "uh" vowels must be made. The "t-sh," as in "chicken," is made by yet another tongue movement to the alveolar ridge, and finally the "yer" concludes the word: *literature*. In the sentence "I like to read modern literature," the word is spoken in about a second. Speech happens so rapidly that the tongue and other articulators overlap in their movements. This overlapping of motor commands and movements is called **coarticulaton.** It leads to **assimilation,** which is the effect one sound has on another when uttered in connected speech. Sounds become more like each other. In effect the sound preceding and following a target one influences its production. Coarticulation and assimilation principles are often used by speech clinicians in articulation therapy for individuals who have trouble making sounds.

Given how rapidly the articulators move, it is not surprising that sometimes a person's tongue can become tangled. Several television shows use outtakes of mistakes that actors make with their lines and scripts. Some weekly television shows routinely show them at the end of each episode. Their popularity is due in part to the humor people find in a person being unable to say a word or phrase.

There are several reasons why a person stumbles through a word or phrase. The primary reason some words and phrases are harder to say than others has to do with programming (see apraxia of speech). If the program of the motor act of speech is irregular or unusual, the articulators are not accustomed to their movements. Other reasons for a tangled tongue include self-consciousness, attempting to speak too rapidly and too precisely, distraction, and even the laws of physics. In some words and phrases, the tongue must move rapidly from one extreme position to another, and the laws of motion and inertia make the movements difficult. (See Box 4.4.)

Etiology of Articulation Disorders

Given the complexities of the neurological and muscular activities in speech production, it is not surprising that many human maladies can cause articulation disorders. It is important to know the **etiology,** or the cause, of an articulation disorder for effective treatment. For example, if weak muscles cause an articulation problem, then the treatment will be different than if it was caused by delayed language. Literally thousands of diseases, injuries, birth defects, and **syndromes** can cause articulation disorders. However, most etiologies can be classified into articulation disorders resulting from (1) deafness or hearing loss, (2) structural defects of the articulators, (3) motor speech disorders, (4) delayed development, (5) auditory perceptual and sensorimotor deficiencies, and (6) emotional distress. Dialect and accent also influence articulation.

BOX 4.4 • *Tongue Twisters*

Tongue twisters are good examples of the difficulties people have in rapidly moving their articulators, particularly the tongue. Try saying the following as rapidly as possible and note the programming and movement difficulties:

Rubber baby buggy bumpers
Six thick thistle sticks
She sells seashells by the seashore.
Red leather, yellow leather
Strange strategic statistics
I picked a peck of pickled peppers.
I slit the sheet, the sheet I slit; and on the slitted sheet I sit.

When you say them slowly and attend very carefully to tongue and lip movements, they can be articulated clearly and precisely.

Deafness or Hearing Loss

Hearing is often called the second sense, the primary one being vision. However, when it comes to learning speech sounds, hearing is the primary sense. The sense of hearing is fundamental to learning not only speech sounds but also *everything* related to verbal communication. No better example of this is the fact that children will learn any language to which they are exposed.

Suppose two different families adopt identical twins. If a family in Japan, who speaks only Japanese, adopts one twin, the child will grow up learning that language. If the other twin is raised in a family that speaks Apache, he will learn only that language. The sounds of a language a child is exposed to are the ones he will produce. But what about children who are born deaf?

Children who are born completely deaf hear no sounds; they live in a world of silence. Deaf children will go through some of the stages of speech and language development that hearing children go through (see Chapter 5). Both hearing and deaf children begin life with a *birth cry*. Also, both go through stages of *undifferentiated crying*, where knowing what they want is difficult based on the type of cry. Both hearing and deaf children go through *differentiated crying*, where parents can tell if the child is hurt, hungry, or wet, based on the cry. This stage is one of the first true forms of communication between babies and their parents. Mothers can recognize five or six different types of cries in their children. *Cooing* is also something both hearing and deaf children do, but beyond this stage they part company in their speech development. Children born deaf begin the next stage of language development called *babbling*. However, they will have little progression beyond this stage without special therapies and educational programs.

When it comes to children who have some functional hearing, classified as **hard-of-hearing,** three factors determine how well they will learn speech sounds. The first factor is the age at which the hearing loss occurred. If the hearing loss (or deafness) occurs after the age of 10 years or so, then most of the speech sounds will have already been learned. Certainly, the hearing loss will affect articulation, but—because they have already heard and learned speech sounds—the effect on articulation development will be less significant.

The second factor to be considered is the frequency of the hearing loss. In many ways, when it comes to articulation development, "what goes in, comes out." What children hear *clearly* is likely to be produced *correctly*. If the hearing loss is limited to the higher frequencies in the speech range, then they will not clearly hear those sounds. Consequently, they will likely learn and use the lower frequency sounds, such as "ah," /b/, and "ra." Because hard-of-hearing children can hear the lower-frequency sounds, they are more likely to learn and correctly use them. Conversely, if the hearing loss is only in the lower frequencies, then high-frequency sounds, such as /s/, "sh," and /f/, are likely to be learned and used.

The third factor in hearing loss and articulation acquisition is the degree of loss. A mild hearing loss, one in which there is only a minor difficulty in understanding the speech of others, will have less effect on articulation development than a severe one. As a rule, the more severe the hearing loss, the more articulation development will suffer.

As you can see, hearing loss and deafness can have significant effects on speech and language development, especially articulation acquisition. It is important that hearing be evaluated early and regularly in children.

Structural Defects of the Articulators

Several structural defects can result in articulation disorders. Structural defects refer to articulators that are insufficient, malformed, or damaged, so their ability to shape the compressed air coming from the lungs is impaired.

As discussed in Chapter 3, cleft lip and palate are birth defects that can impair voice and articulation. Cleft lip and palate affect the structure and function of the articulators in several ways, depending on the severity of the birth defect. First, a cleft palate results in an opening between the oral and nasal cavities, causing distorted sounds, resonance abnormalities, and nasal emission. Second, when the cleft includes the lips and dental arches, speech sounds produced by them can be impaired. The ultimate effects of a cleft lip and palate on articulation depend on the success of plastic and dental surgeons to repair the orofacial anomaly and the therapies provided by a speech–language pathologist. Together, surgeons and therapists often obtain normal or near-normal speech in individuals with cleft lip and palate. Today, because of advances in surgeries and therapies, this birth defect need not cause permanent speech problems. People born with them can become television anchors like Tom Brokaw and actors like Stacy Keech and Cheech Marin.

The palatal vault also houses the tongue when the mouth is closed. A person can have an **insufficient palatal vault.** It is too shallow, small, or shaped irregularly and can cause articulation and resonance problems. An insufficient palatal vault also causes dental problems in some people. Because the palatal vault is not large enough to accommodate the tongue, it pushes against the back of the teeth when the mouth is closed. This constant pressure causes the teeth to protrude and creates a malocclusion. Malocclusion is a misalignment of the teeth and is a structural–functional cause of articulation disorders.

Another structural defect of the articulators is having an abnormally sized tongue. **Microglossia** is a tongue that is too small and occurs in a small number of individuals. **Macroglossia,** a tongue that is too large in relation to the oral cavity, is common in individuals who have Down syndrome.

Down syndrome, named after an eighteenth-century physician who studied this chromosome disorder, is also known as chromosome 21–trisomy syndrome; it has several physical and mental features (see Chapter 5). People with Down syndrome often have macroglossia, and—because of the abnormal tongue—speech is usually slow and indistinct. With therapy many Down syndrome individuals can obtain intelligible, near-normal speech. In addition, some people with Down syndrome undergo tongue surgery to reduce its size.

There are several types of dental malocclusions and malpositions of the teeth, and they can have varying effects on a person's ability to make speech sounds. Jumbled teeth, particularly the front ones, can impair dental valving of the airstream. Some children lose their temporary, or deciduous, teeth too early because of trauma or disease and go for many months, even years, without these important sites of articulation contact. As a result, they misarticulate their dental sounds and may require articulation therapy, sometimes even after the deciduous teeth are replaced by the 32 permanent ones.

The **lingual frenulum** is a short cord of tissue running from the bottom of the tongue to the middle of the floor of the mouth. You can see it in a mirror by opening your mouth while trying to touch your nose with your tongue. A shortened lingual frenulum, or being "tongue-tied," is a structural cause of an articulation disorder. In the past, many articulation disorders, and even stuttering, were attributed to a person being tongue-tied. Actually, having an abnormally short lingual frenulum that interferes with articulation is rare. The mobility of the tongue must be significantly reduced by a shortened lingual frenulum to impair speech. The amount the tip of the tongue must elevate in speech is small, and the lingual frenulum must be *very* short to result in elevation and mobility problems. "Clipping" it to improve speech is often unnecessary. When this surgery is done, it should be accompanied by articulation therapy.

Orofacial surgeries for cancer can result in articulation disorders. Cancers of the jaw and lips are common in individuals who use smokeless tobacco. One of the treatments for these cancers is surgery, which can cause structural articulation deficits. Some patients undergo a complete or partial **glossectomy,** or surgical removal of all or part of the tongue. Obviously, articulation can be impaired when all or part of the tongue is surgically removed, but therapy is often helpful in regaining the ability to produce speech.

Fractures and other traumas to the head can result in structural articulation disorders. Any fracture or trauma that impairs the structure and function of the articulators can impair both static and dynamic articulation. Some fractures, such as with the temporal mandibular joint (the joint where the lower jaw connects with the skull), require that the jaws be temporarily wired together. Obviously, speech articulation is impaired during this time, but after 6 weeks or so, the wires are removed and the patient can talk normally. In movies, people prone to this type of fracture are said to have a "glass jaw." Most fractures and traumas of the head and face that affect the speech articulators result in temporary speech problems.

Motor Speech Disorders

There are two general categories of motor speech disorders: apraxia of speech and the dysarthrias. Both are neurogenic communication disorders and are discussed in detail in Chapter 7. However, because they can disrupt articulation, they will be reviewed briefly in this section on the etiology of articulation disorders.

Motor speech disorders result from damage to nerves and muscles that control speech. They can be caused by strokes, head traumas, and many diseases such as multiple sclerosis, muscular dystrophy, amyotrophic lateral sclerosis, and Parkinson's disease. Motor speech disorders can interfere with articulation in five ways.

First, articulation can be disrupted at the conceptual level, where the idea behind the utterance is formulated. The motor aspects of verbal thought driving the speech act are created and clarified. A disorder at this level is called **ideational apraxia** of speech and is seen in patients with Alzheimer's disease, certain types of head trauma, and other diseases and disorders that can affect the motor aspects of language expression. The second level is where the plan for the speech act is formulated. The plan is called the *articulatory program.* At this level, the entire articulatory act from beginning to end is planned. The movement of each articulator, including its timing, speed, and strength, is formulated. The third level is the execution of the articulatory program. Here, nerves and muscles of the articulators are sent the commands necessary for the utterance. A disorder at the second and third levels is called **apraxia of speech.** It has been traditionally thought that in most people it is a result of damage to part of the frontal lobe of the brain called **Broca's area.** However, current brain imagery research has shown that the articulatory plan may also occur in other areas of the brain (Wise, Greene, Büchel, & Scott, 1999).

The fourth level involves the nerves supplying, directly or indirectly, the muscles of articulation. Once the articulatory program has been conceptualized, planned, and executed, motor **neurons** must carry the complex commands to the muscles. The fifth level in the motor speech act occurs at the muscle level. Here the muscles alternately contract and relax to move the articulators. Damage at these two levels causes muscles to be rigid, weak, and/or ill coordinated and result in one or more of the dysarthrias. The **dysarthrias** are six types of neuromuscular speech disorders that can occur because of damage to the fourth and fifth levels of motor speech production.

Articulation therapy for the motor speech disorders depends on the type of impairment and level of dysfunction. Apraxia of speech therapy has different goals and objectives than therapy for dysarthrias. The goal of articulation therapy for apraxia of speech is to help patients gain control in conceptualizing, planning, and executing their tongue movements, whereas therapy for dysarthria involves creating more forceful, coordinated, and precise articulation movements.

Delayed Development

Children do not master the sounds of their language rapidly. It takes most of the first decade of life to learn all the speech sounds of language. In speech–language pathology, there are two seeming divergent views regarding delayed speech sound development (Culbertson & Tanner, 2001a). One of these views is the sensorimotor approach. In the sensorimotor approach, speech sounds are thought to develop at predictable ages due to several maturation factors, especially auditory perceptual and fine motor skills. The other is the **phonological approach,** which regards speech sound development as the discovery and fusion of syllable-formation principles. Some authorities use the term *articulation disorders* when referring to difficulty producing speech sounds and the term *phonological disorders* when referring to difficulty with phonological rules (Davis & Bedore, 2000). Other authorities simply call them *phonology* and *phonetic disorders*, respectively. There may be a genetic component to some articulation disorders: "Approximately 20–40% of children with speech and language disorders have positive family histories for disorders" (Lewis & Freebairn, 1997, p. 45).

The sensorimotor approach has been the treatment of choice and employed by clinicians for several decades. Clinicians using this approach to articulation disorders examine phonemes in the child's repertory and compare them to charts or tables that list the age of acquisition of each speech sound in large samples of children.

The age normative data are often contained in charts or tables that list the phonemes and corresponding developmental ages. As a rule, in articulation development, the sequence of learning sounds is invariant, but the ages at which children learn them are highly variable. This means that there is a general predictable *order* in the sounds that are learned, but normal children may vary, by as much as a year or more, in *when* they learn them. Figure 4.4 shows the ages associated with consonant–phoneme acquisition (Tanner, Culbertson, & Secord, 1997).

In the sensorimotor approach, two factors are important when considering whether a child is mastering her sounds at the expected ages. First, the clinician must know whether the norms being used mean the sound is produced correctly in all positions of words. To have met the norms for mastery of a particular sound, does the child need to produce it correctly

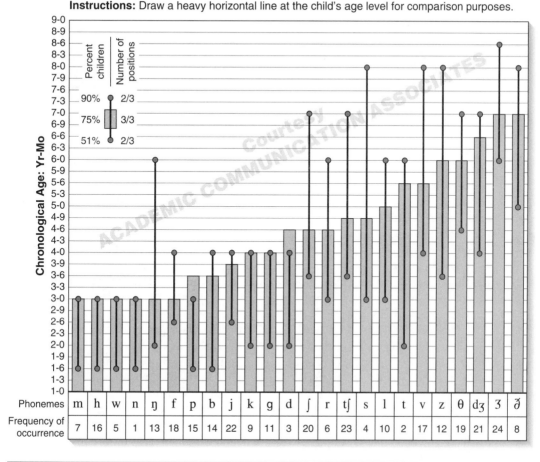

Instructions: Draw a heavy horizontal line at the child's age level for comparison purposes.

FIGURE 4.4 *Consonant Acquisition Norms*

Source: D. Tanner, W. Culbertson, and W. Secord, *The Developmental Articulation and Phonology Profile*. Copyright 1997. Courtesy Academic Communication Associates.

in the initial, medial, and final positions of words? (See the section Evaluating Articulation and Phonology Disorders.) Or do the norms only indicate when the child has mastered the sound in the initial position or in two positions of words? The second consideration is what percent of children had acquired the sound in a particular chart or table. This is known as the *criterion for mastery*. Some charts and tables use a 51% criterion mastery level, whereas others use 60%, 75%, or 90%. For accurate diagnosis of articulation disorders using the sensorimotor method, it is necessary to know the percent of mastery and in how many positions of words. Once it has been decided that a particular child is delayed in his mastery of a sound, therapy is provided to bring him up to expected age norms.

Phonology is the rule-governed way by which humans produce the sounds of language. As such, phonology is one aspect of language. Many specialists in the field of communication sciences and disorders feel that the mispronunciations of certain school-age children are manifestations of delayed or arrested phonological development. This phonological approach treats such mispronunciations as language, rather than speech articulation disorders. In the phonological approach, the mispronunciations are thought to result from delay in acquisition of the phonological rules or processes of the standard adult language. Children with a phonological disorder develop immature processes in attempts to approximate adult phonology. Rather than evaluating and teaching each phoneme individually, a *phonological process*—which may affect several sounds—is taught while simultaneously extinguishing immature phonological processes. The role of clinicians in the phonological approach is to help children discover adult phonology through assimilation of adult phonological processes. In so doing, children "master" adult phonology, and their articulation becomes normal. Approaching phonological development from such a linguistic orientation does not deny a role for sensorimotor function. Indeed, mastery of adult phonology likely depends on physical maturation: "While recognizing that phonological development follows a predictable sequence for most children, we believe there is wide individual variation in the abandonment of immature syllable formation strategies, and that a major factor underlying this variation is neuromuscular maturation" (Culbertson & Tanner, 2001b, pp. 28–30). Several approaches to the phonological analysis have differing degrees of success in remediation (Yavas, 1998). Phonological rules and their approximate ages of extinction are provided in Figure 4.5 (Tanner, Culbertson, & Secord, 1997).

The speech displayed by the Warner Bros. cartoon characters Elmer Fudd and Tweetie Bird illustrates how both approaches can be used to understand problems with articulation. Elmer Fudd's w/r substitution can be viewed in the sensorimotor sense. Given his chronological age, he should have mastered the /r/ sound in all three positions. He is delayed in /r/ sound acquisition. Tweetie Bird, on the other hand, substitutes /t/ for /k/ and /d/ for /g/, which is the process of replacing front consonants for back ones. This is the phonological process of *velar fronting*. In therapy Elmer would be taught the perceptual and motor skills to articulate correctly the /r/ sound, whereas Tweetie would be taught more mature phonological rules using several sounds as examples.

Auditory Perceptual and Sensorimotor Deficiencies

Auditory perception is the ability to sense the important, salient parts of something heard. It is the mental awareness of a sound and the organization of sensory data received through the ears. Auditory perception is knowing what to attend to and what to ignore. It is the learned ability to detect and attend to important aspects of auditory stimuli. In perception the important parts of the sensory information are called the **signal,** and that which is ignored is called the **noise.** Signal and noise are in all of the senses (see Box 4.5); the closer two or more signals are in their characteristics, the harder it is to perceive differences in them.

Learned auditory perception is the foundation to musical abilities. If you have learned to play a musical instrument, you have developed the auditory perceptual skills to appreciate more about its sound than does someone who has never played it. Violinists, for example, attend more clearly to the violins in a concert. They appreciate the quality, strength, and range of the violinists' performance because of years of training auditory perception (see Box 4.6).

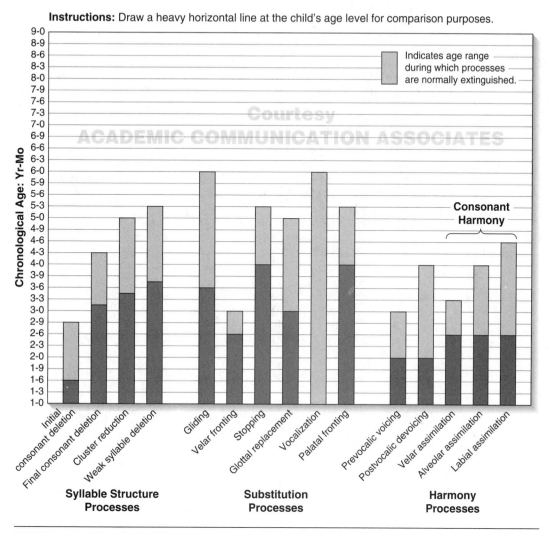

Instructions: Draw a heavy horizontal line at the child's age level for comparison purposes.

FIGURE 4.5 *Phonological Process and Approximate Ages of Extinction*

Source: D. Tanner, W. Culbertson, and W. Secord, *The Developmental Articulation and Phonology Profile.* Copyright 1997. Courtesy Academic Communication Associates.

Auditory perception is necessary for the development of articulation. Children, as they learn the sounds of their language, must distinguish subtle acoustic differences between them. Many children do not produce sounds correctly because they do not auditorially perceive the differences between similar ones. This was shown in *The World According to Garp*, when Garp's son was unable to distinguish "ow" from "ode" in "undertow" and "under toad." Children who have confused auditory perception often make in-class substitutions. An in-class substitution is producing a phoneme that is similar in acoustic energy to the correct one.

BOX 4.5 • *Other Forms of Perception*

Visual perception allows the organization of visual data and permits attention to learned, important aspects of reality that come in through the eyes. An example of visual perception is the ability to perceive differences in trades and handicraft. The skilled carpenter, for example, has highly developed visual perceptual skills. She clearly perceives the differences in high-quality cabinet construction from that which is done poorly. A person with no experience with carpentry—thus with little learned visual perceptions about how lumber must be cut, routered, sanded, and so on—would not be able to detect fine differences that separate superior carpentry from the mediocre. The same visual perceptual skills hold true for the bricklayer, painter, roofer, and other skilled workers. Years of practice develop these visual perceptual skills and permit the awareness of minor differences between high- and low-quality construction.

Perception with the sense of touch permits experienced clothiers to perceive fine differences in the texture of cuts of cloth. People who read by the Braille method have higher developed perceptions of the saliency of raised dots than people who do not have the ability to read through the sense of touch. Connoisseurs of fine wines have higher developed perception of taste and smell than do novices. They can appreciate the body, flavor, and bouquet of wines through the senses of taste and smell. Some wine connoisseurs can tell the vintage of several wines, the regions where the grapes were grown, and even how long they have been aged. Because of his cultured palate, James Bond can even appreciate the differences between shaken and stirred martinis. Actually, *palate* as used here is a figure of speech; there are no taste buds on the hard or soft palate.

These errors involve similar place and manner of sounds—for example, labials for labials, glides for glides, or fricatives for fricatives. Recall, the closer two signals are in nature, the harder it is to perceive their differences. Children who have auditory perceptual articulation disorders may produce the /w/ for the /r/ sound or the /s/ for the "sh" one. Their auditory perceptual abilities have not developed enough to allow perception of the fine acoustic differences between similar sounds. Because they perceive little or no differences in these sounds, articulation is done incorrectly. Children with both speech and language difficulties tend to have poorer speech-processing abilities when compared with normal controls and children with speech-only difficulties (Nathan, Stackhouse, & Goulandris, 1998).

Therapy for these types of articulation disorders involves training the individual to perceive the differences between the error and correct sounds. Auditory discrimination training must be taught first so that the person hears the differences. Only after the development of auditory perception of the correct sounds does the therapy involve working with the child on the fine motor skills needed to make them. (Auditory discrimination training is discussed in detail in the section Treatment of Articulation Disorders.)

Emotional Distress

Sometimes, when children are abused, neglected, and subjected to extreme environmental stress, they regress to a more secure psychological state. *Regression* is a psychological defense mechanism employed in situations of extreme distress. Frequently, this secure psychological

BOX 4.6 • *The Gatekeeper*

The thalamus is an important part of the brain, particularly regarding perception. It is sometimes called the "gatekeeper" because it allows some information coming from the senses to reach conscious perception while denying it to other sense information. You can see the gatekeeping function at work now as you are reading this book. As you are reading this, you are not aware of how your shoe feels on your right foot. Only until you read this do you allow conscious awareness of the sensation of your sock or stocking, the tightness of your shoe, and the way your toes are squashed together. The gatekeeper allowed the sensations of your shoe to become conscious. Until then, they were unconscious. You can also do this exercise with how a pencil feels in your hand, glasses on you nose, belt around your waist, and tongue inside your mouth.

state was one that occurred at a much earlier age. As a result, this psychological regression is accompanied by an obvious speech and language regression. The child who regresses to the psychological state of the 2-year-old also may talk like a toddler. As a result, extreme stress and the child's reaction to it can be a casual factor in articulation disorders.

Three important factors are necessary to attribute an articulation disorder to emotional distress and regression. First, the child must have previously been producing speech at a significantly more mature level. Normally developing children do not regress to previous stages of development. Second, many children who regress in their articulation development have this regression preceded by a complete cessation of speech. They stop talking altogether and become **mute** for a period of time. Third, in articulation disorders resulting from emotional distress, a psychologically devastating event occurs before the regression in articulation abilities. The regression in articulation abilities is a symptom of a deeper, important emotional problem, and a psychological referral is warranted before initiating articulation therapy.

Dialect and Accent

There are no substandard dialects; all rule-governed cultural variations in the production of speech and language are normal. Differences in dialects are not speech pathologies because everyone has a dialect. The United States has many dialectical variations, and they give richness and diversity to the language. Most news anchors on the major broadcast networks use the Standard American Dialect, and it is the most common one in the United States. Table 4.3 provides a partial list of dialects found in the United States. Some are only recognizable by a few people familiar with a particular region of the country. Dialect and accent differences began with the first settlers and are more apparent in the eastern part of the United States (Alvarez & Kolker, 1987).

In the media and literature, the words *dialect* and *accent* are often used interchangeably. Technically, they are different. Because of auditory perceptual factors, people who speak with an **accent** have the phonetic traits of their native language carried over into a second language. Accents happen because people learn to perceive differences between sounds that signal differences in meaning within their languages. For example, in English, there is a

TABLE 4.3 *A Partial List of Dialects and Accents in the United States*

African American	Dutch American	Queens
Appalachian	Eastern	Southern
Boston	Hillbilly	Texas
Boston Brahmins	Kentucky	Upstate New York
Bronx	Korean American	Vietnamese American
Cajun	Manhattan	Virginia
Canadian	Mexican American	Wisconsin
Chicago	Mississippi	Yonkers
Cowboy	New England	
Dakota	Ohio	

significant semantic difference in the sounds "sh" and "ch," as in the words *share* and *chair*. In Spanish, however, the difference between these sounds is not enough to signal a difference in meaning between any two words. Therefore, Spanish speakers often experience difficulty perceiving the differences between "ch" and "sh," in word pairs such as *chin* and *shin*, and *chew* and *shoe*. The accent carryover gives a typical Spanish flavor to certain aspects of speech: "He cut the hair off his shin (chin)" and "Have you seen my chew (shoe)?"

People who speak with a **dialect** use a specific form of pronunciation and vocabulary that are spoken in a given geographical area, culture, or education and social class. With regard to pronunciation, several dialects substitute the /f/ phoneme for the voiceless "th" sound: "Will you go 'wif' me." Other dialects often do not distinguish between the vowels "ih" and "eh" as in *pin* and *pen*; they are both said as "pin." The vocabulary differences are often remarkable. In Appalachian and other rural dialects, a person might ask, "Have you seen my 'clodhoppers,'" when trying to find her shoes. Other examples of vocabulary differences include calling a "milk shake," a "cabinet"; "rubber band," a "gum band"; "schlep," for "to carry"; and "snickelfritz," for a "rowdy child" (Alvarez & Kolker, 1987).

Some individuals prefer to reduce or eliminate their dialect and accent. For example, a broadcaster may want to reduce or eliminate a southern accent. Many dialects and accents also connote socioeconomic status in much the same way that the Cockney dialect is portrayed in the film *My Fair Lady*. In the United States, a southern dialect often connotes ignorance and racism, as Jimmy Carter found in his presidential campaign (Alvarez & Kolker, 1987). The great orator Martin Luther King, Jr., had speech patterns that were minimally influenced by dialect. Individuals may want dialect and accent reduced or eliminated to support attempts at social and economic upward mobility. Barbara Walter's w/r substitution is less apparent now than in previous years, maybe as a result of formal articulation therapy or dialect reduction.

Evaluating Articulation and Phonology Disorders

There are four reasons for evaluating articulation and phonology disorders. First, an evaluation is conducted to determine whether a disorder exists. This is particularly important in children. Parents sometimes bring their children to speech and hearing clinics, suspecting an articulation disorder when in fact one does not exit. Some parents have unrealistic expectations about how rapidly articulation should develop. In schools, speech–language pathologists routinely screen all kindergartners, first graders, or second graders. In this type of testing, a *screening articulation test* can be given rapidly and efficiently to determine whether additional testing is necessary. Usually, in this kind of test, a child simply describes a pictorial story, and the clinician listens for articulation errors. If the child has intelligibility problems or has errors in sound production that should have been mastered, then he is referred for additional testing. A screening test does not evaluate a pathology; it simply determines the need for additional testing.

Second, an evaluation is conducted to determine etiology. As discussed previously, knowing the cause of an articulation disorder in order to properly select the best treatment is important. Although the general principle in all articulation therapy is the same—to get the person to produce speech sounds more precisely—articulation disorders resulting from different etiologies require various treatment approaches. For example, articulation therapy resulting from a structural defect, such as dental malocclusion, requires a different approach than if the disorder was phonologically based.

Third, an evaluation is conducted to analyze which sounds are defective and to what degree. The nature, number, and characteristics of the articulation errors are evaluated in detail, to yield a composite description of a person's speech articulation at a given point in time. Children and adults may be assessed during conversation, while naming or describing pictures, or while reading words and sentences. Including samples of conversational speech in the assessment is also important. The spontaneous sample of speech ensures that the person produces a range of sounds in a variety of contexts for phonological analysis. During articulation testing, having the person simply repeat the test stimuli after the examiner says them is not a good idea. Repeating a test sound, syllable, or word does not give an accurate indication of how the person habitually talks.

Sometimes, a deep articulation test is administered to assess each error sound in a variety of phonetic contexts. In *deep articulation testing*, the phonetic context in which the error sound is correctly produced is identified. Deep testing can provide important therapeutic information to help the individual produce the error sounds correctly.

Fourth, an evaluation is conducted to design an appropriate treatment program and to prepare goals and objectives. Long- and short-term objectives, including the methods that will be used to achieve them, are written. Speech–language pathologists working in school settings are required to write these goals, objectives, and methods for every student in the program. They are called *individualized education plans (IEPs)* and are mandated by federal legislation. Federal law guarantees all children the right to an education program that is appropriate for their needs. The student and her parents regularly meet with the special education team to discuss and review the IEP.

Individualized education plans must include the following (Tanner, 1997):

1. Projected dates for initiation of services
2. Anticipated duration of services
3. The extent to which the child will be able to participate in regular classroom activities
4. A statement of the child's present level of educational performance

5. A list of short-term and long-term goals
6. A statement of annual goals
7. Appropriate objective criteria and evaluation procedures to determine whether the objectives are being met

Articulation Testing

Several commercial articulation tests are available to assist clinicians in evaluating articulation disorders. Most tests use pictures for children and written words for adults to elicit the speech sample. During the articulation test, the individual names a picture or reads a word containing the target sound. When the person says the stimulus word, the clinician records whether the sound was said correctly. If there was an articulation error, then the clinician shows what type of error was made. Articulation errors are generally classified as distortions, omissions, and substitutions and are tested in three positions of words: *initial, medial,* and *final.* This is the describing of articulation errors in the *three-by-three system.*

A **distortion** is a sound that is not made clearly and succinctly, although the clinician can identify it. A good example of a distorted sound occurs in cleft palate speech. A person with a cleft palate sometimes produces a sound with too much nasality. The hypernasality usually occurs on sounds produced with pressure buildup, such as /p/ or /t/. When the sound is made, although it can be identified, it is distorted with hypernasality. When a clinician recognizes a sound but does not believe it was produced succinctly, it is labeled a distortion. Technically, a distortion is the substitution of a nonstandard sound—one that is not a recognized phoneme of the language. On the test form, the clinician writes "dist" to indicate that the sound was distorted. Some test protocols list the nature of the distortion by indicating "dist-nasal" for a sound distorted by hypernasality. Other tests suggest listing the severity of the distortion by indicating "Dist-1," "Dist-2," and "Dist-3," to indicate increments in the severity of the articulation error.

When the person does not say one of the sounds in a word, it is called an **omission.** Omissions can occur in the initial, medial, or final positions of words. For example, when an individual says "__abbit" for "rabbit," he has omitted the /r/ phoneme in the initial position. Saying "chur__" for "church" is the omission of the "ch" sound in the final position. On the test form, the clinician writes "om" in the space provided, which indicates the positions of words: initial, medial, and final.

When a recognizable sound is substituted for another one, it is called a **substitution.** Like distortions and omissions, substitutions also occur in the initial, medial, and final positions of words. The following are examples of common phoneme substitutions and the way they are clinically identified:

"fum" for "thumb"	/f/ for /θ/ substitution initially
"dun" for "gun"	/d/ for /g/ substitution initially
"cawot" for "carrot"	/w/ for /r/ substitution medially
"buthes" for "brushes"	/θ/ for /ʃ/ substitution medially
"dod" for "dog"	/d/ for /g/ substitution finally
"nipe" for "knife"	/p/ for /f/ substitution finally

Beyond phonetic errors of distortions, omissions, and substitutions, some individuals add a sound to a word. Additions are different from substitutions. In a substitution one sound is replaced by another. In an **addition** the word has all of the necessary sounds, but an additional one is added to it. Additions are complication errors that often occur in motor speech disorders and will be discussed in Chapter 7.

Additional Diagnostic Information

Besides evaluating the phonetic aspects of articulation, a phonological analysis is usually conducted, especially on individuals with multiple articulation errors. As noted previously, a phonological disorder involves producing sound errors due to incomplete learning of the rules of usage. In a *phonological analysis*, the speech sample is examined in several contexts to derive the rule-governed structures in the individual's speech.

Oral diadochokinesis is also assessed. A diadochokinetic rate is how rapidly a person can engage in repetitive movements. An oral diadochokinetic rate is how fast a person can move articulators. This is typically assessed by having the person produce "pa, ta, ka" in rapid succession. Oral diadochokinetic rate assessment provides general information about the strength, speed, and mobility of the articulations.

When evaluating patients with the neuromuscular disorder dysarthria, it is sometimes necessary to determine where the speech-valving mechanism is impaired. The clinician finds the valving sites (e.g., tip-alveolar or bilabial) that are impaired and works on the groups of muscles responsible for their actions.

In individuals with several articulation errors, a test of *speech intelligibility* can be administered. Intelligibility is the ability of the person to make herself understood. "Intelligibility is affected by the type of articulation error. Distortions are most easily understood, followed by substitutions and then omissions which are considered the most immature sounding of these errors" (Hall, Oyer, & Haas, 2000, p. 33). Usually, intelligibility is assessed from a spontaneous speech sample, although tests can determine intelligibility from elicited samples. Speech intelligibility is usually provided in a percent, or it is ranked as high, medium, or low. When intelligibility is not affected, the articulation disorder is considered a cosmetic one. If speech can be understood completely but the error draws negative attention to the speaker, the speech error is obtrusive. As a rule, articulation errors that impair intelligibility of the speaker have a higher priority for therapy than cosmetic ones.

Stimulability testing determines the degree to which a sound can be produced with models, cues, and prompts. Some individuals have trouble making the target sound even when they slow down or try to produce it in isolation. A sound produced in isolation is one made alone without other sounds occurring before or after it, and it is not affected by coarticulation or assimilation factors. When a person cannot physically produce the target sound, he is called nonstimulable. The stimulable person can make the sound when provided with a verbal model, cues, and prompts on how to say it. This can be done by showing the individual where to place the articulators when making the target sound. Stimulability testing also can be done in syllables and words to provide a measure of consistency of the person's errors.

No articulation evaluation would be complete without an orofacial examination and a hearing screening. The *orofacial examination* involves looking at the structure and function of the articulators. The status of a person's face, dentition, palates, tongue, lips, and jaw is examined for physical defects and functional abnormalities. A hearing screening is given to eliminate hearing loss or deafness as a cause of the articulation disorder (see Chapter 6).

Treatment of Articulation Disorders

Several therapies are available for articulation disorders. The following are general articulation therapies, with a brief description of their goals and methods.

Articulation Therapy for Hearing Loss and Deafness

Therapy for articulation disorders resulting from hearing loss and deafness is done in conjunction with aural rehabilitation. **Aural rehabilitation** is an educational process that uses the existing expressive and receptive modalities to improve functional communication. It is conducted in the **total communication approach** that uses any or all communication methods (sign language, speech reading, written, oral) to improve communication in the hearing impaired or deaf person (see Chapter 6). To improve articulation, visual, tactile, and residual auditory feedback are employed to gradually improve speech sound production. For example, the clinician may place the individual's hand on her throat, to sense vocal cord vibration for voicing cues, while she visually models the sound. Several interactive computer programs can provide visual feedback regarding the precision of sounds being made.

Articulation Therapy for Structural Defects of the Articulators

Therapy for structural defects of the articulators depends on which articulators are defective and to what degree. The structural limitation of the articulator must be determined before goals can be set. For example, if the tongue is limited in its range of movement, therapy is designed to improve excursion and articulation precision. With structural defects of the articulators, therapy is sometimes done in conjunction with surgery and placement of prosthetic devices.

Articulation Therapy for Motor Speech Disorders

Articulation therapy for motor speech disorders involves two goals, depending on where the motor speech process breaks down. If the breakdown occurs at the conceptual or programming levels, therapy involves planning and control of the articulators. The goal is to get the individual to conceptualize, create, and execute the motor plan for the articulators. In effect the person is taught to gain control of his articulators. If articulation breaks down at the neuromuscular level, the goal of therapy is to improve strength, mobility, coordination, and precision of articulatory gestures. (Specific therapies for motor speech disorders are discussed in Chapter 7.)

Articulation Therapy for Auditory Perceptual and Sensorimotor Deficiencies

Unlike the phonological approach, where children are taught phonological rules using more than one sound as examples, traditional articulation therapy involves working on one phoneme at a time. In this approach, the sensorimotor aspects of phoneme production are taught by using auditory perceptual training and articulation drills to learn correct production of the error sound. Auditory perceptual training usually precedes production activities.

Auditory perceptual training gives the individual the discrimination abilities to perceive the differences between sounds, particularly similar ones. At this aspect of the treatment approach, no emphasis is placed on sound production; the goal is to train the ear, not the tongue. The person is taught to perceive differences in her error sound in a variety of contexts. Once this is done, then the individual is taught the fine motor skills to produce it.

As discussed earlier, nonstimulable individuals have trouble producing the error sound because they are physically incapable of it. They cannot make the sound either in isolation or in more complicated contexts such as in words and phrases. Stimulable individuals can produce it; they have the neurological and physical abilities to do so. However, they lack the attention or motivation to do so. When provided with auditory and visual cues—when someone shows them the appropriate tongue and lip placement and gives cues about how the phoneme is supposed to sound—they can produce the sound correctly. The person who is nonstimulable requires special techniques, which involve shaping and using coarticulation, to learn to produce the sound correctly in isolation.

Once the person can produce the sound in isolation, the next step is gradually to increase the complexity of the speech productions. Drill is an important part of this procedure. The standard procedure is to begin with production of the target sound in syllable contexts. For example, if the target sound is /s/, the individual is drilled on it bracketed in various vowels until it is produced correctly in these contexts. The next goal is to advance to making the sound in simple words. The individual is taught to produce the sound in the initial, final, and medial positions in words. Commercially available word lists, which clinicians use in these activities, are available. The final aspect of the production phase involves production of the target sound in short phrases and during conversation. Here, the clinician reminds the individual when to produce the sound correctly and rewards appropriate behaviors.

Habituation, or carryover, is the final phase of the therapy. It involves having the individual produce the sound correctly during school activities and at home. Teachers and parents are usually enlisted to serve as monitors for this activity. In addition, the clinician speaks with the child and chooses topics that "tax" his attention. The goal is to teach the individual to concentrate on the topic while still producing the sound correctly.

Other Articulation Therapies

Several syndromes, diseases, and disorders may require special considerations and the use of one or more of the preceding articulation therapies. Articulation disorders resulting from or occurring with such conditions as autism, schizophrenia, organic brain syndrome, head trauma, and Alzheimer's disease often require multiple approaches to intervention.

Articulation therapy in these cases is incorporated into the total cognitive, linguistic, and psychological management of the underlying disorders. Changing the effects of dialect and accent in teenagers and adults is difficult because those articulatory patterns are firmly established. The goal of accent and dialect reduction in adults is often limited to improving intelligibility and communicative effectiveness (Owens, Metz, & Haas, 2000).

Treatment of Phonological Disorders

For individuals whose articulation disorder results from delayed development of the phonological rules of language and who have several articulation errors, the phonological approach is appropriate. In the phonological approach, speech samples are examined in several contexts to determine rule-governed structures. To move the individual to adopt a more mature phonological level, the clinician targets a small number of words to teach the new pattern. *Auditory bombardment activities*, in which the child is barraged with words having the particular phonological process, helps her awareness of the process. Drills on the production of the words also help the child practice using the process. The individual internalizes and generalizes it to all sounds affected by the phonological process. No single approach is appropriate for all children with disordered phonology, and clinicians should select from a range of different approaches (Dodd & Bradford, 2000). Individuals with delayed phonology often have other deficiencies in language, especially reading, spelling, and language achievement measures, suggesting a relationship between spoken and written language (Lewis & Freebairn, 1997). Consequently, phonological goals should be integrated into other language development activities.

Literature and Media Stereotypes

Is a w/r substitution inherently comical? Does Cindy's lisp make her a more vulnerable and endearing character on *The Brady Bunch*? Would the cartoon characters Elmer Fudd and Sylvester the Cat be as funny if they spoke articulately? Why does the image of Barbara Waa Waa interviewing the president of the United States have comedic value? Why does a young boy's confusion over the words "undertow" and "under toad," and "graduate student" and "gradual student" give charm and depth to his character? Do "ladies men" lisp? Based on a person's speech patterns, why are assumptions made about education, power, sexual preference, status, and maturity?

Literature and media frequently use articulation disorders, accents, and dialects to develop characters and for their comedic value. Many adults in today's society have grown up laughing at the antics of speech-disordered cartoon characters. The humor found in Barbara Walters' speech pattern can be traced in part to hearing the same articulation patterns uttered by Elmer Fudd during his comical cartoon antics. The same is true of sophisticated James Bond ordering a martini, with the speech pattern similar to Sylvester the Cat. A lisping womanizer is humorously contradictory *(The Ladies Man)*.

Screenwriters use accent and dialect to reinforce stereotypes of their television and film characters. Whether the person is a "good ole boy" from the Deep South, drawling on and on, or an intense, hurried New Yorker schleping groceries to her apartment, dialect and accent are important in character development. They are as important to developing their persona as are the costumes they wear or the cars they drive. Having money, power, and status is synonymous with using clear, articulate speech patterns. Conversely, rural and other dialects are used to connect the character to the soil and little money, power, and status. In movies the typical gardener to the California wealthy speaks with a heavy Spanish accent. It would be "out of character" for him to speak without it.

Articulation patterns, whether they are remnants from childhood speech development gone astray or the result of an accent or dialect, give richness to the language of the speaker. Society is quick to draw stereotypical assessments of people based on their articulation patterns. And like many stereotypes, some are probably based in fact for groups of people but invalid for every individual. Because of literature and media, articulation disorders, accent, and dialect are considered by many to be a reflection of an individual's intelligence, social status, and maturity.

Summary

Articulation and phonology disorders impair the production of speech sounds. Several causes of articulation disorders include structural defects, improper learning, hearing loss, deafness, and perceptual factors. The goals, objectives, and methods of treatment depend on the etiology of the articulation disorders. Dialect and accent are not technically considered articulation disorders, although some speakers may want them reduced or eliminated. Several types of articulation patterns do not impair communication and only draw attention to the speaker. Whether these differences in speech articulation should be considered disorders is a controversial topic in communication sciences and disorders. Articulation, accent, and dialect give information about the speakers' socioeconomic status and education.

Study Questions

1. Why does a lisp, slur, or drawl diminish the intent and potency of a verbal statement?

2. List the hard, soft, fixed, and mobile articulators.

3. What is the International Phonetic Alphabet, and why is it used?

4. Compare and contrast *manner* and *place* of articulation.

5. What is *intelligibility*?

6. What factors affect hearing loss and articulation development?

7. What is the *lingual frenulum*?

8. Compare and contrast the *sensorimotor method* and the *phonological approach* to articulation therapy.

9. Describe *auditory perception*.

10. What is the difference between *dialect* and *accent*?

11. List the information that must be supplied on an individualized education plan (IEP).

12. Give an example of a w/r substitution in the medial position of a word.

13. What is *oral diadochokinesis*?

14. What are some of the stereotypes society draws from a male who lisps? Why do these stereotypes exist?

Suggested Reading and Video

Alvarez, L., & Kolker, A. (1987). *American Tongues*. New York: Center for New American Media. This is an excellent video with examples of dialects and accents from across the United States.

Culbertson, W., & Tanner, D. (2001). Clinical comparisons: Phonological processes and their relationship to traditional phoneme norms. *Infant-Toddler Intervention, 11*(1): 15–25. This article discusses the phonological and traditional methods of viewing articulation disorders in children.

Dodd, B., & Bradford, A. (2000). A comparison of three therapy methods for children with different types of developmental phonological disorder. *Int. J. Lang. Comm. Dis., 35*(2): 198–209. This article explores different therapy approaches to children with phonological disorders.

Hall, B. J., Oyer, H. J., & Haas, W. H. (2001). *Speech, language, and hearing disorders: A guide for the teacher*. Boston: Allyn & Bacon. This book, designed for teachers, has a comprehensive review of articulation disorders with an emphasis on school-age children.

Wise, R. J. S., Greene, J., Büchel, C., & Scott, S. K. (1999). Brain regions involved in articulation. *Lancet, 353*: 1057–1061. This study, published in a major medical journal, challenges the long-held view that motor speech programming is a function only of Broca's area of the brain.

5

Language Development and Disorders

Chapter Preview
Language, the foundation of society, has allowed humans to become the dominant creatures on the planet. Learning language is a massive undertaking, but one done naturally by normal children. In this chapter you will learn five common aspects that go into a definition of language. There is a discussion of linguistic competence and performance. The cognitive, linguistic, and social–communication aspects that are important to the diagnosis and treatment of language disorders are reviewed. There is also a general summary of important milestones of childhood language acquisition. The role that language plays in intelligence is also discussed. Various factors that can cause language delay and disorders are examined. Finally, there is an analysis of the literature and media stereotypes associated with people who have language delay and disorders.

"Born to talk." Few things in life come as naturally or easily as talking. Every normal baby born into this world embarks on a long journey of learning and using language; each person is wired for it. All normal men, women, and children have the neurological foundation to learn, use, and enjoy any language to which they are exposed. Country, race, gender, religion, or culture does not matter. Learning language is as natural as our first breath of air. For most children, learning the complexities of language is second nature. They learn the form and structure of language as easily as in what context to use it. Even though language acquisition comes so naturally, its complexity is not diminished. Learning language is a massive undertaking, one that takes years to gain competency, and it is probably never really "mastered" by even the greatest screenwriters, orators, playwrights, and novelists.

Because language is so common, we sometimes underestimate its importance. We forget the powerful role it plays in our everyday lives. Language is the foundation of society. There would be no libraries and corporate offices without it. The legal system, from the wording of contracts to jury deliberations, require language. Without language there would be no Shakespearian plays. The role of language in religion, all religions, is paramount. After all, in the beginning was the "Word." Relationships are created and nurtured by it. There is a

Literature, Media, and Personality Profiles

What's Eating Gilbert Grape

Film critic Joan Ellis, of the *Chicago Sun-Times,* calls *What's Eating Gilbert Grape* a story of despair that is buoyed by the decency of its characters. It stars Johnny Depp as Gilbert Grape, a tortured young man living in rural Iowa, who must deal with his morbidly obese mother and care for his mentally deficient brother, Arnie. Arnie Grape is played by Leonardo DiCaprio, who manages to create a character that is mentally deficient, lovable, and interesting. In the film, Arnie loves to climb the town's water tower, an illegal, dangerous, and attention-getting act. The love and concern Gilbert has for his brother is a central theme of the movie. The film and screenplay are adapted from a novel written by Peter Hedges. Directed by Lasse Hallstroem and produced by Paramount Pictures, *What's Eating Gilbert Grape* was released in 1993.

Nell

Nell is a story about a woman raised by her speech-impaired mother. She grows up in the backwoods of North Carolina, totally isolated from others. Because of her isolation, Nell speaks a unique language, one understood only by her. The film is an exploration of language, socialization, values, and ambition and revolves around the relationships of three people: Nell, a doctor, and a psychologist. The film explores Nell's encounter with the outside world and the reality of socialization. The film, directed by Michael Apted, stars Jodie Foster as Nell, Natasha Richardson as psychologist Paula Olsen, and Liam Neeson as Dr. Jerome Lovell. The movie was shot in the Smokey Mountains, and their beauty was captured by cinematographer Dante Spinotti. The screenplay, written by William Nicholson and Mark Handly, is based on the play *Idioglossia* (idioglossia is a made-up, unique language).

Chris Burke

Actor Chris Burke is a remarkable person. He was born with Down syndrome, and doctors advised his parents, Frank and Marian Burke, to institutionalize him. Fortunately for millions of people who grew to love his character on the ABC television series *Life Goes On,* they chose to ignore that advice. The television series, first broadcast in 1989, ran until 1993. It was the first major television show to have a star with Down syndrome. Burke was nominated for a Golden Globe Award for his role as Corky Thatcher and has also received a Youth in Film Award. He has even had a New York City public school named in his honor. Burke, with friends Joe and John DeMasi, has released several albums of uplifting and inspiring music. He is a supporter of the Very Special Arts program that brings the arts to people with physical and mental disabilities. He continues to act and has had several guest-star roles. He has appeared on *The Commish, Touched by an Angel,* and *Heaven and Hell.* He is a spokesperson for the National Down Syndrome Society. His autobiography, *A Special Kind of Hero,* was published by Bantam Doubleday Dell in 1992.

Rain Man

Rain Man is a film about an autistic savant. Directed by Barry Levinson, it stars Dustin Hoffman as Raymond, "Rain Man," Babbitt, and Tom Cruise, as his brother Charlie Babbitt. In the movie, Charlie learns that his recently deceased father has left his autistic brother, one he never knew existed, a large estate. The film is about the road trip where Charlie and Raymond travel to California by car to claim the inheritance. During the trip, the audience is treated to some of the autistic savant's amazing abilities. One ability entailed memorizing an entire phone book. Hoffman, who did a laudable job in portraying the emotionally distant, mentally deficient character, studied extensively for the part. He watched hours of tapes about savants, talked to professionals, read scientific papers, and visited several patients and their families. *Rain Man* was written by Barry Morrow, produced by Mark Johnson, and released by Metro-Goldwyn-Mayer/United Artists (MGM/UA). Hoffman received the Academy Award for Best Actor in *Rain Man*.

Sling Blade

In the disturbing movie *Sling Blade*, Karl Childers is a mentally deficient man whom his parents severely abused. He was kept in a shed for most of his early life. At age 12, Karl was committed to a psychiatric hospital for killing his mother and her lover with a gardening tool called a "sling blade." When middle-aged, Karl is released to his hometown and befriends a 12-year-old boy, Frank. Doyle, an alcoholic roommate of Frank and his mother, reignites Karl's violent tendencies.

The pace of the film is described as slow, largely due to Karl's speech pattern and processing time. Billy Bob Thornton was nominated for Best Actor for his portrayal of Karl Childers and won the Academy Award for Best Adapted Screenplay. It also stars Dwight Yoakam, Lucas Black, J. T. Walsh, John Ritter, Natalie Canderday, and Robert Duvall. Written and directed by Billy Bob Thornton, it was released in 1996 by Blue Angel Films.

Forrest Gump

Forrest Gump, released in 1994 by Paramount Pictures, was directed by Robert Zemeckis and produced by Wendy Finerman, Steve Tisch, and Steve Starkey. Starring Tom Hanks in the title role and Robin Wright, Gary Sinise, Mykelti Williamson, and Sally Field, it is the endearing story about the life of a mentally "slow" person during the turbulent 1960s and 1970s. Forrest Gump lives an exciting life. He manages, through impressive visual effects, to meet famous people of the times, like Elvis Presley, John F. Kennedy, John Lennon, and Richard Nixon. Forrest Gump goes to war, runs a marathon, and becomes a commercial fisherman. The film depicts how this innocent and kind person viewed those turbulent times. The soundtrack of sixties and seventies songs became as popular as the movie. The philosophical Forrest Gump utters two now-famous statements about the uncertainties of life and the nature of mental deficiency: "Life is like a box of chocolates; you never know what you're going to get" and "Stupid is as stupid does." Tom Hanks received the Academy Award for Best Actor in *Forrest Gump*.

Of Mice and Men

John Steinbeck's *Of Mice and Men* was published in 1937 by Covici, Friede, Inc., and subsequently by Viking Press and Penguin Books. Set in the Salinas Valley of California, it is the story of two ranch hands. The two main characters are George Milton and Lennie Small. Lennie is a large man with low intelligence. *Of Mice and Men* is a study of the bonds of friendship, dreams, mental deficiency, and coping with a cruel word. The book has been adapted into a play and an opera. The most recent movie version stars John Malkovich and Gary Sinise and was released in 1992 by MGM/UA. John Steinbeck (1902–1968) is noted for his powerful descriptions of the downtrodden and oppressed. He received a Pulitzer Prize Fiction Award for *The Grapes of Wrath* and, in 1962, was awarded the Nobel Prize for Literature.

language to aviation, philosophy, psychology, and medicine. Some philosophers believe the structure of language constrains our thoughts, whereas others believe it gives us unlimited means to explore the universe. Without language, our complex, industrialized society would grind to a slow crawl. Language is essential to education, so there would be no colleges and universities without it. The thoughts on this page would be unwritten and unread without language.

Unfortunately, some children and adults suffer from language delay and disorders. For reasons that range from environmental depravation to profound mental deficiency, some individuals have delayed or disordered language. These problems with the acquisition and use of language can be part of a specific learning disability and be limited to minor reading, writing, or understanding difficulties. They can also be all pervasive and render the child mute, isolated, and alone.

Defining Language

Defining *language* is no easy task; there is no universally accepted definition of the word. The reason for the difficulty in defining *language* is the fact that it is complex and multidimensional. It is the highest mental function performed by the human brain. Some definitions are narrow, whereas others attempt to capture the essence of language in all its complexity. There are five necessary aspects to any definition of language (Table 5.1).

First, language is a *socially shared code*. There are more than 10,000 languages and dialects in the world, and they are products of individual societies. Language is a code or a system for representing ideas, events, things, and feelings. The people in a society who speak a particular language agree to the system or code for communication.

TABLE 5.1   *Five Aspects to a Definition of Language*

Aspect	Description
Socially shared code	Socially accepted system for representing ideas, events, things, and feelings
Symbolic	Ideas, events, things, and feelings represented by a symbol or series of symbols
Arbitrary	The symbol–referent relationship on which a language society randomly agrees
Modalities	Communication through speech, writing, reading, gestures, and auditory comprehension
Rule governed	Grammar for the form, content, and usage of language

Second, language involves symbols. A *symbol* is a representation of something else. A good example of a visual symbol is a flag. The U.S. flag is a cut of red, white, and blue cloths, made up of stars and stripes. When people see it, they think of the country it represents. People have strong emotional responses to symbols, especially flags. The flag of a country represents all its aspects. It can also be used to express unity, as was demonstrated after the tragedy of September 11, 2001. Words, too, are symbolic. Whether they are written, gestured, or spoken, they stand for an idea, event, thing, or feeling. The relationship between the symbol and what it refers to—the **referent**—is the essence of meaning.

A philosophy of dealing with symbols, especially words, is called *general semantics.* It helps people understand the relationship between words and their meanings, and not just to react to them. It promotes a relativistic view of word meanings. A statement made in general semantics is that the "map is not the territory." This means that the word is different from the idea, event, thing, or feeling. For example, the flag is not the country; destroying a flag is not the same as destroying the country it represents.

Third, the symbols used in language are *arbitrary.* No set rules dictate the creation of words and what they mean. The sound or letter combinations that make up a word are purely arbitrary. Early in the development of a language society, a sound or a series of sounds uttered by people over time came to mean the idea, event, thing, or feeling to which they were referring. The same arbitrary rules of semantics hold true for new words that become part of languages each year. Because early societies were isolated from one another, differences arose in what the sound combinations referred to, and some languages use sounds that others do not use. This isolation of language societies accounts for the many different languages and dialects of the world.

Not all people believe in this evolutionary view of language. Creationists believe that the biblical parable of the Tower of Babel explains the reason for the varied languages of the world. In the creationist view, before attempting to build the Tower of Babel, only one language was spoken by the people of the world. To prevent the building of the tower, God created different languages. The word *babbling* grew from this parable.

Fourth, the definition of language concerns its various forms. There are several **modalities,** or avenues, that communication can take, and they are separated into **expressive language** and **receptive language.** When expressing ourselves through language, we use speech, writing, or gestures. We **encode** our thoughts into spoken words, written letters, or expressive gestures. On the receiving end, those spoken words, written letters, or expressive gestures are **decoded** by the listener. Of course, people can express themselves in other ways. Artists, mathematicians, and musicians also communicate using paintings, equations, and music. The wry smile on the *Mona Lisa*, $E = mc^2$, and the rapidly changing notes in "Flight of the Bumble Bee" also communicate. Some scholars believe that even paintings and symphonies have, at their core, a basis in language.

Fifth, when defining language, consider the fact that it is *rule governed.* All languages have rules that govern the way we combine and use the symbols. The word **grammar** is an all-encompassing term for those rules. These rules involve the form, content, and usage of language. The form that language takes is its phonological and syntactical systems. **Phonology** deals with the rules governing the way speech sounds are organized and sequenced in language (see Chapter 4). **Syntax** relates to word order and the rules for organizing sentences. **Semantics** is the content of language and concerns the meanings of words—the symbol–referent relationship.

An important aspect of language is the role it plays in verbal thought. Inner language, internal monologues, or inner speech is the act of communicating with oneself. Verbal thought is the use of words and word meanings during thinking. The nature of verbal thought and the role it plays in **cognition** is the subject of debate, sometimes called the *language–thought* controversy. Some scholars believe that language simply allows for the expression of ideas and concepts; others are convinced that thought and language are inseparable. The role language plays in thought is different for children and adults. In children, language probably serves more to represent and express concrete thoughts. In adults, especially during abstract thinking, language and some kinds of thought are inseparable. One thing is for certain in both children and adults: *Language facilitates thought and thought facilitates language.*

Linguistic Competence and Performance

Two important aspects to language are competence and performance. **Linguistic competence** is the knowledge of the rules of language: its grammar, semantics, phonology, and syntax. It is the basic information that people have about their language that is necessary to speak and understand it. **Linguistic performance,** on the other hand, is the actual usage of language; it is how people use linguistic competence.

An example of the difference between competence and performance is the game of chess. Chess has rules about how to move the pieces; it is a complicated game. The queen has the most movement capabilities, whereas the pawns are extremely limited in direction and the number of spaces they can move. Knights must be moved in an "L" fashion, and the bishops can be moved only diagonally. Rooks, and even the king, whose goal it is to capture, have specific rules governing their movements. Besides the number and direction of movements, a chess player must know other rules about how to capture a piece or avoid being captured. A competent chess player knows all the rules of chess.

It is the performance of a chess player that often determines who wins the game. Grandmasters and novices may know all the rules of the game, but grand masters will easily defeat novices because they efficiently translate the rules into victory. Grand masters use the rules of chess extremely efficiently and productively. Like chess, linguistic competence and performance involves knowing the rules and being effective and productive in using them.

Cognitive, Linguistic, and Social–Communication Systems

Three aspects to evaluating and treating language delay and disorders in children are cognitive prerequisites, linguistic form and structure, and social–communication development. They can be assessed directly by conventional tests given to the child. They can also be evaluated indirectly by interviewing parents and teachers (Tanner, Lamb, & Secord, 1997).

The term cognitive prerequisites refers to the thought processes that underlie language. The clinician determines the child's understanding of how things relate to one another, the use of symbols, and the ability to solve problems. Linguistic systems include the combination of sounds into words, grammatical inflections, and the creation, organization, and understanding of sentences. Linguistic development encompasses both reception and expression. Social–communication development refers to the functional processes that underlie language; it is the way language communicates the needs, desires, feelings, and ideas of the speaker. The clinician assesses the intent and effectiveness in the child's use of spoken language. In the diagnostic process, the speech–language pathologist determines the child's level of performance, compares it with expected milestones and practical limitations, and then provides appropriate intervention. The relationship between these three areas of development is strong and serves as a basis to an integrated program of therapy.

Pragmatics

Included in the discussion of social–communication development are the pragmatics of language. They are a set of sociolinguistic rules that include the speech act but also govern the discourse structures in which speech acts are embedded (Norris, 1998). **Pragmatics** deals with the communicative context and the environment in which language occurs. Owens, Metz, and Haas (2000, p. 186) list the following as the most common pragmatic language characteristics of children with language disorders:

- Difficulty answering questions or requesting clarification
- Difficulty initiating or maintaining a conversation, or securing a conversational turn
- Poor flexibility in language when tailoring the message to the listener or repairing communication breakdowns
- Short conversational episodes
- Limited range of communication functions
- Inappropriate topics and off-topic comments; ineffectual, inappropriate comments
- Asocial monologues
- Difficulty with stylistic variations and speaker–listener roles
- Narrative difficulties
- Few interactions

Children with pragmatic language problems are impaired in their understanding and use of language in various speaking situations. According to Owens (1995), children with pragmatic language problems wait for the environment to act in some way, and then they respond. They rarely ask questions because making mistakes and being corrected is easier.

Assessing Language in Children

When assessing a child's cognitive, linguistic, and social–communication performance, comparing chronological age to tested mental or developmental age is necessary. A person's chronological age is determined by subtracting his birth date from the date when the assessment is conducted. For example, if a child is born on January 1, 1998, and the date of assessment is January 1, 2002, his chronological age is 4 years and 0 months (4-0) (see Box 5.1). The chronological age is compared with the developmental age in a particular area of language ability.

There are two theories about how to view language delay and disorders. The *neutralist approach* assumes that if a person's performance on a test is significantly lower than other

BOX 5.1 • *Compute Your Chronological Age*

You can determine your chronological age in years, months, and days. Place the current date in the space provided and subtract your birth date from it. If you have to borrow, be certain to convert months, years, and days. Use the following as an example:

	Year	Month	Day
Current Date:	2002	10	21
Your Birth Date:	1983	11	27
Chronological Age:	18	11	24

	Year	Month	Day
Current Date:			
Your Birth Date:			
Chronological Age:			

children of the same age, then she has a language delay or disorder (Gillam, Marquardt, & Martin, 2000). "The word *neutralism* has been applied to this position because formal language tests are *neutral* on the importance of considering social norms and expectations in identification" (Gillam et al., 2000, p. 412).

The *normativist approach* values social norms and focuses on the consequences of a language delay or disorder on the individual (Gillam et al., 2000). This approach considers language disorders to be a defect in the development of the form, content, or use of language (Fey, 1986). According to Fey, if the language delay or disorder negatively affects the person's vocational, educational, psychological, or social life, then he should receive language therapy. Whereas the neutralist approach looks at the child's success on tests, the normativist approach considers the effects of the disorder on the child's everyday interaction. "A growing number of clinicians combine the neutralist and the normativist approaches to identifying language disorders" (Gillam et al., 2000, p. 413). They look both at test scores and on the limitations caused by the language disorder when considering the need for therapy.

Teachers, Language Delay, and Disorders

The role that teachers play in assessing whether a particular child is developing speech and language normally should never be underestimated. Teachers can provide a valuable source of information about a child's cognitive, linguistic, and social–communication development. Asking a child's teacher the following questions can provide valuable diagnostic information (Tanner, Lamb, et al., 1997, pp. 52–56):

In your professional opinion, do you believe that the child has a delay in speech and language development?

Is the child able to understand questions as well as other children in the classroom?

Does the child follow instructions as well as other children in the classroom?

Do you believe that the child's understanding of vocabulary is adequate for his or her age?

Is the child able to remember information presented in classroom instruction as well as most other children in the class?

Is the child able to understand new information as well as most other children in the class?

How well does the child get along with other children?

Does the child cooperate with the other children in games and other activities?

Does the child have difficulty asking for help when it is needed?

Does the child have word-finding problems? Does the child have frequent problems selecting the correct word to be spoken?

Does the child wander from topic to topic when talking?

Are sentences spoken by the child of the appropriate length and complexity for his age?

Is the child's use of grammar similar to that of other children in her age group?

During reading and writing, how well does the child perform compared to the other children in his age group?

Experienced teachers have the benefit of having taught many students. As a result they intuitively know when a student is not understanding or using language normally. Although they may not be able to identify the specific cognitive, linguistic, or social–communication deficiency, they can serve as important screening sources. Their observations can indicate whether a child should be evaluated for a language delay or disorder. Early intervention is important because language disorders can be long lasting. Stothard, Snowling, Bishop, Chipchase, and Kaplan (1998) found that if a child's language difficulties are still present at age 5 years, 6 months, she is likely to have language, literacy, and educational difficulties throughout childhood and adolescence. However, if the child's language difficulties are largely resolved by that time, the outlook for spoken language development is better—and the earlier the detection of language delay, the better. Ward (1998) found that if language delay is detected in the first year of life and intervention provided, these children are less likely to require speech and language therapy at the age at which children are usually referred for it.

Individuals with Disabilities Education Act

President Bill Clinton signed the reauthorization of the Individuals with Disabilities Education Act (IDEA) in 1997. IDEA (Public Law 101-476) is a continuation and refinement of PL 94-142, which was enacted in 1975. Public Law 94-142 was the first national legislation that guarantees students with disabilities the right to a free and appropriate public education. It, and several other laws enacted in the past four decades, specifies the nature and type of services that can be provided to the disabled, including those with learning and language disabilities. IDEA specifically prohibits the use of culturally discriminatory tests to determine the presence or absence of a communication disorder. The law also prohibits a child with a learning disability from being discharged from special services because of behavioral problems.

Language Development

A person's communication development, from the birth cry to speech and language competence, is a remarkable journey. It is an amazing time of neurological, mental, and physical growth. Researchers from several disciplines have studied this time of rapid development extensively. Speech and hearing scientists, linguists, physicians, educators, and professionals from other disciplines have observed, tested, and tracked the steps and stages of language acquisition. To date what we have is a rather good picture of the normal process of language development. We know that by the time normal children are 7 or 8 years old, most of their language structure is established. Of course, we continue to learn new words all of our lives, but many aspects of language competency are established relatively young. Continuing with the example of chess competency and performance, by the time normal children enter school, they will have learned most of the rules of the game. With language development, most normal children pass through the sequential steps and stages on the road to language competence. These stages have been carefully cataloged and charted and can be used to decide whether a particular person is learning language at the expected ages. They can provide a profile of language development for diagnostic and therapeutic purposes (Tanner, Lamb, et al., 1997; Tanner & Lamb, 1984).

It has been said that we are born with a brain that is a "blank slate." Little knowledge about the nature of the world has been programmed into the newborn's brain. A newborn's behavior is almost exclusively reflexive. Sucking, crying, grasping, and random movements of the arm, legs, and head are noted. The newborn's crying is reflexive. No different patterns of crying appear until approximately 1 month of age. Gradually, the child begins to develop different types of crying, and the parents, particularly the mother, can soon distinguish five or more types of cries. For example, a mother can tell by the nature of the cry whether her child wants to be changed, held, or nursed or feels pain. The baby's crying and the mother's reactions are the first social forms of communication.

Cooing and babbling are vocalizations involving vowels and consonants. *Cooing* is the sound made by babies when one or more vowels are combined. *Babbling* consists of consonant–vowel syllables. Babies engage in these behaviors because they enjoy making the sounds and the way the sounds feel in the mouth and throat. Occasionally, during cooing and babbling, sounds that appear to be words may be combined, but they are just random combinations. Babies interact with their parents by other means, too. Laughing and smiling in response to playful activities by the parents are delightful first signs of social communication.

Between the ages of 9 and 18 months, a normal child begins to use single-word utterances. This is true of all normal children and for all languages. Typically, the first word is a *phonetic duplication*, such as "Mamma" or "Dadda." For parents the emergence of the first word is a major communication milestone. When their child says his first words at the approximate age of other children, most parents breathe a sigh of relief. To many parents the appropriate emergence of first words is an indication that all is well in speech and language development. At this time the child also begins to understand words such as "no," "up," and "bye, bye" and can follow easy one-step commands. The child often overgeneralizes a particular word; for example, she might call all males who are about the same age as her father, "Daddy." Many embarrassed mothers in supermarkets have found it necessary to correct their children when they point to several males and call them "Daddy."

Parents observe a child's developing cognition by the things he does and does not do (Tanner, Lamb, et al., 1997). For example, a 2- to 4-month-old baby will watch a rattle being hidden under a blanket, but will not lift it to find the toy, and will make sucking movements before a nipple is placed in his mouth. As he matures mentally, a child will start to use toys correctly, such as winding up a car to make it go or pulling a string to make a doll talk. The ability to find hidden objects shows important cognitive maturation. Later in his cognitive development, a child can categorize, place things in rank order, and engage in symbolic play. To determine whether a child has developed normal language, interviewing parents or direct testing can determine several cognitive prerequisites. A child develops higher linguistic and social–communication abilities only when the appropriate cognitive prerequisites have been mastered.

Linguistic development continues at a rapid rate. At about the age of 2 years, a child begins to make two-word utterances, and her receptive vocabulary improves to the point where she can name many objects in the house, friends, and relatives (Tanner, Lamb, et al., 1997). A child gradually gains more complex grammar and syntax abilities, both for expression and understanding. Vocabulary continues to develop, and at about age 6 or 7, a child produces and understands linguistic structures similar to those of an adult. Parents see the growing mastery of linguistic systems as the child goes from two-word utterances, such as "Mommy bottle," "Ball roll," and "Fall down," to more complex constructions. A child increases the length and complexity of utterances as she is able to say, "I want my bottle," "The ball is rolling," and "The picture fell down." She gradually learns to follow complex commands and uses tenses and contractions correctly.

A child's emerging social–communication development is seen in the ways he interacts with others and when playing games (Tanner, Lamb, et al., 1997). He uses language to satisfy his increasing number of desires and needs. A child goes from narrating aloud what he is doing to being able to think the words to himself. Parents note changes in a child's play patterns as he develops more sophisticated social–communication abilities. At about 2 or 3 years of age, children, when playing with each other, will talk among themselves, but it will not be interactive. They will engage in turn-taking, but they have completely different topics of conversation (see Box 5.2). Later, their conversations become more adultlike with appropriate topics and subject changes. At about the age of 6 or 7, most children interact well enough with others to play cooperatively and follow group rules. They can talk about their feelings, plan for the future, and give logical rules for doing things. At about the age of 6 or 7, normal children can communicate needs, desires, feelings, and ideas in an adult fashion. In school they can participate in "Show and Tell" without problems and enjoy the activity (Tanner, Lamb, et al., 1997).

The focus of language development in school-age children changes from semantics and pragmatics to written language in both input and output (Owens, 1998). During the rapid

BOX 5.2 • *Collective Monologue in Two Children*

In a collective monologue, two children may appear to be having a conversation. They engage in turn-taking, use gestures, and have eye contact, but there is no real exchange of information. For example:

Steven	**Jeffery**
"My daddy has a new pickup."	"Kittens play with string."
"It is red."	"We have a yellow kitten."
"It has a toolbox."	"There are two white ones, too."
	"The mother is white and yellow."

growth of language in preschoolers, they learn all aspects of language, but most development is seen in learning words and their meanings. By 20–30 months of age, preschoolers have a vocabulary of about 100 words and can comprehend most adults if they speak slowly and simply (Van Riper & Erickson, 1996). By the time children enter school, receptive and expressive vocabulary has increased dramatically. (See Box 5.3.) The acquisition rate of language slows during the school years and is more subtle (Owens, 1998). Schoolwork in the higher grades involves more reading, writing, and formal use of language. Both semantic and pragmatic use of language are developed well into adulthood. Even in older adults, refining the syntactical, grammatical, and phonological aspects of language continues, as they learn new rules of construction or refine ones learned incorrectly. Also continuing to develop throughout adulthood are the social–communication aspects of language and knowing the way that language communicates needs, desires, feelings, and ideas.

BOX 5.3 • *Vocabulary Learning and Usage*

When a speech clinician works with a child who has delayed vocabulary, she must first develop the child's understanding of words and concepts before she can expect him to use them correctly in sentences and phrases. Clinically, vocabulary understanding precedes expressive usage. For example, if someone asks you to use the word *aileron* in a sentence and you do not know the meaning of the word, you cannot correctly use it, no matter how hard you try. However, if it is explained that an aileron is part of an airplane's wings that helps bank and turn it when the pilot moves the steering apparatus, you have learned the meaning of the word. Now, you can construct correct appropriate sentences such as "The aileron was broken, and the airplane crashed" or "The ailerons caused the airplane to bank very sharply."

Intelligence and Language Development

Discussing language development and disorders without considering a person's intelligence is impossible. Many children with a language delay or disorder are not mentally deficient and in fact may have superior intelligence. However, mental deficiency and language delay and disorders often occur concurrently. Intelligence is the totality of a person's mental abilities. It includes the abilities to learn, think rationally and logically, solve problems, abstract, and interact productively and successfully with the environment. A ratio in which a person's mental age is divided by her chronological age measures intelligence. The score is called an *intelligence quotient* (IQ); the average score is 100. People whose scores are higher or lower than the mean, as measured in standard deviations, are grouped as advanced or reduced in IQ scores. A *standard deviation* (SD) is a statistical measure that expresses how far a score deviates from the mean. About two-thirds of the population have intelligence scores that fall 1 SD above and below the average; this is often called the range of normal. Most IQ scores reflect both verbal and nonverbal (performance) abilities. Intelligence plays an important role in both normal and abnormal language development.

"I don't believe in intelligence tests." Many college students, when they first study IQ testing, make that statement. The statement does not mean that they do not believe that IQ tests exist but simply reflects their concern that reducing such an important part of a person's life to a score is fraught with errors. People who are critical of intelligence testing are understandably concerned that these tests are not accurate. They wonder about their validity, reliability, and potential for bias:

• *Validity* is the extent to which a test does what it purports to do. A valid test measures what it says it does. An IQ test that is proved to be valid accurately measures a person's ability to learn, think rationally and logically, abstract, solve problems, and is only one of many predictors of how well he will succeed in life. In test construction there are several ways of determining a test's validity.

• *Reliability* is the dependability of a test, the consistency of the scores over repeated test administration. A reliable IQ test produces the same results when given to the same person at different times, or by different forms or sections of the same test. Reliability of a test can be compared to the reliability of a friend. A reliable friend is one who is consistently a friend. A reliable test is also consistent.

• Many people fear that IQ tests are biased. They suspect that people who speak certain languages or who are from different cultures than the mainstream population on which the tests were designed will not do well. Because of the test's *bias*, their scores will not reflect their true intelligence, and society will make improper judgments about them as individuals and as a group.

Intelligence testing has been around for a long time, and most tests have provable track records when administered and interpreted properly. Like all tests they can be used in careless and even unethical ways. However, tests like the Stanford–Binet, the Wechsler Adult Intelligence Scale, and the Wechsler Intelligence Scale for Children are used widely and

provide valuable and accurate results. These and other tests are important parts of the determination of whether a child is diagnosed as mentally impaired or has retarded development.

Mental Deficiency

One of the causes of language delay and disorders is mental deficiency. Mental deficiency,
like intelligence, is difficult to define. A main consideration in determining whether a person
is mentally deficient is whether her IQ is significantly below average. This usually means that
the person's IQ falls 2 SD below the mean on a valid and reliable IQ test. According to
Owens (1995), a score of 68 or below would meet this part of the definition and encompasses
about 3% of the population. This yields about 9 million people in the United States that
would meet this aspect of the definition of mental deficiency. Besides having a subaverage
score on a standard IQ test, the person must also have an impairment in *adaptive behaviors*,
which includes personal independence and social responsibility (Owens, 1995).

To be classified as mentally deficient, the reduction in intelligence should occur during
the developmental period, which is considered below the age of 18 years. Some adults suffer
brain injuries and subsequently score low on IQ tests and have reduced adaptive functioning.
Although certainly impaired and deficient in mental functioning, because their injuries did
not occur during the developmental period, they would not be considered mentally retarded.

According to Owens (1995) and Grossman (1983), the severity of mental retardation
ranges from mild to profound, and 89% of the population of people with mental retardation
are classified as *mildly* impaired. They usually live and work independently and often have
families. About 6% of mentally deficient people have *moderate* impairments. They are often
capable of some semi-independence at work and in residence. Those with *severe* mental retardation are capable of learning some self-care skills and do not totally depend on others. They
account for about 3.5% of the population of mentally challenged people. *Profoundly* retarded
people are capable of learning some basic living skills but require continual care and supervision. They often have multiple disabilities and represent 1.5% of the retarded population.
Sometimes, *borderline*, *educable*, *trainable*, and *custodial* retardation are used to describe, respectively, the preceding degrees of mental retardation.

The causes of mental deficiency range from environmental depravation to severe birth
defects. Lack of stimulation can cause mental retardation during the developmental period.
Several syndromes can cause mental retardation. The mother's excessive alcohol consumption during pregnancy causes fetal alcohol syndrome (FAS). Mental retardation and a host of
other mental and physical defects can result from this syndrome. Head trauma, diseases, and
anoxia during delivery can result in mental deficiency. For some people, it is easier to understand mental retardation resulting from head trauma. In the 1992 movie *Of Mice and Men*,
George Milton fabricated the story that his friend, Lennie Small, was retarded because he
was "kicked in the head by a horse" when he was a youngster. Other organic causes of mental
retardation include genetic disorders such as Down syndrome. The effects of Down syndrome on mental development can be seen in the popular actor Chris Burke. Mental deficiency can be caused by virtually any disorder, disease, or trauma that occurs during the
developmental period, results in a significant subaverage mental performance, and impairs
adaptive behavior.

The severity of mental deficiency is the most important factor influencing language development. As a rule, the more extensive the mental retardation, the more language development will suffer. In the mild or borderline category, a wide range of language impairments is associated with deficient mental development. Sometimes, people in the mild or borderline category are described as "slow." Forrest Gump was depicted as being in the mild, borderline category. In this film, he had an adequate vocabulary and used grammar normally. However, his overall processing time was slower than normal, he appeared to be more concrete, and he displayed problems with the social use and appropriateness of language (pragmatics). His concrete attitude was an endearing aspect of his personality. The film used it to give him an innocent, straightforward view of the times. In the film, Forrest Gump was blessed by a low IQ when expressing his views about the turbulent times in which he lived.

Moderately mentally deficient individuals often speak with shortened length of utterances. They have difficulty following complex commands, and both expressive and receptive vocabulary is limited. Their grammar, syntax, and phonology are often arrested and typical of preschoolers. Severely retarded individuals, people considered only trainable, often speak in only one- or two-word utterances. Their comprehension is also severely impaired. The language of these children and adults is limited to expression of immediate wants and needs. People who are profoundly mentally deficient—those who require custodial support—usually have no functional oral communication abilities. Some are mute. Communication, if attempted at all, is done with gross gestures, grunts, and other sounds. (Their speech is typical of Nell's during the initial confrontation with her in the cabin.)

Pervasive Developmental Disorders

According to Nicolosi, Harryman, and Kresheck (1996), *pervasive developmental disorders* (PDDs) are characterized by impairments in the development of social interaction, verbal and nonverbal communication skills, and imaginative activities. Although a high variability in these behaviors occurs from child to child, there is a marked restriction in activities and interests. These disorders occur as often as 15 per 10,000 live births, and they are 4 times more common in boys than girls (Hirsch, 1998). The *Diagnostic and Statistical Manual of Mental Disorders* of the American Psychiatric Association (1994) lists several categories of PDDs and describes their symptoms. "Depending on the severity of a child's disorder, the behavior might be labeled as autistic-like, or the child might be said to have varying levels of severity of PDD" (Owens et al., 2000, p. 175). According to Nicolosi et al. (1996), the age of onset in PDD is before the age of 3 years, and the younger the child, the more associated features are likely to be present. Associated features include abnormalities in cognition, posture, sensory input, motor behaviors, sleeping, eating, mood and the tendency to engage in self-destructive behaviors. An extreme pervasive developmental disorder, and the one with most public recognition, is autism.

Autism.   In the past this disorder was thought to be caused, at least in part, by poor parent–child interactions. Today, it is accepted that *autism* is organically based, a result of neurological or biological functioning of the child (Wetherby, 2000; Haynes & Shulman, 1998). A link may exist between autism, prenatal infections, and the immune system (van Gent, Heijnen, &

Treffers, 1997). As with most PDDs, parents note autistic behaviors when the child is young, particularly in the way he interacts with them. There is little if any true social interaction. "Often, parents are treated as things or, at best, no different from other people" (Owens et al., 2000, p. 176).

Wetherby (2000) describes the language and communicative characteristics of children with autism and PDDs. These children have limited or no speech development, and there are inconsistent or hypersensitive responses to auditory stimuli. Some children are oblivious to speech and environmental sounds. There is limited comprehension of verbal and gestural communication, and these children tend to be on a concrete level. Communication is used primarily for meeting immediate needs. They have unconventional verbal behaviors including immediate and delayed echolalia. (**Echolalia** is the repetition of that which has recently been spoken—that is, automatically repeating or "parroting" something that has been heard.) Perseveration is present and associated with incessant questioning. (**Perseveration** is the automatic continuation of a response—that is, sensory and motor responses that persist for a longer duration than what would be warranted by the intensity and significance of the stimuli.) There are voice-quality and prosodic abnormalities, difficulty with conversational and narrative discourse skills, and problems in the use of space during communication. The communication limitations seen in children with autism and PDDs are closely related to challenging behaviors, such as difficulty in expressing intentions and protesting.

In some children the severity of autism or PDDs lessens with age (Owens et al., 2000). Most children with autism and PDDs require continuous care: group homes, sheltered workshops, and institutionalization. (In the film *Rain Man*, Raymond Babbitt was institutionalized. His brother, Charlie, found how demanding caring for him was during the road trip to California.)

Environmental Deprivation

Depending on the extensiveness of the environmental depravation, a child's language may range from subtle gaps in cognitive, linguistic, and social–communication development to complete **mutism.** Some children are denied attention from one or both parents but are not subjected to abuse and extreme neglect. With others the environmental depravation, and the effects on the child's language development, can be devastating:

> We knew one little girl whose mother was a drunkard with whom no child could identify as she staggered around the house, dirty, cursing, and in half collapse. We have worked with children too hungry, too weak or too tired to talk and had to take care of these basic needs before they had a chance to learn. The county sheriff once brought us three almost-wild children from a hut in a swamp only a few miles from Kalamazoo. The father was retarded and a junk scavenger who fed them when he could. The mother had abandoned them. The tale is too incredible to put in a textbook, but these three nonspeaking children in the observation room were animal children. Yes, there are environmental conditions that deter speech development. (Van Riper & Erickson, 1996, p. 187)

Owens (1995) reviewed and summarized the research on language characteristics of neglected and abused children and found that phonology and receptive vocabulary are similar to nonabused children. Typically, these children have reading and auditory comprehension problems, limited expressive vocabulary, and shorter, less complex utterances. Language delay and disorders are most apparent in the pragmatic category. Abused and neglected children tend to have poor conversational skills, the inability to discuss feelings, shorter conversations, and fewer descriptive utterances. Language is used primarily to meet immediate wants and needs; there is little social and affective use of language. Parents who are intellectually limited, emotionally disturbed, or depressed may understimulate their children (Haynes & Shulman, 1998). Neglected and abused children are tragic examples of the detrimental effects that lack of love and stimulation have on normal language development.

Does poverty lead to environmental depravation and delayed and disordered language in children reared in those homes? Not necessarily. Many poverty-ridden homes are rich in love, environmental stimulation, and communication. Unfortunately, *extreme* poverty is associated with a lack of optimal language learning, especially in the early years. Hart and Risley (1995) found substantial variation in language stimulation and learning in young children from low socioeconomic levels when compared to those reared in families with more education and higher income levels. Parents in professional families used more words and utterances per hour and were generally more encouraging than were families on welfare. These and other actions and inactions by lower socioeconomic families were strongly linked to lower early vocabulary growth and subsequent school performance. Malnutrition and dental, vision, hearing, and other health factors also contribute to suboptimal conditions for language development in poverty homes. (In *Sling Blade*, isolation and confinement to a shed contributed to Karl's lack of mental development.)

Some children who are deprived of meaningful verbal interaction from parents and peers develop idioglossia. Idioglossia is a unique language, one that is clearly not identifiable with an existing one. *Idioglossia* was the title of the play on which the movie *Nell* was based. *Nell's* lack of normal cognitive and language development was because of her mother's stroke-related speech disorder and her complete isolation from other children and adults in the Smokey Mountains. In addition to being severely delayed in cognitive, linguistic, and social–communication functioning, Nell had developed her own language. It was meaningful to her, but not to others.

Idioglossia is sometimes called "twin speech" because twins sometimes develop their own language. This is more likely if they have grown up together with little interaction with other children (see Box 5.4). Idioglossia is a natural occurrence when children, who do not necessarily need to be twins, have little exposure to others and thus no model for language of their community.

Learning Disabilities

Learning disabilities are a heterogeneous group of disorders that are thought to be a result of a central nervous system dysfunction. According to Miniutti (1991), 15% of the children with learning disabilities have motor learning and coordination problems, and more than 75% have difficulty learning and using symbols. According to Wiig and Secord (1998), the *language disorder syndrome* is the most common type of learning disability. Nicolosi et al. (1996)

BOX 5.4 • *A Case of Idioglossia*

Two Navajo children moved to a small town and were enrolled in a Head Start program. They were very close in age to each other. They had spent most of their lives under the supervision of their maternal grandmother in a very remote region of the Navajo Indian Reservation in northern Arizona. The first years of their lives were spent tending to sheep and interacting exclusively with each other. The grandmother was quiet and rarely engaged in communication with the children. When they enrolled in Head Start, they were given comprehensive speech and language evaluations. The results showed that they had developed their own language, one that was quite advanced. Their utterances were lengthy and had complex grammar. They stood out in the Head Start classroom when they would ask questions, engage in dialogue, and play games with each other using this unique language. They were provided with intensive speech and language therapy and discouraged from using their language. Ultimately, they were separated at school. One was enrolled in the morning Head Start session, and the other in the afternoon. This was necessary because they refused to interact with other children when they were together in the same classroom. Over time, the idioglossia faded and the children acquired the language spoken in their new home. For these children, therapy was much like teaching English as a second language.

report that learning disabilities are all-encompassing diagnoses that include children who have perceptual handicaps, brain injury, minimal brain dysfunction, dyslexia, and developmental aphasia. It does not include children who are mentally deficient or have problems with vision or hearing. Speech–language pathologists who work in special education classes and resource rooms usually see children with language disorder syndrome. Although they may see them only for their communication disorder, children with learning disabilities are often treated by a team of educational professionals.

Attentional deficit disorder with or without hyperactivity (ADD/ADHD) syndromes are commonly diagnosed neurobehavioral disorders (Wiig & Secord, 1998). Children with ADHD appear to be constantly in motion and seem to have an endless amount of energy. Of course, many children are active, full of energy, and seem to be constantly in motion. However, only 5% of all children meet the criteria for hyperactivity, and it occurs 9 times more often in boys than it does in girls (Sattler, 1988). Children classified with ADHD tend to be impulsive, distractible, talkative, and constantly moving their hands and feet (see Box 5.5). They have short attention spans, although sometimes they appear to compulsively engage in certain motor acts. According to Hayes and Shulman (1998), children with ADHD have *metacognitive deficits.* These problems in "thinking about thinking" affect their social and academic behaviors. They lack introspection and reflection. These children appear not to appreciate the causes and effects of certain actions, or they are impervious to them.

Dyslexia and dysgraphia are reading and writing disorders associated with language-learning impairments. **Dyslexia** is a reading disorder due to no known neurological, emotional, environmental, intellectual, or perceptual problem and results in reading comprehension and word-recognition abilities 2 years below age expected levels (Vellutino, 1979).

BOX 5.5 • *A Case of Attention Deficit Hyperactivity Disorder*

One child who had ADHD attended a stuttering camp. He had been on medication but was taken off it before coming to the camp. The result was an exacerbation of hyperactive symptoms, or a "slingshot effect." During the 8-day period, he created many problems for the staff and was disliked and avoided by the other campers. He would lose interest in the individual and group therapy activities. At times he appeared not to understand the rules of the social activities and therapies. He would rarely take turns during conversations and would interrupt the staff during counseling sessions. When working on tools to improve his fluency, he would be easily distracted by other campers or the sights and sounds of the camp. He was always fidgeting and squirming. It appeared that he could not contain his energy. Of the children who attended the camp, he made the least improvement in speech fluency because of his hyperactivity and almost complete inability to concentrate and attend to the task at hand.

Dyslexia is associated with poor phonological awareness and reduced listening comprehension (Catts, 1996). Dyslexic children have difficultly with letter reversals and inversions. For example, they may confuse *b* for *d* or *p* for *b* or completely draw a blank when trying to recognize the significance of a letter. Comprehension of even short written statements is often poor. **Dysgraphia** is a problem encompassing both the motor and symbolic aspects of writing. With this disorder, children have difficulty putting their thoughts on paper. Written thoughts are poorly expressed both in content and with the construction of letters. Dyslexic and dysgraphic children, however, often have normal or higher tested IQs. Both disorders, which often persist into adulthood, are problems with written symbols and reflect an underlying problem with language.

Dyslexia and dysgraphia are also seen in aphasia in adults (see Chapter 8). However, the specific learning disabilities of dyslexia and dysgraphia are not typical of the reading and writing problems occurring in patients with aphasia. In aphasia the graphic problems are part of the syndrome of language disorders as a direct result of the language centers of the brain being damaged. Although the reading and writing problems associated with language-learning impairments may be seen in other disabling conditions, they are not a direct result of them.

Literature and Media Stereotypes

Forrest Gump—a unique movie featuring a character with mental deficiency—removed many previous negative stereotypes attributed to people with delayed mental development. Forrest Gump, as portrayed by Tom Hanks, is a kind, thoughtful, and interesting person. The film characterizes his mental slowness as an advantage that helps him navigate through the complex, controversial, and difficult times of the 1960s and 1970s. The message of the movie is that success and happiness are found in viewing the world through the eyes of an "innocent," one not complicated by too much thinking about events. Forrest Gump is a lovable character with the needs, desires, and fears shared by most people. Most important, the movie plays on his abilities rather than his disabilities. Actor Chris Burke has also been in the forefront of showing the capabilities of people with mental deficiencies.

Unfortunately, *Sling Blade* has the effect of portraying mentally deficient people as dangerous and even capable of premeditated murder. This movie feeds the stereotype held by some people that mental illness and mental retardation are the same. Certainly, some mentally deficient people are homicidal, but they are the exception, not the rule. Karl Childers is a complex character whose homicidal tendencies are a result of abuse, neglect, desperation, and mental retardation. He shares some of the likable characteristics of Forrest Gump but has a destructive personality. In the final scenes of the movie, the audience believes that his murdering the abusive Doyle is an act of desperation. Because of his mental deficiency, Karl cannot find a better solution to the abuse. In his simplistic view of the world, the only option of stopping the cycle of abuse was murder. In the book *Of Mice and Men*, Lennie's retardation made him unable to appreciate his strength.

The films *Rain Man* and *Nell* deal effectively with severe language disorders and delay. Both Dustin Hoffman and Jodie Foster do remarkable jobs in portraying the language patterns of people with autism and idioglossia. Hoffman's portrayal of the autistic savant Raymond Babbitt, who is one of the most interesting characters to emerge in recent films, is accurate and compelling. Even today, people remark that someone has "gone Rain Man" when they become obsessed and compulsive. The chemistry and evolving relationship between the brothers is one of the best aspects of the film. The brotherly relationship between Gilbert Grape and his brother Arnie is also an endearing aspect of the film *What's Eating Gilbert Grape*. The role that language plays in connecting with the world is a primary theme of the movie *Nell*.

One of the most pervasive myths screenwriters propagate about mental deficiency is the way they unrealistically portray the speech and language patterns of people with severe mental retardation. Frequently, the audience knows the person is retarded only by her slow speech. The character may have an IQ of only 60, but she will have long, complex utterances with sophisticated grammar, syntax, and phonology. Her ability to abstract, solve complex problems, and relate to the world is often normal, even advanced. Certainly, some mentally deficient people are capable of sophisticated language, albeit with slow speech. However, most people with significant mental deficiency have reduced form and function of language. Conversely, some people with slow speech may be superior in intelligence, as was the case of Stephen Hawking, during the early course of his amyotrophic lateral sclerosis. The use of speech rate as the only indication of mental retardation is often inaccurate and replete with inaccurate stereotypes.

Severe language delay and disorders can render a person unable to communicate about people and things, but these communication disorders can also muzzle the human spirit. This places a special responsibility on the shoulders of those who write about them, Authors—be they academics, novelists, playwrights, essayists, journalists, or dramatists—have a special accountability. They must portray these people accurately and compassionately and, in doing so, emphasize their abilities, tenacity, courage, mettle, and resolution of being. Whether the story revolves around the brotherly love between Gilbert and Arnie Grape, the emotional isolation of the Rain Man, Karl Childers' desperate homicidal tendencies, Lennie Small's dangerous physical strength, or the glowing optimism and innocence of Forrest Gump, writers must grant eloquence of expression to those incapable of it. John Steinbeck,[*] in his Nobel Prize for Literature acceptance speech, commented about the role of the writer with regard to the human spirit:

> Literature is as old as speech. It grew out of human need for it and it has not changed except to become more needed. The skalds, the bards, the writers are not separate and exclusive. From the beginning, their functions, their duties, their responsibilities have been decreed by our species . . . the writer is delegated to declare and to celebrate man's proven capacity for greatness of heart and spirit—for gallantry in defeat, for courage, compassion and love. In the endless war against weakness and despair, these are the bright rally flags of hope and of emulation. I hold that a writer who does not passionately believe in the perfectibility of man has no dedication nor any membership in literature.

Summary

Language is a difficult concept to define, and several factors are necessary to any definition of the word. The board game of chess provides an example of the difference between language performance and competence. There are three systems to evaluating and treating language delay and disorders in children: cognitive, linguistic, and social–communication. Parents and teachers play important roles in the evaluation and treatment process. Major causes of language delay and disorders in children include mental deficiency, autism, environmental depravation, and learning disabilities. Literature and media, which often promote commonly held myths, are powerful forces influencing public opinion about these disorders.

Study Questions

1. List and discuss the necessary aspects to any definition of language.

2. Compare and contrast the evolutionary and creationist view of language.

3. What is the *language–thought controversy?*

4. Discuss linguistic performance and competence.

5. What is the normativist approach to language delay and disorders?

6. How does *babbling* differ from *cooing?*

7. Discuss cognitive, linguistic, and social–communication functioning in preschool children.

8. What is *validity, reliability,* and *bias* with regard to intelligence testing?

9. What aspects must go into classifying a person as mentally deficient?

10. Discuss the features that lead to a diagnosis of pervasive developmental disorder.

11. What is *idioglossia?*

[*]For more about John Steinbeck, check out his biography on the World Wide Web: http://www.steinbeck.org

12. What are some inaccurate ways that literature and media characterize people who are mentally deficient?

13. List common characteristics of children who have a pragmatic language disorder.

Suggested Reading

Stothard, S., Snowling, M., Bishop, D. V. M., Chipchase, B. B., & Kaplan, C. A. (1998). Language-impaired preschoolers: A follow-up into adolescence. *Journal of Speech, Language, and Hearing Research, 41*: 407–418. This article reports a longitudinal study of adolescents with a preschool history of speech–language impairments and provides valuable information about determining prognoses.

Ward, S. (1998). An investigation into the effectiveness of an early intervention method for delayed language development in young children. *International Journal of Language and Communication Disorders, 34*(3): 243–264. This study, conducted in England, shows the importance of early intervention in treating young children who have language disorders and delay.

6

Hearing Loss and Deafness

Chapter Preview

In this chapter, you will learn about the sense of hearing and the professionals involved in the study and treatment of hearing, hearing loss, and deafness. The range of human hearing will be explored, and you will discover the evolutionary basis to it. Hearing is a process of energy transformation, and you will learn the acoustic, mechanical, hydraulic, and electrochemical aspects to it. Several types and causes of hearing loss are discussed in this chapter. You will understand how to test for them and many of the treatments and therapies available to help the deaf and hard-of-hearing. You will explore the age-old philosophical question: If a tree falls in the forest and there is no one there to hear it fall, does it make sound? Finally, you will learn how some people take pride in their deafness and the social implications of this cultural movement.

Birds chirping
A screaming siren
The "lub-dub" of a beating heart
A baby's laugh
Whispered terms of endearment
Coffee percolating
Directions on how to get from here to there
A Mozart waltz

People with normal hearing often take for granted the sounds of the world. Hearing, like other aspects of our health, is only sorely missed when lost. We are born into a world of sound, live our lives surrounded by it, and sometimes feel bombarded by it. The sounds of speech need to be heard if we are ever naturally able to speak them. Hearing provides us with a constant contact with reality. Even while sleeping, the ears are alert to environmental sounds, ever vigilant to danger. Our sense of hearing jars us from the sleepy netherworld, immediately enabling us to respond to the shriek of a child or a subtle scratching at a door. We are so accustomed to being awash in sound that absolute quiet can be distressing. The

Literature, Media, and Personality Profiles

Children of a Lesser God

Released in 1985 and directed by Randa Haines, *Children of a Lesser God* is a love story and was nominated for five Academy Awards. It stars William Hurt as an unconventional speech teacher at a school for the deaf. He manages to motivate and inspire his students but cannot connect with Sarah Norman (Marlee Matlin), who—although graduating with honors from the school—is cynical, bitter, distant, and works at a menial job. Hurt's character, James Leeds, has unconventional ways of reaching his students that are frowned upon by the administration. Predictably, Leeds falls in love with Norman. *Children of a Lesser God* provides a glimpse into the complexities of young love compounded by deafness. Audiences love *Children of a Lesser God* because of the chemistry between Hurt and Matlin, the use of sign language, and speech reading. It is a wonderful, intimate window into the world of the deaf. In real life Matlin's hearing is limited to 20% in her left ear (with amplification provided by a hearing aid). She can read lips, sign, and speak. Matlin received the Academy Award for Best Actress in *Children of a Lesser God*.

Arnold Palmer

Arnold Daniel Palmer, born on September 10, 1929, in Latrobe, Pennsylvania, first started golfing when he was 4 years old. He won the first of five West Pennsylvania Amateur Championships when he was only 17. He went on to become a leading collegiate player and turned professional in 1954, winning 60 PGA Tour victories. Palmer is director or owner of several golf organizations and businesses and is also a major stockholder of ProGroup, Inc., a sporting goods company that manufactures and markets golf equipment, which bears his name. He has received many honors and golfing awards. He is also a pilot and holds one aviation record. Arnold Palmer has a moderate hearing loss, which hearing aids partially correct.

Heather Whitestone McCallum

In 1995 Heather Whitestone McCallum became the first Miss America in history with a disability: deafness. Born in Dothan, Alabama, in April 1973, she was 18 months old when she lost her hearing because of a reaction to medication. She is totally deaf in her right ear and profoundly deaf in the other one. She learned to speak through the educational program Acoupedics, a type of aural rehabilitation. A deeply religious person, McCallum considers her relationship with God to be the most important aspect of her life. She attributes her faith in God to giving her the strength to fulfill her dream. Her beauty and grace, despite her deafness, provide a role model for many young women.

The Heart Is a Lonely Hunter

Carson McCuller's first novel, *The Heart Is a Lonely Hunter*, is about four people who confess secrets to a deaf and mute person in a small southern town before World War II. The book explores the plight of the emotionally and physically disabled, the status of Blacks, and the angst of young people during that period. The characters include a suicidal deaf person who is unable to speak, an alcoholic, and a black physician. McCuller wrote *The Heart Is a Lonely Hunter* when she was just 23 years old, and it was first published in 1940. It is available from Bantam Books.

The film by the same title was released in 1968. It was directed by Robert Ellis Miller and stars Stacy Keach (see Chapter 3), Cicely Tyson, Alan Arkin, and Sondra Locke. The film carefully follows the book in both plot and character development. It realistically depicts the loneliness and alienation of the characters. *The Heart Is a Lonely Hunter* was nominated for two Academy Awards.

Nanette Fabray

Although four operations and hearing aids have restored Nanette Fabray's ability to hear, she continues to be an advocate for the rights of people with disabilities. A tireless actor, comedian, singer, and dancer, she has had a hearing disorder for most of her life. Fabray, who has been called a "joyful humanitarian," is the recipient of the President's Distinguished Service Award for her international leadership in advocating for the disabled.

Fabray has received two Donaldson Awards for the Broadway musical *High Button Shoes* and has won a Tony and three Emmy Awards. She regularly appeared on the television comedy *Coach*. She has done many radio, newspaper, and television interviews, informing the public of the needs of the disabled. She has been the commencement speaker at Gallaudet University.

Leslie Nielsen

Leslie Nielsen, who has a hearing loss and wears hearing aids, is well known as the star of *The Naked Gun* movies. He also has had memorable film roles in *Peyton Place, Dracula . . . Dead and Loving It, Spy Hard,* and *Airplane!* He has been in more than 50 movies and many television shows including the crime series spoof *Police Squad*. Born on February 11, 1926, in Regina, Saskatchewan, he was raised in the Yukon. Nielsen studied at the Academy of Radio Arts in Toronto and then moved to New York City.

Florence Henderson

The perennial mom of the television series *The Brady Bunch*, Florence Henderson's hearing was restored with corrective surgery for a disorder known as otosclerosis, a hardening of the structures in the middle ear. Born on February 14, 1934, in Dale, Indiana, Henderson has appeared in *Naked Gun $33\frac{1}{3}$; Holy Man; Little Women; The Tonight Show; Roseanne; Murder, She Wrote; Hart to Hart;* and *The Muppet Show*—to name a few. She has starred, of course, in *The Brady Bunch* reunion shows, including the *Brady Bunch Movie, A Very Brady Christmas, The Brady Brides,* and *The Brady Girls Get Married*. Henderson is a tireless actor and media personality.

Rush Limbaugh

Rush Limbaugh had the largest audience of any radio show in the early 1990s. The ultraconservative talk-show host is known for his inflammatory diatribes against liberals, feminists, and Democrats. He has approximately 20 million listeners weekly. His audience includes "ditto-heads" who agree with any statement made by the occasionally portly talk-show host. In 1991 *The Rush Limbaugh Show*, a television program with the same ultraconservative theme, was released. It was produced between 1992 and 1996.

In October 2001, Time.com announced, "The mouth that roared has lost its ears." Initially, Rush Limbaugh was totally deaf in his left ear and could only "recognize" sound in his right one. According to Time.com, Limbaugh suffers from autoimmune inner-ear disease. In this possibly genetic disorder, the body's own immune system attacks the normal, healthy tissue of the inner ear. Effective treatments for this sensorineural hearing loss

(continued)

Literature, Media, and Personality Profiles (continued)

include steroid therapy and surgical implants. He has since had a cochlear implant with good results. Limbaugh jokingly has noted that the cloud of deafness had a silver lining: He no longer had to listen to the liberal media's nonsense.

The Miracle Worker
The Miracle Worker, released in 1962 and directed by Arthur Penn, stars Anne Bancroft, Patty Duke, and Victor Jory. The film, based on the Broadway stage play, was nominated for five Academy Awards; Anne Bancroft won an Academy Award for Best Actress, and Patty Duke won an Academy Award for Best Supporting Actress.

   The story is about the life of Helen Keller. Scarlet fever left her blind, deaf, and mute at a young age. Frustrated at her disabilities, she would have uncontrollable rages that frightened her family. With the help of her devoted and persistent teacher, Anne Mansfield Sullivan, Keller gradually learned sign language and how to connect with the world. *The Miracle Worker* is a captivating study of patience, love, and support, and the miracle that is communication.

complete absence of sound is like something comforting has been taken from us. Sound informs, alerts, irritates, and calms the beast within. Sound is the vibration of the world, the perception of its energy. Hearing, from the external ear to the centers of the brain responsible for perception and interpretation of sound, is a marvelous sense. People deprived of sound from birth and those who have lost it later in life are tributes to human adaptation. From speech reading to sign language, the deaf and hard-of-hearing embody the human ability to adapt to a silent world.

The Study and Treatment of Hearing Disorders

Several professions are involved in the study and treatment of the ear, hearing loss, and deafness. Three medical specialities are involved with hearing. **Otology** is a medical specialty limited to the diagnosis and treatment of ear disorders. **Otolaryngology** is a specialty in diseases and disorders of both the ear and throat. **Otorhinolaryngology** is a specialty in the diagnosis and treatment of disorders and diseases of the ear, nose, and throat; it is also called an ENT (ear, nose, and throat) specialty.

   In the education professions, **teachers of the hearing impaired** educate deaf and hard-of-hearing people. They have extensive training in methods of teaching the deaf and hard-of-hearing, as well as individuals with multiple disabilities. They are often special education teachers who have completed course work related to educating hearing-impaired students. Teachers of the hearing impaired usually have their own classrooms or teach at special schools.

   Audiology is involved in the assessment and nonmedical treatment of people with hearing disorders. Audiology got its start as an independent clinical discipline at the close of

World War II (Martin, 1997). Trained to evaluate the nature and identify the type of hearing loss, audiologists use sophisticated and sensitive instruments that can locate the site of injury or type of disease causing the hearing loss or deafness. They also engage in aural rehabilitation, which helps improve a person's ability to communicate. Audiology specialities include pediatric, medical, rehabilitative/dispensing, educational, and industrial (Bess & Humes, 1995).

Speech–language pathologists also work with the deaf and hard-of-hearing. As a member of the special education team, the speech–language pathologist helps the deaf and hard-of-hearing learn to make speech sounds. Visual, tactile (touch), and auditory feedback is used to help the student learn new sounds and to make existing sounds clearly. The speech–language pathologist also works on language development and other aspects of communication.

Table 6.1 shows the professionals and their responsibilities in evaluating and treating people with hearing disorders.

The Range of Human Hearing

Hearing is a highly evolved sense that grew out of a survival need. For humans the frequency range of hearing is between 20 and 20,000 cycles/second (Box 6.1). Cycles/second is also referred to as **hertz** (Hz). Frequency of vibration is perceived as **pitch.** As the frequency of vibration increases, so does the psychological perception of pitch. Frequencies below 20 Hz are perceived as vibration, and those above 20,000 Hz are **ultrasonic;** they are above the human range of hearing. Dogs and cats, for example, can perceive frequencies higher than humans can. Speech is composed of energy principally below 4000 Hz. Most of the energy of

TABLE 6.1 *Professionals and their Responsibilities in Evaluating and Treating People with Hearing Disorders*

Professional	Responsibility
Audiologist	Specialist who assesses and provides nonmedical treatment of hearing disorders
Otolaryngologist	Physician who specializes in diseases and disorders of the ear and throat
Otologist	Physician whose practice is limited to the ear
Otorhinolaryngologist (ENT)	Physician who diagnoses and treats disorders and diseases of the ear, nose, and throat
Speech–language pathologist	Specialist who helps the deaf and hard-of-hearing learn speech and language
Teacher of the hearing impaired	Specialist who educates deaf and hard-of-hearing people

BOX 6.1 • *Evolutionary Basis to Hearing*

The frequency range of human hearing is a result of millions of years of evolution. The 20–20,000-Hz range has evolved because those frequencies were important to the survival of animals of our size. Being able to hear those frequencies alerted prehistoric humans to danger and permitted them to hunt small animals successfully. The range of human hearing also evolved because it is important to understanding speech, which itself played an important survival function.

speech is around 2000 Hz. Some speech sounds, such as /s/, /z/, and "th," are high-frequency sounds that are in contrast to lower-frequency sounds having lower bands of energy.

The psychological perception of the force of vibration is **loudness.** As the amplitude, or intensity, at which matter is displaced increases, so does loudness. As the force of the molecular displacement increases, the individual has a subsequent increase in the perception of loudness. Loudness is measured in **decibels.** The abbreviation for decibel is dB and literally means one-tenth of a **bel,** which is a unit of sound. (The *B* in dB is capitalized in reference to Alexander Graham Bell for his contributions to the study of sound and hearing.) Very soft sounds, such as breathing, are about 10 dB of loudness. Extremely loud sounds, about 140–160 dB, are the noises produced by jet airplanes at takeoff and chain saws. A rock 'n roll band in a dance club produces a typical loudness level of 120 dB (Durrant & Lovrinic, 1995). As discussed later in this chapter, exposure to loud noise can cause irreparable damage to hearing.

Hearing and Energy Transformation

There are many ways of exploring the human hearing mechanism. One of the most interesting ways to look at hearing is as the process of energy transformation. Sound begins as molecular vibration in air, acoustic energy, and is transformed into mechanical energy by the eardrum and bones of the middle ear. At the cochlea the vibration becomes hydraulic energy and, finally, electrochemical energy in the nervous system and brain. Hearing is disrupted when there is a breakdown at any stage of energy transformation.

Acoustic Energy Stage

Sound requires vibration of a medium. The medium can be any substance capable of vibration at a sufficient frequency and intensity to be detected by a hearing mechanism. Although a person can detect sound by placing an ear to a railroad track, for example, air is the most efficient medium. Air is extremely elastic. It can be distorted and easily return to its original shape. Billions and billions of air molecules surround us and are in contact with the eardrum.

A good way of understanding acoustic energy transmission is to compare it with waves in a pond of water. If a pebble is dropped into a calm pond, it disrupts the water with a splash.

Waves of water are sent away from the point of impact. One wave rises and falls, another does the same, and this continues until a wave laps the shore. The first wave impacts the next wave, the next wave contacts another one, and so on, until there are many waves lapping on the shore. What is transmitted though the water is energy in the form of water ripples. It is important to remember that the first mass of water, the one closest to the pebble, does not actually reach the shore. It moves a short distance from the pebble and goes back and forth. It is energy that is transmitted from the pebble that finally reaches the shore.

A similar form of energy transmission occurs when an individual claps his hands in a quiet room. Energy is displaced outwardly from the point of impact. The mass of air molecules closest to the hands impacts another mass of air molecules, that impacts another, and so on, until acoustic energy is transmitted to a listener's ears. This impact and bouncing back of masses of air molecules are called compressions and rarefactions. The compression stage occurs when air molecules are compressed from their resting position. **Rarefaction** occurs when distance decreases from their neutral, or resting, position. The mass of molecules in the room compresses and rarefacts until energy is transmitted to the listener. During the compression stage, pressure increases because air molecules are more densely compacted. The air pressure is lower during the rarefaction stage because the molecules are farther apart from their resting, or neutral, position. Sound moves as a wave on progressive points of compression of the air molecules. Sound waves are high- and low-pressure changes traveling though the medium of air. Figure 6.1 shows molecules of air compression, rarefaction, and subsequent high- and low-pressure changes.

The mass of air molecules vibrate at a certain frequency and intensity. The frequency of vibration is the number of pressure changes, or compressions and rarefactions, that occur in a period of time, usually 1 second. The intensity, or amplitude, of vibration is how much force is applied. The movement of the mass of molecules, their frequency and intensity, corresponds to the vibrations occurring at the source. They vibrate at a frequency and intensity that coincide to the source of the molecular displacement. Energy is displaced throughout the room. Although the preceding example is a hand clap in a quite room, the source of the acoustic energy can be a snapped finger, a dropped pencil, or two lips producing a bilabial speech sound. Acoustic energy is the first stage in the process of energy transmission that leads to hearing. At this level, sound is acoustic energy. See Box 6.2 for a philosophical discussion of sound energy.

Mechanical Energy Stage

The acoustic energy of the vibrating air molecules is transformed into mechanical energy at the middle ear. The middle ear is the space between the **tympanic membrane** (eardrum) and the cochlea is about the size of an aspirin (Figure 6.2). The **external ear** (pinna or auricle) channels the acoustic energy in the medium of air to the middle ear. In humans the external ear is the least functional hearing structure (see Box 6.3). In other animals, independent movement of the external ear structures helps localize sound. (For example, a horse has the ability to independently move its ears. One ear can be directed to the front, while the other is directed to the side or back. This independent movement of the ear helps the animal localize sound.) The ear canal is a cylindrical S-shaped passageway about $\frac{1}{2}$ inch in length. The tym-

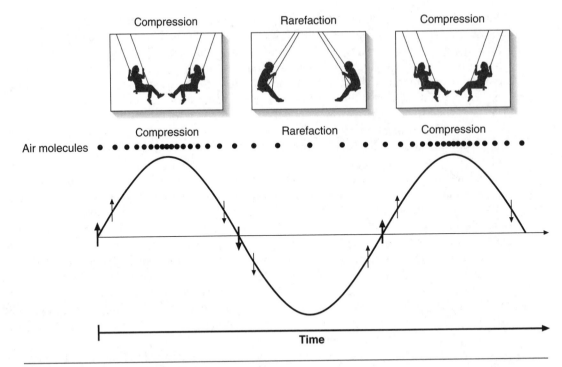

FIGURE 6.1   *Energy Transmission*

Source: W. Perkins & R. Kent, *Functional Anatomy of Speech, Language, and Hearing.* Copyright 1986. Reprinted by permission by Allyn & Bacon.

panic membrane, which is in direct contact with the atmosphere, vibrates in concert with the air molecules, thus transforming acoustic into mechanical energy.

Attached to the tympanic membrane are the three smallest bones in the human body: the **ossicles.** The ossicles—the **malleus, incus,** and **stapes**—are also known as the hammer, anvil, and stirrup; they get their names because of their shapes. The malleus is attached to the tympanic membrane, and the incus is connected to the malleus. The stirrup, in contact with the incus, is also connected to the oval window at the opening of the inner ear. Because the ossicles are connected to the tympanic membrane, they too vibrate at a frequency and intensity that correspond to the molecular vibrations.

Because people go from regions of high pressure to areas of lower pressure, and vice versa, pressure in the middle ear must be equalized to that of the outside atmosphere. When this happens, there is the sensation of the ears "popping" (see Box 6.4). This is due to the tympanic membrane being slightly pushed out or pulled in because of the pressure equalization. The eustachian tube makes this equalization of pressure possible. Simply put, the **eustachian tube** is a duct, or passage, between the middle ear and the back of the throat (*nasopharynx*). The eustachian tube also allows drainage of the fluids from the middle ear when a person has a head cold or other illness. To help the equalization of pressure, a person can yawn, chew gum, or swallow; these activities help open the eustachian tube.

BOX 6.2 • *If a Tree Falls in the Forest . . .*

Professors of philosophy often ask their students abstract questions to stimulate thought and to ponder the complexities of the universe. Philosophical questions such as "How many angels can dance on the head of a pin?" and "Can God create a rock he cannot lift?" and "What is the sound of one hand clapping?" are asked to get students to think about the limits of language and the constraints of traditional thought. "If a tree falls in the forest and there is no one there to hear it fall, does it make sound?" is a question often asked in philosophy courses to explore the nature of life perceptions and experiences.

Common sense tells us that a tree falling in a forest would make a whooshing sound as it falls through the air, and there will be snapping and cracking sounds as its branches break. A thud would happen when the full weight of the tree trunk hits the ground. These sounds would happen no matter whether human, bird, or animal ears were there to hear it fall. Although common sense suggests that the falling tree makes sound, the philosophical implications are much greater.

The human ear can detect frequencies of vibration between 20 and 20,000 Hz, and these vibrations must be of a sufficient intensity to be registered as sound. That is the hearing range of the human ear. Frequencies of vibration below 20 Hz and those above 20,000 Hz are beyond the range most human ears. When the tree falls in the forest, the whoosh, snapping, cracking, and thud sounds that are heard only consist of the intensities and frequencies allowed by the human ear. To other animals, the sound of the falling tree is different. It may contain higher or lower pitches and sound quieter or louder in some of the frequencies. It depends on their hearing range and sensitivity.

If the forest were void of humans, birds, and animals, would sound be created? The tree would certainly disrupt air molecules as it falls and hits the ground. The falling tree would create acoustic energy. Nevertheless, because there is no tympanic membrane, ossicular chain, cochlea, cranial nerve VIII, and auditory cortex to transform molecular disruptions into electrochemical energy, there will be no subjective experience of sound; there is only the *potential* for sound. Of course, there is the obvious philosophical issue of how different conscious entities perceive the universe, and even if it would exist if there were no one to perceive it. This age-old philosophical query is used to prompt exploration of these types of debatable issues. However, from a scientific perspective, the tree actually does not produce sound when it falls in the absence of a hearing mechanism. All that is produced is acoustic energy with the potential of being perceived as sound.

Hydraulic Energy Stage

Hydraulic energy is transmitted through a fluid medium. (This type of energy is how the brake system on an automobile works. Pressure changes in the brake fluid cause the brake shoes to stop the car.) Sound transformation from mechanical to hydraulic energy occurs at the cochlea. The **cochlea,** the end organ of hearing, is a snail-shaped structure about the size of a pea (Figure 6.3). The cochlea also contains the semicircular canals, which are responsible for the ability to maintain balance. The fluids in the inner ear are called endolymph and perilymph (Durrant & Lovrinic, 1995). A convenient way of remembering the function of the cochlea is to compare it to the eyes: *The eyes are to vision as the cochlea is to hearing.*

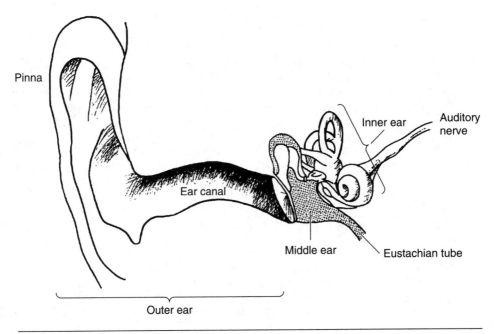

FIGURE 6.2 *The Human Ear*

Source: W. Perkins & R. Kent, *Functional Anatomy of Speech, Language, and Hearing*. Copyright 1986. Reprinted by permission by Allyn & Bacon.

The sensory part of the cochlea is the **organ of Corti.** It plays an important part in the sensation of hearing because it contains the hair-cell nerve endings that move and vibrate. It is believed that different pitches are produced through stimulation of nerve endings at different areas of the cochlea. Low frequencies are detected in the higher ends of the cochlea, and higher frequencies are received in the areas closest to the stapes. The fluid in the cochlea is

BOX 6.3 • *Sound Localization*

Even though the external ear is the least functional hearing structure, humans have excellent abilities to tell the direction of a sound. You can test this ability with a friend. Have your friend stand approximately 30 feet away from you in an unused classroom. Instruct your friend to move quietly to different parts of the classroom and clap his or her hands while your eyes are closed. Then point to the direction from which you believe the sound is coming. Even with your eyes tightly closed, you can tell the direction of the hand clap. When you open them, you can see the accuracy of your directional hearing. This phenomenon occurs primarily because the sound is louder in one ear than the other. If you put an earplug in one of your ears and do the same exercise, you will see that localizing the hand clap is more difficult.

BOX 6.4 • *Pressure Changes*

Individual coffee creamers provide illustrations of the effects of pressure changes on closed containers. Some brands of coffee creamers are produced in the United States at places low in elevation or at sea level. Then they are shipped to higher elevations. When they get to cities with higher elevations such as Denver, Albuquerque, Reno, Salt Lake City, or Flagstaff, the air pressure will be much greater in the containers than the atmospheric pressure. As a result, the top of the creamer will bulge outwardly, and air will escape when it is opened. This phenomenon can also be observed with ice cream containers.

set into motion by the movement of the tympanic membrane and ossicles, which themselves are vibrating in concert with air molecules. The function of the cochlea is not completely understood by speech and hearing scientists and is part of the theory of audition. At this stage of the process of hearing, sound is hydraulic energy.

Most people, when hearing their voices on a tape recorder, remark that they "don't sound like themselves." Speech heard on a tape recorder sounds foreign and different from what we are accustomed to. This is true even when the tape recorder has little distortion and accurately records the speech signal. The primary reason for this difference is due to bone

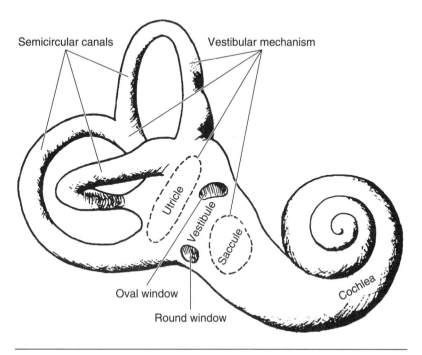

FIGURE 6.3 *The Human Cochlea*

Source: W. Perkins & R. Kent, *Functional Anatomy of Speech, Language, and Hearing.* Copyright 1986. Reprinted by permission by Allyn & Bacon.

conduction. **Bone conduction** is the transmission of sound to the inner ear via the vibrations of the bones of the skull. When speaking, a person gets feedback from both air and bone conduction. However, when listening to a taped recording of her speech, the person hears only through air conduction and does not receive bone-conduction feedback.

Electrochemical (Neural) Energy Stage

The movements of the inner-ear fluid stimulate the nerve endings in the cochlea. When the movements reach a certain threshold, the sensory information is transformed to its final form: electrochemical, or neural, energy. These impulses are sent to an area of the brain called the **auditory cortex** via cranial nerve VIII.

Humans have spinal and cranial nerves. Thirty-one pairs of spinal nerves enter and exit the spinal column. The **cranial nerves,** which are above the spinal nerves, are important for vision, hearing, and other senses. There are pairs of cranial nerves, one for each side of the body. Cranial nerve VIII is also called the *auditory–vestibular nerve* because it carries information about hearing and balance to the brain. The cranial nerve VIII enters the **brainstem** at a structure called the *pons*. From the pons the information is sent to other structures of the brain that ultimately allow the perception and interpretation of sound. At the neural level, sound is electrochemical energy.

Auditory perception is an important aspect of this stage of hearing. As discussed in Chapter 4, auditory perception is the ability to attend to the salient, or important, aspects of hearing, while ignoring the rest. Humans learn to attend to those things that are important, the **signal,** and to ignore the unimportant, the **noise.** Not all information received through hearing is brought to a conscious level. Once the important aspects of the signal are perceived, the auditory signal is decoded in the auditory cortex of the brain. Sounds are associated with other information stored in the brain.

In summary, the process of hearing begins as acoustic vibration. A force sets air molecules in motion. They begin vibrating, or oscillating, and energy is projected outwardly from the source. The listener's tympanic membrane is in direct contact with air molecules, and it, as well as the ossicular chain, vibrates at a frequency and intensity that corresponds to the source. The fluid in the cochlea also vibrates in concert with the middle-ear structures, and neurological impulses that travel to the auditory cortex of the brain are set off. Sound is a process of energy transformation that begins as sound waves and then becomes mechanical, hydraulic, and electrochemical impulses. Any break in the chain of events can disrupt the process.

Hearing and Speech Acoustics

Before discussing different types of hearing disorders and their treatments, describing some of the important aspects of the **acoustics** of speech is first necessary. Hearing loss and its effects on the person's ability to communicate is fundamentally related to the acoustics of speech. The makeup of the speech signal directly affects which sounds will be heard and understood. In addition, it is necessary to know about speech acoustics to understand how amplification helps people detect and perceive the speech signal.

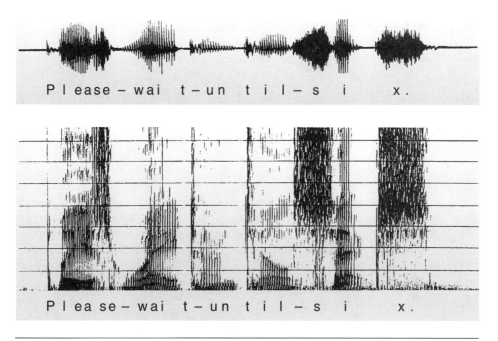

FIGURE 6.4 *Sound Spectrogram*

Source: W. Perkins & R. Kent, *Functional Anatomy of Speech, Language, and Hearing.* Copyright 1986. Reprinted by permission by Allyn & Bacon.

The sounds of speech are fleeting and intangible. We cannot point to a sound or other part of ongoing speech. Scientists and clinicians use graphic representations to see speech sounds. The speech sound wave can be represented in many ways, and one of the most informative pictures of speech is the sound spectrogram. Sometimes called a "voice print," the sound spectrogram is a graphic representation of speech and other sounds by time, frequency, and energy. As Figure 6.4 shows, the frequencies of the signal are represented as horizontal lines. Each vertical striation represents one opening and closing of the vocal cords. They occur regularly and appear different from sounds that are not voiced. Voiceless sounds are aperiodic and nonrhythmic repetitions as seen at the end of the spectrogram (above the x) in Figure 6.4. Figure 6.4 shows the time of the speech event along with the bottom of the spectrogram. The darkened bands on the spectrogram are called **formants,** and they represent high-energy areas of the speech signal. They are a result of **resonance,** which is the amplification of some aspects of the signal due to sympathetic or forced vibration of the air in the oral-tract cavities. Together, these and other aspects of **spectrography** provide a visual representation of speech.

Types of Hearing Loss

The three general categories of hearing loss are conductive, sensorineural, and central (Table 6.2). Some authorities further divide these categories into smaller subgroups, but for the

TABLE 6.2   *General Categories of Hearing Loss*

Category	Description
Conductive	Damage or impairment of the external or middle ear
Sensorineural	Damage or impairment of the cochlea and/or cranial nerve VIII
Central	Damage or impairment to the central auditory nervous system

purposes of this introductory book, these three general categories of hearing loss are examined. Conductive hearing loss occurs because sound energy is disrupted at the level of the external or middle ear. Sensorineural hearing loss occurs because of damage to the cochlea and/or cranial nerve VIII. When there is damage to the central auditory nervous system, the hearing loss is called a central auditory processing disorder.

Conductive Hearing Loss

Any defect, disorder, or disease that obstructs the energy transmission in the outer or middle ear can cause conductive hearing loss. Common outer-ear pathologies include impacted wax, foreign objects, and inflammatory diseases of the external ear canal.

Cerumen, the wax-like substance produced in the external auditory canal, protects the ear canal by capturing foreign bodies and preventing irritation. A gradual wax buildup in the external canal is normal and natural. The external canal, a self-cleaning mechanism, naturally cleans itself of excess wax. However, some people use swabs and other probes to remove the wax from the external ear canal for hygienic purposes. Unfortunately, sometimes this can compact the wax and create an obstruction. This obstruction disrupts the acoustic energy transmission and results in a conductive hearing loss. Commercially available solutions can be used to soften the impacted cerumen. However, having an otologist remove the impacted wax is sometimes necessary.

For decades, medical professionals have warned children: "Never put anything smaller than your elbow in your ear." Obviously, this means that they should put nothing in the external ear canal because of the damage that can occur. However, many children are sometimes tempted to place eraser heads, pebbles, beads, paper, raisins, corn, and other foreign bodies in their ear canals. These objects can damage the tympanic membrane, irritate the external canal, and create a conductive hearing loss. They can also become lodged and may need to be removed by an otologist.

Otitis is an **inflammation** of the ear. Inflammation of the external ear is called *otitis externus.* Inflammatory skin conditions can create an obstruction along the external canal. The inflammation can be so extensive as to block the energy transmission to the tympanic membrane. *Swimmer's ear* is an irritation in the external ear caused by frequent exposure to water and the chemicals found it. Swimmer's ear can also cause itching and scratching and the subsequent possibility of infection.

Middle-Ear Dysfunction and Conductive Hearing Loss. "The development of the middle ear must have been one of evolution's most splendid engineering feats. The middle ear carries sound vibrations from the outer ear to the inner ear by transferring the sound energy from the air in the outer ear to the fluids of the inner ear" (Martin, 1997, p. 233). Middle-ear disorders can include defects or diseases that disrupt the mechanical energy transmission to the cochlea. One of the most common causes of middle-ear dysfunctions is a rupture of the tympanic membrane, which can be ruptured by foreign objects that penetrate it, by sharp blows to the head, and by extremely loud noises. Usually, perforations of the tympanic membrane are small and heal on their own. However, repeated perforations or scarring of the tympanic membrane can reduce its movement and sensitivity.

Otitis media is an inflammation of the middle ear. When the eustachian tube does not function properly, there can be a buildup of pressure in the middle ear. With no way to equalize the pressure, the tympanic membrane can burst. Sometimes, a fluid buildup impedes the movement of the ossicular chain; this condition is called *serous otitis media.* Negative middle-ear pressure can also result from eustachian tube dysfunctions.

Sometimes, a patient must undergo a myringotomy. A **myringotomy** is a procedure in which a tube is placed in the tympanic membrane to allow drainage and equalization of pressure. This medical procedure is sometimes recommended for individuals, particularly children, who have chronic otitis media and significant conductive hearing losses. Controversy is ongoing about the medical necessity and benefit of myringotomies for children suffering from frequent ear infections. Some medical specialists believe they are helpful; others are convinced that they are unnecessary.

Otosclerosis is a disease that causes a disruption of mechanical energy in the middle ear. Otosclerosis produces a hardening of the bone affecting the middle-ear capsule, and this hardening impedes the movements of the ossicular chain. The cause of otosclerosis is not known, but there probably is a genetic predisposition to it. A surgical procedure known as a stapedectomy can be successful in treating the disorder. A *stapedectomy* is the removal of the stapes and replacement of it by a prosthetic device. (A stapedectomy was successful in helping actor Florence Henderson regain her hearing.)

Sensorineural Hearing Loss

Damage to the inner ear and/or the auditory nerve can cause **sensorineural hearing loss.** According to Martin (1997), the function of the inner ear is to transduce the mechanical energy in the middle ear into a form of energy that can be interpreted by the brain. Congenital defects, tumors, head traumas, syndromes, and diseases can damage the inner ear and auditory nerve. Certain drugs can also damage them. One of the most common causes of sensorineural hearing loss is prolonged exposure to loud noise. Farmers who spend long hours on noisy tractors, workers in loud factories, and musicians who play their music too loudly are at risk for sensorineural hearing loss (see Box 6.5). Even concert-goers and people who listen to loud music through headsets can harm their hearing due to excessive sound exposure.

Presbycusis and Meniere's disease are two conditions that can dramatically affect hearing. **Presbycusis,** the loss of hearing associated with old age, is the degeneration of the cochlea that occurs over time. More common today because people are living longer,

BOX 6.5 • *Hearing Education and Awareness for Rockers*

Hearing Education and Awareness for Rockers (HEAR) is a nonprofit organization dedicated to educating and increasing the awareness of noise exposure to musicians and music fans. It was formed by Kathy Peck, bass player for the San Francisco punk band The Contractions, and Flash Gordon, M.D., a San Francisco physician. It was established after Peck suffered hearing damage while playing at the Oakland Coliseum in the 1980s. Support for this organization has come from Lars Ulrich of Metallica, Ray Charles, Lee Ranaldo from Sonic Youth, and Les Claypool of Primus. Professional organizations and media businesses such as MTV, *Guitar Player* magazine, the American Speech-Language-Hearing Association, the American Academy of Otolaryngology, and the National Association of Music Manufacturers, to name a few, have also provided support for HEAR.

presbycusis is a gradual deterioration of the inner ear. Also the result of living in a noisy society, it is more common in industrialized countries.

Meniere's disease is caused by an increase of fluid pressure in the inner ear and is associated with vertigo and tinnitus. **Vertigo** is a dizziness and falling sensation. (*Vertigo* was also the title of a thriller film by Alfred Hitchcock.) Patients with Meniere's disease have difficulty maintaining balance while walking, standing, or even sitting. They are often nauseated because the balance centers are part of the inner ear. Surgeries and medications are used to treat Meniere's disease.

Tinnitus is often described as a high-pitched ringing in the ear. However, tinnitus can also include buzzing, humming, and other unwanted sounds. Martin (1997) lists other adjectives describing tinnitus: *crickets*, *roaring*, *hissing*, *clanging*, and *swishing*. Pete Townshend, of the rock group The Who, suffers from tinnitus. Townshend is also a contributor to Hearing Education and Awareness for Rockers (HEAR). He provided a $10,000 donation to help HEAR get started (see Box 6.5).

Central Auditory Processing Disorders

Central auditory processing disorders are known by several names: **central auditory defects, cortical deafness, pure-word deafness, auditory agnosia,** and **acoustic agnosia** are labels sometimes given to these disorders. Usually, hearing is normal for pure tones, but sounds are not recognized or perceived properly. In children, central auditory processing disorders are applied to those whose use and recognition of language is not age appropriate and/or is inconsistent with their intelligence (Martin, 1997).

Damage to the auditory cortex of the brain and the tracts leading to it can cause central auditory processing disorders. Strokes, tumors, head traumas, brainstem compressions, diseases, and developmental irregularities can cause a central auditory processing disorder. Unlike receptive aphasia, where the patient has difficulty processing and comprehending all avenues of language, central auditory dysfunctions are usually limited only to the auditory modality (see Chapter 7). These disorders are often considered a part of aphasia or agnosia.

Particularly in patients with severe aphasia, it is difficult to separately diagnose and treat central auditory processing disorders.

Hearing Assessment

The importance of early detection of hearing loss and deafness cannot be understated. In the film *Children of a Lesser God*, Sarah Norman's deafness was not discovered until she was 7 years old. Consequently, she was diagnosed as mentally retarded because of her lack of speech and language development. Sometimes, in real life, children who are deaf or hard-of-hearing are misdiagnosed as mentally deficient, but this misdiagnosis was more common in the past than it is today. Currently, many hospitals routinely screen newborns for hearing loss and deafness (Yellin, Culbertson, Tanner, & Adams, 2000). In November 1999, the U.S. Congress passed the Newborn Infant Hearing Screening and Intervention Act, which provides grants to develop infant hearing screening and intervention programs. This act should continue to improve methods of early detection of hearing loss and deafness in newborns.

About 50% of sensorineural hearing losses in children occur after the newborn period, requiring ongoing screening and evaluation services (Billings & Kenna, 1999). Children are screened for hearing disorders in schools, speech and hearing clinics, and pediatrician offices. A child who fails a screening is referred for comprehensive hearing testing conducted by an audiologist. Because hearing loss in the elderly usually develops slowly, many older persons do not get hearing tests and treatment at the first signs of the disorder. It is common for older persons to deny their hearing problems and attribute them to people mumbling or not talking loud enough. Many hearing aid dispensers, audiologists, and clinics offer free hearing screening for the elderly.

A screening hearing test is different from a comprehensive audiological evaluation. As noted in Chapter 4, the purpose of screening is to detect the presence of a problem. If a problem is detected, then the patient is referred for a comprehensive battery of tests. A **comprehensive hearing test** determines the type and severity of the hearing problem and includes treatment recommendations. Audiometric measurement can determine the degree of hearing loss, estimate the location of the lesion causing the problem, judge the extent of the disability produced by it, and help establish habilitative or rehabilitative objectives (Bess & Humes, 1995).

Otoscopic Examination

An **otoscope,** an instrument with a light source, is used for examining the external ear and tympanic membrane. After the otoscope's probe is placed in the individual's ear, the examiner looks for impacted wax, foreign bodies, and other defects or deviations of the ear canal. The tympanic membrane is also examined for ruptures and other irregularities.

Pure-Tone Audiometry

In **pure-tone** audiometry, various frequencies are tested at differing loudness levels to determine the patient's hearing thresholds. The *threshold* is the loudness levels necessary to hear a particular tone. The results of pure-tone audiometry are placed on an **audiogram,** which is a graphic chart used to record pure-tone air-conduction and bone-conduction thresholds. The patient's thresholds are shown by the minimum intensity level obtained at each tested frequency. On a typical audiogram, the frequencies are listed along the top of the chart and range between 125 and 8000 Hz. The loudness levels are shown down the sides of the audiogram and range from –10 to 120 dB. The tones are presented to the patient wearing earphones or sitting in a soundproof booth. The examiner marks the minimum decibel level for each tested frequency. For **air-conduction testing,** a red *O* indicates air-conduction responses in the right ear, and a blue *X* indicates the results in the left ear.

   Bone-conduction testing is conducted by placing a vibrating **oscillator** on the patient's **mastoid process,** a part of the skull behind the ear. By setting this bone into vibration, the inner ear is stimulated while bypassing the structures of the middle ear. **Masking,** the process of placing noise in the opposite ear being tested, is sometimes necessary to prevent the good ear from hearing the sounds being presented to the tested ear. When a patient hears better by bone conduction when compared to air conduction, he is said to have an **air–bone gap.** An air–bone gap suggests that the site of the hearing problem is in the external or middle ear (a conductive hearing loss) because the better bone-conduction thresholds are a result of bypassing the structures of the middle ear. Bone conduction testing is less common now due to technical advances in hearing testing.

   To obtain pure–tone thresholds, the tones are first presented at comfortable and easily detected loudness levels, and then the decibel levels are gradually decreased. When the patient does not indicate that she heard a particular sound, the loudness levels are increased and decreased in gradual steps until the threshold is learned. This step-by-step process systematically determines the lowest decibel level at which the patient can hear pure tones for each tested frequency. It is sometimes called the *ascending-descending method.* At the conclusion of pure-tone testing, there is a graphic representation of the patient's hearing thresholds for both ears.

Speech Audiometry

Speech audiometry is a method of testing hearing by adjusting loudness levels of the speech signals. The speech of the examiner can be used or stimuli can be presented from a tape recorder. A speech audiometry test is conduced in a soundproof booth. This type of audiological test can be delivered through earphones or through a sound field using a loudspeaker. "Using speech audiometers, audiologists set out to answer questions regarding patients' degree of hearing loss for speech; the levels required for their most comfortable and uncomfortable loudness levels; the range of comfortable loudness; and perhaps most important, their ability to recognize the sounds of speech" (Martin, 1997, p. 113). Current advances in technology have made this test, as well as other audiological tests, automated.

Acoustic Immittance Audiometry

Acoustic immittance audiometry automatically compares the acoustic energy flowing into and reflected out of the ear. Immittance is a combination of impedance, sound energy reflected from the tympanic membrane, and admittance, the energy that is admitted to the middle ear

(Gillam, Marquardt, & Martin, 2000). **Impedance** is the opposition to energy flow. **Acoustic immittance audiometry** measures that resistance in the middle ear and is used in detecting conductive hearing disorders. A handheld probe is placed against the ear, creating a seal between it and the tympanic membrane. Sound and air-pressure changes are used to measure the status of the middle ear. The objective of this test is to assess the energy reflected in the ear canal. If more energy is reflected, the tympanic membrane and/or the ossicular chain are less **compliant** (the state of flexibility and responsiveness of a structure) than normal, suggesting a problem at the mechanical energy stage of the hearing process.

Part of impedance audiometry testing is assessing the **acoustic reflex,** an involuntary, protective reaction. This reflex action is sometimes called the *stapedial reflex* and is the contraction of the stapedius and tensor tympani muscles in response to loud sounds. About 85 dB will produce the stapedial reflex in people who have normal hearing. Not only does acoustic reflex testing provide information about the middle ear, but in some instances, it can also provide information about the electrochemical stage of the hearing process.

Evoked Response Audiometry and Otoacoustic Emissions

Evoked response audiometry (ERA) is the assessment of the electrochemical energy stage of hearing. In this procedure, electrodes are placed on the patient's head, and electrochemical discharges associated with hearing certain sounds are recorded. Electrochemical discharges give important information about the cochlea, cranial nerve VIII, and brainstem. Evoked response audiometry can be helpful in determining the hearing abilities in infants and adults who cannot respond to traditional testing.

Otoacoustic emission testing (OAE) also helps determine the status of the cochlea, cranial nerve VIII, and brainstem structures. Otoacoustic emissions are echoed sounds created by the expansion and contraction of a normal cochlea and are used in newborn screening programs (Yellin et al., 2000). These sounds are detected by sensitive instruments and analyzed by a computer. This test is also helpful in determining whether a person is feigning a hearing loss or if it is caused by psychogenic factors.

Aural Habilitation and Rehabilitation

Aural habilitation is provided to individuals, primarily children, who have never developed speech and language skills because of their hearing disorder. In contrast, **aural rehabilitation** is given to individuals who have lost their hearing in later life after they have learned speech and language. The goals of both therapies are to help individuals improve their abilities to communicate by developing new skills and abilities and strengthening existing ones. Amplification, auditory training, speech reading, and manual communication are the primary therapies available (Table 6.3).

Most patients with hearing disorders benefit from amplification provided by hearing aids. For some patients, the amplification eliminates the communication disorder. For others, hearing aids help restore some of the ability to hear, but additional therapies are necessary to optimize communication. **Hearing aids** are simply small amplifiers, which work like microphones and amplifiers used at concerts. A hearing aid consists of a microphone that detects

TABLE 6.3   *Aural Habilitation and Rehabilitation*

Therapy	*Description*
Amplication	The use of small amplifiers that make the signal louder and direct it into the ear canal
Auditory training	A treatment that increases the general awareness of sound, including auditory discrimination abilities
Speech reading	The reading of lips, body, and facial gestures to comprehend speech
Manual communication	The use and understanding of sign language and finger spelling

sound, electronically amplifies it, and directs the louder signal into the ear canal. There are several styles of aids, including those worn behind the ear, in eyeglasses, on the body, or completely within the ear. Many hearing aids have special settings that help the listener adjust to different hearing environments. Digital technology has dramatically improved the quality and efficiency of hearing aids. For many, hearing aids significantly improve the sensation and perception of sound, sometimes for the first time. According to Martin (1997), there is considerable variability in the enthusiasm children display for amplification. Sometimes, the sudden presentation of sound can be frightening, and the ear mold, receiver, or cord can be confusing and annoying.

In **auditory training** the patient is taught to perceive new sounds that are provided by amplification and surgical and medical treatments. Auditory training is particularly important in children, and its goal is to increase general awareness of sounds and improve **auditory discrimination** abilities. Auditory discrimination therapies range from discrimination of gross environmental sounds to learning the ability to perceive small acoustic differences between similar sounds (see Chapter 4).

Speech reading is more than recognizing certain sounds by the way the lips create them or by "lip reading." In speech reading, body and facial gestures are also read to understand the speech of others. Even the best speech readers cannot understand 100% of what others are saying. However, speech reading, especially when combined with amplification, can dramatically improve a person's ability to understand the speech of others.

Manual communication, often called *sign language*, is the use of the fingers and hands to communicate. Finger spelling, sometimes called *dactology*, and signs are the language symbols used in communication. Whether to use sign language has been a controversial topic among the deaf population. One faction believes that sign language is the "natural" language of the deaf and it should be taught to the exclusion of all other forms of communication. They consider it their native language. Sign language is not just the literal translation of another spoken language; it is a true language unto itself with unique semantic and grammatical structures. The obvious limitation of learning only sign language is that the person can communicate only with other people who know it. The other faction believes that only speech and lip reading should be taught to children. This is often more difficult, demanding, and time-consuming, and not all children learn how to speak or lip-read well. Between these two extremes are the proponents of the **total communication approach** in which children are taught all forms of communication and use whatever means of expression and understanding available to them.

Medical and Surgical Treatment

Several medical and surgical interventions can combat hearing loss and deafness. Surgical procedures to repair the tympanic membrane and ossicular chain are increasingly more common and effective. Many new drugs are effective in treating ear diseases and disorders. New chemotherapies are effective in reducing or eliminating tumors affecting the hearing mechanism. Research regarding the reproduction of destroyed hair cells in the cochlea is also ongoing (Larkin, 2000). One of the most exciting medical treatments is the cochlear implant.

Cochlear implants are becoming more common and efficient, but they are far from restoring normal hearing in previously deaf individuals. In a **cochlear implant,** electrodes are placed in the existing cochlea and attached to a microphone. Although cochlear implants are in their early stages of development, they show promise in helping many people with profound hearing losses or deafness to regain some of their hearing. At present, they are indicated only for certain people and conditions (Munson, 1999).

This medical progress, however, has come with a social cost. Cochlear implants, and their ability to restore hearing, have caused a rift in some families. "Sound and Fury" is an MSNBC *Dateline* report about one such division that occurred in a family in New York City. It involves the conflict and division in a family about a cochlear implant and the subsequent restoration of a child's hearing. The documentary is available on tape and also on the Net: http://www.msnbc.com/news/478714.asp.

Literature and Media Stereotypes

Individuals with voice, articulation, language, and motor speech disorders and those people who stutter are often portrayed in media and literature in an unfavorable light. Certainly, there are exceptions, but as a rule, stigma is associated with communication disorders. These disorders are often viewed simplistically, and the people with them are subjected to teasing, ridicule, and rejection. Defective speech patterns often delegate the population of communication-disordered individuals to inferior status and position. The underlying assumption of the rehabilitation goal, besides minimizing the disorder, is to remove the stigma of their defect and to enable them to be like the mainstream population. Society perceives them as striving for social inclusion through rehabilitation.

These stereotypes and assumptions also hold true for many individuals who are hard-of-hearing and deaf. Many movies, television shows, and books use deafness and hearing loss for comedy purposes. Television situation comedies and skits maximize the confusion and humorous outcomes created by a hearing disorder. For example, one of the most humorous uses of hearing loss was with Gilda Radner's character "Roseanadana" on the television show *Saturday Night Live,* when she questioned public outcry over "endangered feces," instead of "endangered species." In an episode of *Frasier*, his father's temporary hearing loss created several sexual misunderstandings. On *Seinfeld*, George and Kramer bumble speech reading to eavesdrop on a conversation at a party. In the blockbuster movie *The Patriot*, comedy relief from the bloodshed of the Revolutionary War occurred when a soldier said "I come to call on Ann" and his request was misinterpreted. Ann's father, holding an "ear trumpet" (an amplifying cone) to his ear said, "Of course, you call yourself a man."

Contrary to conventional wisdom and assumptions, among the deaf are individuals who do not want social inclusion with the mainstream hearing–verbal population. They desire manual communication. Rather than believing their deafness is a stigma, they consider it a positive social trait. They are happy being members of the deaf culture, take pride in it, and are perfectly content with their communication abilities. These members of the deaf community reject hearing and speech and voluntarily limit their communication to people conversant with finger spelling and sign language. For society, their attitude creates the same kind of dissonance seen when other supposedly inferior subgroups openly embrace their differences and take pride in them. From homosexuals to certain racial groups, when there is a rejection of societal negative stereotypes and pride shown about them, dissonance and confusion are often reflected in media and literature. The film *Children of a Lesser God* only partially addresses this alternative view of deafness. To date no book or film has adequately and accurately depicted the positive view of some deaf people who choose to isolate themselves from the hearing and verbal mainstream.

At the core of their isolationism is the power of language to define their culture. Much like the French-speaking Canadian province of Quebec and certain ethnic groups in the United States, some deaf people seek and demand segregation based on language. These individuals who communicate with manual communication have created a true community, a social subgroup, where the so-called normal population must learn their language if they are to be welcomed into and delighted by the many facets of the deaf culture.

Summary

Hearing is a marvelous sense, and the range of human hearing evolved from a survival need. Several professionals are involved in its study and treatment. The process of hearing can be viewed as a transformation of energy: acoustic, mechanical, hydraulic, and electrochemical. A disruption at any level of energy transformation can result in hearing loss or deafness. Hearing testing involves several types of tests including otoscopic examinations, pure-tone, acoustic immittance, and speech audiometry. The treatment for hearing loss and deafness range from aural habilitation and rehabilitation to cochlear implants. Some members of the deaf community refuse treatment, prefer manual communication, and revel in the deaf culture.

Study Questions

1. List and discuss the responsibilities of the professionals involved in the study and treatment of the ear, hearing loss, and deafness.

2. What is the range of human hearing, and how did it develop?

3. What is the psychological perception of loudness, and how is it measured?

4. Describe the acoustic energy stage in the transmission of sound.

5. Describe the mechanical energy stage in the transmission of sound.

6. Provide both the technical and lay terms for the bones of the middle ear.

7. Describe the hydraulic energy stage of the transmission of sound.

8. How can the cochlea be compared to vision?

9. Describe the electrochemical (neural) energy stage of the transmission of sound.

10. List and discuss the types of hearing loss.

11. What is *vertigo*?

12. What is *acoustic impedance audiometry*?

13. Discuss the primary therapies in aural rehabilitation.

14. How does literature and media portray people with hearing loss and deafness?

Suggested Reading

Larkin, M. (2000). Can lost hearing be restored? *Lancet, 356*: 744. This article, published in a major medical journal, addresses current advances in medicine and technology to restore hearing loss and deafness.

Martin, F. (1997). *Introduction to audiology* (6th ed.). Boston: Allyn & Bacon. A comprehensive, general review of audiology.

Munson, B. (1999). Myths and facts about deafness. *Nursing 99, 29*(12): 84. A short summary addressing some of the myths about hearing loss and deafness.

7

Motor Speech Disorders and Dysphagia

Chapter Preview

Two categories of motor speech disorders are discussed: apraxia of speech and the dysarthrias. These disorders are distinct and separate from aphasia, which is a language disorder and is covered in Chapter 8. Apraxia of speech is a motor programming deficit for voluntary and purposeful speech acts; one characteristic of this speech programming disorder is automatic speech. Patients with automatic speech can sometimes say a problem word or phrase when they give it little forethought. You will learn about oral and limb apraxia, which are nonspeech programming disorders. The dysarthrias affect the motor speech process of respiration, phonation, articulation, resonance, and prosody. You will learn their symptoms and the objectives of treatment. Many diseases and disorders that can cause dysarthria also impair a patient's ability to chew and swallow, a disorder called dysphagia. You will learn how this disorder has become the responsibility of speech–language pathologists and how it is evaluated and treated. Finally, you will learn societal stereotypes about people with these disorders and how they are often inaccurate and misleading.

Motor speech production is one of the most complicated physical acts done by the human body. Literally hundreds of muscles and thousands of neurological impulses per second are necessary to create speech sounds. Highly coordinated muscle movements are necessary to drive the five motor speech processes: respiration, phonation, articulation, resonance, and prosody. **Respiration** drives the act of speech by compressing the air in the lungs and allowing it to be gradually expelled through the oral tract. In **phonation** the vocal cords vibrate and give speech its energy and loudness. In **articulation** the vocal tract structures move rapidly from one point to another, fine-tuning the head resonator in the creation of speech sounds. The velum gives some sounds more **nasal resonance** than others. All the time this compressing, shaping, and valving of the airstream is occurring, there is **prosody**—a smooth rhythm, flow, and cadence to speech. The average speaker utters about 250 words per minute, about 4 per second, and each possesses the acoustic properties to be understood by the listener. An injury, disease, or stroke can impair or even eliminate this highly coordinated and sophisticated act.

Thousands of injuries and diseases of the brain and nervous system can cause motor speech disorders. These disorders are nonsymbolic. They are not a result of impaired language and cognition (Darley, Aronson, & Brown, 1975; Darley, 1982). This clear separation of language and motor speech disorders is based on research conduced by Frederick Darley, and others, at the Mayo Clinic in Rochester, Minnesota. Referred to as the Darley model, it divides motor speech disorders into two categories: apraxia of speech and the dysarthrias.

Apraxia of speech disrupts the programming of the muscles of speech production, especially the tongue. The person with apraxia of speech can be thought of as having a "tangled tongue." In apraxia of speech, the person knows what he wants to say, but, because of neurological deficits, he cannot plan and execute the speech act. In mild cases of the disorder, it can be a minor nuisance, resulting in frequent slips of the tongue. Severe apraxia of speech can render a person unable to talk. Apraxia of speech, sometimes called *verbal apraxia*, can be caused by strokes, diseases, and brain injuries.

The **dysarthrias,** a collection of motor speech disorders, result from damage to the **central** or **peripheral nervous systems.** They are sometimes called *neuromuscular speech disorders* because they involve neurons and/or the muscles they innervate. The dysarthrias can affect the muscles of breathing, larynx, soft palate, and tongue. Whereas the person with apraxia of speech has a tangled tongue, the individual with dysarthria can be thought of as having a "paralyzed" one. The illnesses that cause motor speech disorders are often progressive and sometimes terminal. The way some people adapt and cope with motor speech disorders is a tribute to the human will to communicate.

The "Big Three" Neurogenic Communication Disorders

Aphasia, apraxia of speech, and the dysarthrias are the "big three" neurogenic communication disorders (Tanner, 1999a). They are the most common communication disorders resulting from diseases and disorders of the brain and nervous system. (Other apraxias also occur; see the following discussions and Table 7.1.) Sometimes they occur in isolation, but more often than not, two or all three occur in the same patient. In addition, some patients with dysarthria have two or more types occurring simultaneously or have one type of dysarthria change into another over time.

TABLE 7.1 *Three Apraxias*

Type of Apraxia	Description
Apraxia of speech (verbal apraxia)	Problems with planning and sequencing the speech act
Oral apraxia (buccofacial apraxia)	Difficulty in performing voluntary oral, nonspeech muscle movements
Limb apraxia (body apraxia)	Difficulty in purposefully performing a movement with a limb

Literature, Media, and Personality Profiles

Annette Funicello

In the early 1990s, actor and singer Annette Funicello revealed that she has multiple sclerosis (MS). Funicello—born on October 22, 1942, in Utica, New York—became famous for appearing on the *Mickey Mouse Club* as one of the original "Mouseketeers." Between 1959 and 1961, she recorded several hit singles. In the 1960s she starred, with Frankie Avalon, in several California beach movies including *Beach Party*, *Bikini Beach*, and *How to Stuff a Wild Bikini*. She has also appeared on several television shows including *Love American Style*, *The Love Boat*, and *Full House*. In 1995, her biography, *A Dream Is a Wish Your Heart Makes: The Annette Funicello Story*, aired on network television. She is founder and sponsor of the Annette Funicello Research Fund for Neurological Diseases.

Stephen William Hawking

Stephen William Hawking was born on January 8, 1942, in Oxford, England. Many consider him one of the premier mathematicians and theoretical physicists of our time. He obtained his Doctor of Philosophy from Oxford University and is Lucasian Professor of Mathematics at the University of Cambridge. He is a prolific author, with *A Brief History of Time* being a best-seller. He has several honorary degrees and is a member of the United States Academy of Sciences. He has three children.

Hawking was diagnosed with amyotrophic lateral sclerosis (ALS), also known as Lou Gehrig's disease, when he was 22 years old. The disease has slowly become progressively worse, and in 1985 he had a **tracheotomy,** a surgical procedure by which a hole is made in the trachea and a tube inserted to allow breathing. He has required 24-hour nursing care since the surgery. He discusses his progressive speech deterioration and alternate communication system on the World Wide Web:

> Before the operation, my speech had been getting more slurred, so that only a few people who knew me well, could understand me. But at least I could communicate. I wrote scientific papers by dictating to a secretary, and I gave seminars through an interpreter, who repeated my words more clearly.

> Later, a computer expert from California provided him with a program called Equalizer. With this program, he selects words from a series of menus by pressing a handheld switch or by using head or eye movements. The system was also fitted to his wheelchair.

> This system allowed me to communicate much better than I could before. I can manage up to 15 words a minute. I can either speak what I have written, or save it on disk. I can then print it out, or call it back, and speak it sentence by sentence. Using this system, I have written a book and dozens of scientific papers.

> The speech synthesizer has been very important in helping Hawking adjust to his disease. He attributes much of his success with family and work with being able to communicate, despite the severity of the ALS.

> One's voice is very important. If you have a slurred voice, people are likely to treat you as mentally deficient. . . . This synthesizer is by far the best I have heard, because it varies the intonation, and doesn't speak like a Dalek. The only trouble is that it gives me an American accent. However, the company is working on a British version.

Muhammad Ali

Born Cassius Marcellus Clay on January 17, 1942, Muhammad Ali is the first man to hold the title of Heavyweight Boxing Champion of the World three times. He first received worldwide acclaim when he won the Olympic Light-Heavyweight Championship in 1960. In 1964 he won his first professional heavyweight title from Sonny Liston.

In the 1960s Ali converted to the Black Muslim religion and has been a role model for many African American people. Stripped of his title in 1967 for refusing military service in Vietnam, he was allowed to resume his boxing career in 1970. He is noted for his self-confidence, quick wit, and colorful phrases: "Float like a butterfly and sting like a bee" and "I am the greatest." He has Parkinson's disease, probably because of repeated traumatic brain injuries, which has significantly affected his ability to communicate. It has struck his voice and caused it to tremor and be weak. *Ali: An American Hero*, a television show about his life, was broadcast in August 2000. A movie also has been produced about his life and was released in December 2001.

Anywhere But Here

Released in 1999, *Anywhere But Here* is the story of a discontented mother and rebellious, defiant teenage daughter. They move to Beverly Hills to start a new life, which is unstable. The mother, played by Susan Sarandon, is a speech–language pathologist who originally obtains employment in a public school. Later she works in a medical facility with elderly patients. One scene shows her providing therapy to a woman who apparently has apraxia of speech. The patient is provided with models of tongue and lip placement, and she attempts repeatedly to program the sounds and words. Although Sarandon's character is self-centered and self-serving throughout much of the movie, her patience and rapport with the stroke survivor provide a glimpse of her nurturing side. Ultimately, mother and daughter learn relationship boundaries and respect for each other.

Janet Reno

Janet Reno, the first female U.S. Attorney General, was appointed by President Bill Clinton after serving as Attorney General of Florida for five consecutive terms. Born on July 21, 1938, in Miami, Florida, she graduated from Cornell in 1960 with a degree in chemistry. She obtained her law degree from Harvard University in 1963 and practiced law from 1963 to 1971. She has Parkinson's disease and shows characteristic tremors of this disease during her public appearances.

Deuce Bigalow: Male Gigolo

The sophomoric comedy *Deuce Bigalow: Male Gigolo*, released in 1999, stars Rob Schneider and was directed by Mike Mitchell. This film is about a bumbling, inept fishtank cleaner, Deuce Bigalow, who is fired from his job at the Los Angeles Aquarium and finds temporary employment at a luxurious apartment complex cleaning its fishpond. At the apartment complex, Bigalow meets a successful gigolo who must leave town. The gigolo leaves Deuce Bigalow to apartment-sit, and he accidentally destroys an expensive fishtank. To pay for a replacement, he earns money in the sex-for-hire business. One of his dates (or "tricks" as they are called in the movie) is Ruth, a woman with Tourette syndrome, who displays symptoms of the syndrome, including the tendency to swear uncontrollably.

(continued)

Literature, Media, and Personality Profiles (continued)

Kirk Douglas

Kirk Douglas—born Issur Danielovitch on December 9, 1916, in Amsterdam, New York—has been an actor for more than 50 years and has been in over 80 films. A respected and revered figure in the motion picture industry, he has received an Honorary Award by the Academy of Motion Picture Arts and Sciences and is the recipient of the presidential Medal of Freedom, which is the highest honor bestowed on private citizens. Douglas has been nominated for an Academy Award for Best Actor for three films. A stroke survivor, Douglas was the Awards Ceremony Special Guest at the 1999 convention of the American Speech-Language-Hearing Association. Since his stroke, Douglas's ability to communicate has improved significantly. In the movie *Diamonds* (directed by John Asher), Douglas is shown having speech therapy. Throughout the film, which was released in 2000, his speech is easily understood, although he talks slowly and carefully. Douglas, like many people, took the ability to communicate for granted. He comments on the Web about his stroke and the complexities of speech and language:

> You're suddenly aware of how much you take for granted in life. . . . We think something, and we speak it. Now I was like a child: I had to learn all the sounds. You realize how complicated it is. The brain on the left side governs the cheek muscles, the lips, the tongue, the teeth. I thought, wow, how people talk is so complicated!

Aphasia

Expressive aphasia and apraxia of speech often occur together. As discussed in Chapter 8, patients with predominately **receptive aphasia,** sometimes called *Wernicke's aphasia,* have problems reading and understanding the speech and gestures of others. Patients with predominately **expressive aphasia,** sometimes called *Broca's aphasia,* have difficulty speaking, writing, and using complicated gestures to communicate ideas.

Patients with Broca's aphasia experience two types of communication problems. Part of their communication disorder is due to a loss of the expressive language functions of semantics, grammar, and phonology. This is the language aspect of expressive aphasia (discussed in detail in Chapter 8). The motor aspect of expressive aphasia is apraxia of speech, and it relates to the planning and sequencing of the motor speech act. Patients with this motor speech problem remember the words they want to say but have problems getting their speech mechanism to say them. A common symptom of Broca's or nonfluent aphasia (Katz, Bharadwaj, & Carstens, 1999), it is not due to paralyzed speech muscles but is a speech programming deficit.

Apraxia of Speech

Rarely does apraxia of speech occur without aphasia because the motor speech programming and some language aspects of expression are in the same general areas of the brain, **Broca's area** (Figure 7.1). It is found in the left hemisphere of the brain in most right-handed individuals (see Chapter 8). As reported in Chapter 4, the articulatory plan may occur in other

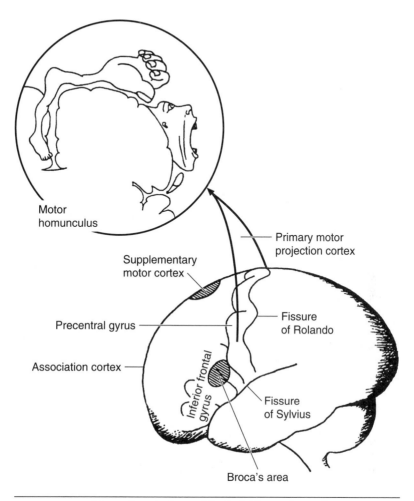

FIGURE 7.1   *Motor Speech Area of the Left Hemisphere of the Brain*

Source: W. Perkins & R. Kent, *Functional Anatomy of Speech, Language, and Hearing.* Copyright 1986. Reprinted by permission by Allyn & Bacon.

areas of the left hemisphere of the brain, specifically the left anterior insula and lateral premotor cortex (Wise, Greene, Büchel, & Scott, 1999). Pure apraxia of speech is also rare because a person's memory for a word is closely tied to how it is uttered. In children, apraxia of speech also presents with poorer discrimination abilities, suggesting a relationship between auditory processing and motor speech programming (Groenen, Maassen, Crul, & Thoonen, 1996). When apraxia of speech occurs independently of a language disorder, it is usually mild. Pure severe apraxia of speech is unusual.

In the film *Anywhere But Here*, Susan Sarandon's character provides therapy to a patient displaying symptoms of apraxia of speech. In therapy, the patient is shown how to make sounds and words by proper placement of the articulators. She is given models and instructions on how to plan and sequence the motor aspects of speech. The patient in this film has apraxic disturbances. The following is typical of a patient with moderate apraxia of speech, describing a picture of a police officer writing a ticket to a frustrated driver:

> The stop, top, uh, prop has told over a very trustrated, uh, frustrated sotorist. You can see that he is strangy . . . angry about the thing. He is trying to splain, estain, erstain, that no speeding. It is futile because the crop, stop, plop, stuhcop is done with it.

Although the patient also displays problems remembering words and using other aspects of expressive language, the main difficulty is planning and sequencing the speech act.

In severe apraxia of speech, patients may be unable to get their breathing and voice production to occur together. They may also be unable to plan and sequence any tongue movement for speech sound production. Patients with severe apraxia of speech can be rendered mute due to problems of programming and sequencing the speech act. (See Box 7.1.)

Apraxia of speech causes patients to confound, complicate, and entangle the speech act. They make mistakes because of overshooting and undershooting the articulators during speech. When *overshooting*, an anticipatory error, the speech error may cause the word *car* to sound like *carp* when the patient tries to say, "Where is the red car parked?" *Undershooting*, a perseveratory error, would cause *dar* to be said for the word *car*. The sounds preceding and following the target word often contaminate proper speech production.

Patients with apraxia of speech also add unnecessary sounds, often the "uh" sound **(schwa),** or substitute one sound for another. An example of an **addition** would be *k-s-ar* for the word *car*. A **substitution** of the /f/ sound for the /k/ one would be *far* for the word *car*. Additionally, patients with apraxia of speech often use fillers during pauses in speech. A **filler** is a sound, syllable, word, or phrase uttered during a pause in speech to counteract the silence. It is usually an attempt to continue talking, so that they will not be interrupted, and to plan the next thing to say. Patients with apraxia of speech struggle when they try to force an utterance. Apraxia of speech and stuttering share several similar symptoms (see Chapter 2). One similarity between apraxia of speech and stuttering is that words with more **propositionality** are harder to say. Words with higher levels of propositionality have more emotion, value, and importance and are more necessary to the utterance.

In apraxia of speech, errors occur more often on consonants than on vowels. Usually, patients have trouble "getting started." In mild apraxia of speech, the first sounds of an utterance are the most difficult to program, and if patients can get them correct, usually the word is completed normally. Most patients with apraxia of speech have trouble repeating the

---

BOX 7.1 • *Normal Speech-Programming Problems*

A way of understanding the type of speech problems seen in apraxia of speech is to compare it with the difficulties saying "problem words." Some people have trouble programming and sequencing their articulators to make words like *specifically, phenomenon, aluminum, supposedly, linoleum, spaghetti,* and *cinnamon.* Patients with apraxia of speech have similar problems programming and sequencing their articulators, but the speech impairment is many times worse, even in mild cases of the disorder.

speech of others. This is one of the more consistent aspects of this motor speech disorder. Many tests of apraxia of speech use repetition of speech as a test to detect the presence and severity of this disorder (Tanner & Culbertson, 1999).

Therapy. Therapy for apraxia of speech involves having the patient learn to program and control the articulators. Visual biofeedback regarding tongue movements has been found to be a helpful therapy (Katz et al., 1999). Because pure apraxia of speech is a nonsymbolic disorder, there is no emphasis on relearning words or their meanings. Because apraxia of speech is not a paralytic disorder, strengthening muscles or improving their range of movements is not an objective. The patient with apraxia of speech learns how to properly program and sequence the sounds of speech.

Automatic Speech. Apraxia of speech occurs primarily on purposeful, voluntary utterances, not automatic ones. Statements made "off the cuff" are not purposeful, nor are they often voluntary. One way of understanding purposeful and nonpurposeful utterances is with typing. Most of the time, when you are typing something, you do not think about each finger movement. This is particularly true on overlearned words such as your name or city in which you live. When you type these words, you are not purposefully programming each finger movement. But when you type a new or lengthy word, you must give more thought to your finger movements. Automatic typing is easier than purposeful typing.

A unique feature of apraxia of speech is the ability of many apraxic patients to produce *automatic speech*. When speech utterances are overlearned or produced with little forethought, many apraxic patients can engage in appropriate speech programming. However, when they purposefully attempt to produce the same speech utterance, the speech programming cannot be produced, and the patient is verbally impotent (see Box 7.2). Automatic speech is often present on well-rehearsed words and phrases. It is also common on profanity. Swear words are often said automatically and involuntarily. Episodes of fluent, accurate speech occasionally occurring in the patient's speech output are clear indicators of the presence of apraxia of speech.

Other Apraxias. Two other types of apraxia sometimes occur in patients with neuropathologies of speech and language. Oral apraxia is like apraxia of speech, except it involves only nonspeech oral tasks like licking or puckering the lips, trying to touch the tongue to the nose, and others. **Oral apraxia,** sometimes called **buccofacial apraxia** (Katz et al., 1999), is difficulty in performing voluntary oral, nonspeech muscle movements. Oral apraxia and

---

BOX 7.2 • *"I Can't Seem to Say 'Maggie'"*

An example of automatic speech is when the patient cannot say a family member's name. She might try repeatedly to say "Maggie." It may sound like this: "aggie," "staggie," "uh-aggie," "raggie." Then, when the patient's attention is elsewhere and there is little thought given to the word, she might say, "I can't seem to say 'Maggie' today."

apraxia of speech often occur together, but sometimes a patient may have only one of these oral mechanism programming disorders.

Limb apraxia, also known as *body apraxia,* is the difficulty of purposefully performing a movement with a limb. These patients have trouble following commands (see Box 7.3). As with all apraxias, the problem is not with understanding the request, nor is it because the limb is paralyzed; the difficulty is in programming the act. These problems with programming body acts extend to using tools and objects and are not a result of frontal lobe damage (Goldenberg & Hagmann, 1998).

The Dysarthrias

The dysarthrias (Table 7.2) are a group of motor speech disorders that can be classified based on the site and nature of damage to the brain and central nervous system (Darley et al., 1975). They are sometimes called *neuromuscular disorders* because they disrupt the muscles of speech and/or the nerves that supply them. They impair, to various degrees, the ability of the human body to compress air, vibrate the vocal cords, and shape speech sounds. The dysarthrias can disrupt respiration, laryngeal functioning, and articulation. Resonance can be impaired because of impaired functioning of the velum and other muscles that close off the nasal passages. The dysarthrias also can impair prosody, the rhythm, melody, cadence, inflection, and emphasis of speech. Although this classification system is accurate for adults, it may not be suitable for acquired childhood dysarthria (van Mourik, Catsman-Berrevoets, Yousef-Bak, Paquier, & van Dongen, 1998). It may be necessary to create a different classification for children with this neuromuscular disorder.

Before exploring each of the dysarthrias, discussing how muscles move body structures is necessary. Two groups of muscles work together to cause movement: *antagonist* and *agonist.* Antagonist and agonist muscles work in opposition to each other. When the antagonist muscles contract, the agonist muscle relaxes, and vice versa. For example, when you want to move your finger toward your body, several muscles contract, bringing their points of origin and insertion closer together. While they are contracting, another group of muscles must relax to allow the movement. When you want to move your finger away from your body, the reverse of the process occurs. This alternating contracting and relaxing permits you to move your finger from front to back several times to nonverbally communicate "come here." Consequently, the only thing a muscle can forcibly do is contract and bring its points of origin and insertion closer together. Although muscle movements can indirectly cause a pushing

---

BOX 7.3 • *Smoking and Automatic Limb Movements*

An example of limb apraxia occurs when you ask a patient to "show me how you light and smoke a cigarette." The patient with this type of apraxia will have difficulty programming the limb muscles necessary to perform the act. He will randomly and haphazardly move the arms and ultimately will be unable to get the cigarette to his mouth. However, when the patient feels the urge to have a smoke and does not give it forethought, he can automatically complete the actions necessary to bring the cigarette to the mouth and light it.

TABLE 7.2   *The Dysarthrias*

Type of Dysarthria	Neurological Deficit
Ataxic	Cerebellum
Flaccid	Lower motor neurons
Hyperkinetic	Extrapyramidal system
Hypokinetic	Extrapyramidal system
Mixed	Multiple systems
Spastic	Upper motor neurons

action, a single muscle cannot forcibly push a structure. This alternating contraction and relaxation of muscles causes movements of the speech production structures. Dysarthria is a breakdown in this process.

When dysarthria occurs in a pure form, the patient has no other types of communication disorders. In pure dysarthria the patient's language is intact, and her ability to program the speech act is unaffected. Some diseases and disorders causing dysarthria can render a person *anarthric* (without speech), while having normal intelligence. An anarthric person can be speechless while having no intellectual deterioration and—in the case of Stephen Hawking—remain brilliant.

Spastic Dysarthria.   A **spastic** muscle is in the state of prolonged partial or complete contraction. This type of dysarthria results from bilateral upper motor neuron damage. Duffy (1995) has identified a type of dysarthria resulting from unilateral upper motor neuron damage. Upper motor neurons regulate and inhibit muscle contraction. When they lose their regulatory and inhibitory functions, muscles go into a state of contraction. Muscles become stiff, move sluggishly, and their range of motion (ROM) is limited.

Range of motion is how far a body part can move. A way of understanding limited ROM is to stand next to a wall and rotate and lift your arm from your side to high above your head. If your arm can go from your side, outwardly, and upwardly to the top of your head, you have normal or complete ROM. However, if the movement is restricted and you can only move it to the level of your waist or neck, then you have reduced ROM.

The effects of spastic muscles on speech production can be dramatic. In severe cases of spasticity, muscles are tightly pulled against themselves all the time. When the muscles of respiration and phonation are spastic, **pitch range** and loudness range are reduced, resulting in monopitch and monoloudness during speech. *Monopitch* is the result of a lack of variation in the frequency of vocal cord vibration, and *monoloudness* is a lack of changes in the loudness levels during speech. Phrasing can also be shortened because of reduced breath support. Phrasing problems are similar to those shown by wheelchair-bound Stevie in the television comedy *Malcolm in the Middle*. Additionally, voice quality can be harsh or hoarse and sound like voice is being forced through the tight muscles of the larynx.

Reduced ROM and weak tongue movements can cause articulation to be sluggish, labored, and indistinct. Sometimes in **spastic dysarthria,** words are prolonged because of the slow, labored movements of the articulators. Spastic and other dysarthrias can also result in assimilated hypernasality. Assimilated hypernasality is too much nasality that occurs during ongoing speech. This is the result of slow movements of the velum in closing off the nasal passage. Although patients can produce sounds with normal nasal resonance in isolation, they will have hypernasality in connected speech because the velum does not move fast enough to prevent it.

Spastic muscles often respond better to slow, gradual attempts to move them. For example, if your arm is spastic and you try hard to move it fast from one position to another, it will have strong resistance. However, if you slowly, gently, and gradually attempt the same movement, it will move with less resistance. The same is true for speech muscles; slow, gentle, and gradual attempts at producing voice and speech result in better movements. This principle is used in therapy to improve the speech of patients with spastic dysarthria.

Flaccid Dysarthria.   In many ways, the opposite of a spastic muscle is one that is flaccid. **Flaccid dysarthria** results from lower motor neuron damage, and the motor unit is impaired. The **motor unit** is the muscle and nerve that innervates it. It is called the *final common pathway* of neurological impulses. All motor commands ultimately go through the lower motor unit to achieve movement. A **flaccid** muscle is weak and limp. If your arm were completely flaccid, you could lift it with your good arm and drop it, and it would swing back and forth, without resistance.

When the respiratory–voice production system is impaired in flaccid dysarthria, the patient is **breathy** or completely without the ability to make voice **(aphonic).** This is because either one or both vocal cords cannot move sufficiently to contact the other one. As was discussed in Chapter 3, **unilateral adductor paralysis** is when one of the vocal cords is either completely or partially paralyzed and there is not sufficient muscle strength and movement for **adduction** (closure). When both vocal cords are paralyzed, it is called **bilateral adductor paralysis.** When patients have the respiratory–voice production system impaired in flaccid dysarthria, sometimes they have audible inspiration and/or inhalatory stridor. Audible inspiration is hearing the air rush in during inhalation, and **inhalatory stridor** is the vibratory component to it. Therapies, in the form of strengthening and mobility exercises to bring the cords closer together, are helpful in regaining the voice. Sometimes, the injection of a solution in the vocal cord to bring it closer to **midline** is also helpful.

When the tongue is affected in flaccid dysarthria, it is often slow and sluggish. This results in indistinct sounds being produced, primarily consonants, that require elevation such as /t/ and /l/. In severe cases of flaccid dysarthria, the patient cannot move the tongue sufficiently to produce recognizable sounds. Therapy involves using existing muscle strength and control to maximize articulation abilities.

Hypernasality and **nasal emissions** are components of dysarthria when the muscles of velopharyngeal closure are affected. Because of muscle weakness or paralysis, the oral and nasal cavities cannot be closed off during speech. This results in too much nasal resonance, hypernasality, and the sound of air rushing out and through the nose (nasal emission). Lack of velopharyngeal closure also contributes to poor intelligibility in some patients because of a reduced ability to create *interoral air pressure,* the buildup of air pressure inside the mouth necessary to make speech sounds. In effect, a leak in the oral cavity through the nose causes reduced air pressure that is necessary for the production of distinct sounds, especially pressure consonants. For patients who have extremely weak speech muscles, this lack of interoral air pressure can significantly reduce their intelligibility. Therapy is often helpful to achieve velopharyngeal closure by strengthening the muscles and improving mobility of the velum. Palatal lifts and surgery are also sometimes indicated. A **palatal lift** is a prosthesis that holds the velum closer to the pharyngeal wall, thus requiring less movement to achieve closure. Surgery is done to lift and move the velum closer to the pharyngeal wall. In addition, in patients whose flaccid dysarthria results from absent or reduced chemicals necessary for muscular contraction, certain medications can be helpful in returning their speech to optimal levels.

Ataxic Dysarthria.   Located at the base of the skull, the **cerebellum** is called the "great modulator" of muscular movements. When the cerebellum and/or the tracts leading to and from it are damaged or destroyed, ataxia results. **Ataxia** can be described as a coordination problem. Ataxic movements are ill timed, jerky, and discoordinated. Although a variety of diseases and disorders can cause damage to the cerebellum, it is often seen in cerebral palsy. There are several types of cerebral palsy, but it primarily involves damage to the motor control system that can result in abnormal muscle tone, discoordination, and other movement disorders. Cerebral palsy may be limited only to motor control functions, or it can also impair cognitive functioning.

   Ataxic dysarthria results from damage to the cerebellar system. It is sometimes called a *prosody disorder* because speech is irregular, jerky, and often accompanied by either too much or too little stress on syllables. **Stress** is the amount of loudness one syllable has compared to another in a word. The stressed syllable is also slightly longer in duration than the others in the word.

   The neurological impulses coming from the brain are exaggerated, and the cerebellum refines them. For example, if you want to pick up a pencil from your desk, your brain must send a series of motor impulses to cause your arm, hand, and fingers to move. Without the influence of the cerebellum, your hand and arm would have exaggerated movements with overshooting and undershooting of movement targets. Without the coordinating effects of the cerebellum, your hand would miss the pencil repeatedly. Your hand would come down too hard or too soft and miss or knock the pencil to the floor. Your movements would appear ham-handed and clumsy, similar to those of a drunkard. The cerebellum refines and coordinates the gross commands coming from your brain and makes them smooth, timed properly, and effective.

   The same type of movement problem occurs with speech articulators in ataxic dysarthria. The tongue overshoots and undershoots articulatory targets. This **coarticulation,** or gestural overlap, reflects biomechanical or motor constraints and higher-level phonetic processing (Hertrich & Ackermann, 1999). Stress is vulnerable to this mistiming of movements. Instead of the correct amount of stress on a syllable, there is too much because of discoordinated and ill-timed movements of respiration and phonation. Speech has an explosive, singsong character. When the damage to the cerebellar system is extensive, intelligible speech becomes impossible.

   In ataxic dysarthria the patient's voice quality is often harsh, due, in part, to the attempts to force normal voice quality. Monopitch and monoloudness are also characteristics of ataxic dysarthria. Although one would expect highly variable pitch and loudness resulting from discoordinated and ill-timed laryngeal muscle movements during pitch and loudness adjustments, this is not always the case. Monopitch and monoloudness in ataxic dysarthria are probably the result of the patient compensating for the cerebellar damage by requiring very few adjustments of the respiratory and laryngeal system.

Whereas the primary treatment for spastic and flaccid dysarthria involves ROM and strengthening exercises, improved coordination and timing are the primary goals for ataxic dysarthria. The patient is taught to be more precise in articulation movements and to attend more to coordination and timing of the articulators.

Hypokinetic Dysarthria.   Hypokinetic dysarthria occurs when there is damage to the extrapyramidal system. The **extrapyramidal system** is a tract of nerve fibers involved in automatic aspects of motor coordination. The extrapyramidal tract is also known as the *indirect motor system* and is important in regulating posture and locomotion. This type of dysarthria is primarily seen in Parkinson's disease, which is a degenerative disorder characterized by tremor, muscular weakness, and slow movements. Parkinson's disease results from a lack of a neurotransmitter chemical called dopamine. Actor Michael J. Fox has early onset Parkinson's Disease.

The speech characteristics of Parkinsonian hypokinetic dysarthria include reduced loudness, monopitch, and monoloudness. The respiratory–laryngeal system is impaired and reduces the power and strength of speech. In severe cases of the disorder, these patients appear feeble, and their speech reflects this weakness. The voice of patients with Parkinsonian hypokinetic dysarthria often tremors and lacks appropriate stress.

The articulation of patients with this dysarthria is often slow and sluggish. Sounds are made imprecisely. In some patients with Parkinsonian hypokinetic dysarthria, there are short rushes of rapid speech. These short rushes of speech are a result of articulatory undershooting due to the dopamine imbalance and is called the *acceleration phenomenon*. Many patients with Parkinson's disease have a masked face where the skin is pulled tight.

Although several anti-Parkinson medications and therapies are helpful, most patients with this disorder still have a speech pathology. Intelligibility is often reduced. There are several causes of Parkinson's disease, including repeated head traumas, such as may be the case of Muhammad Ali.

Hyperkinetic Dysarthria.   Also a disorder of the extrapyramidal system, there are several types of hyperkinetic dysarthrias. *Hyperkinetic* means too much movement, and the movements can be either slow or quick. In slow hyperkinetic dysarthria, patients have slow, unwanted speech movements. In the quick variety, the unwanted movements occur rapidly.

Slow hyperkinetic dysarthria is seen in athetoid cerebral palsy. In this type of dysarthria, the patient has writhing movements of the body, including those of the speech mechanism, which can cause voice and articulation to be impaired. These involuntary writhing contractions affect one muscle after another. They blend into one another. Patients have head and jaw muscle contortions, and their faces appear to grimace. Speech is often weak and distorted. Some patients, those who have more muscular tension in their symptoms, often speak in their upper-pitch range.

Quick hyperkinetic dysarthria is a result of **tics** and jerks of the speech mechanism. They cause unwanted sounds and can interrupt the smooth flow of speech. Tics and jerks of the muscles of speech production can also interrupt phonation and can cause loudness, stress, and pitch to be impaired. Quick hyperkinetic dysarthria is seen in Tourette syndrome. Uncontrolled barking, grunting, and facial grimacing characterize Tourette syndrome, first described by the French physician Gilles de la Tourette. As was shown in the film *Deuce Bigalow: Male Gigolo,* some individuals with this disorder also have uncontrolled swearing called **coprolalia.** The barking, grunting, facial grimacing, and coprolalia can interfere with speech communication. Medications are helpful in reducing these symptoms, as can be the application of some of the techniques used in stuttering therapy to remove unwanted speech patterns.

Multiple (Mixed) Dysarthrias.   The preceding speech pathologies involve only one motor system. More often than not, dysarthrias result from damage to two or more motor systems. This is because strokes, diseases, and other disorders of the brain and nervous system often do not limit their destructive effects to just one aspect of the body. They often damage multiple systems, and the result is **multiple dysarthria.** The types of speech disorders seen in multiple dysarthrias depend on the neurological systems that have been damaged. Two progressive, degenerative diseases are typical of dysarthrias resulting from multiple-system damage: multiple sclerosis and amyotrophic lateral sclerosis.

Multiple sclerosis (MS) is a deteriorating muscular disorder caused by myelin damage. Myelin is a protective connective sheath surrounding the nerve tracts. A good way of thinking of myelin is to compare it to the insulating substance around an electric cord. Several symptoms characterize MS, depending on the sites of the lesions. **Nystagmus,** an **oscillation** of the eyes, is often present. In the majority of patients, the symptoms remit and exacerbate: They come and go spontaneously regardless of treatment regimens.

Over 50% of the patients with MS display dysarthria that is sometimes characterized as scanning speech. Scanning speech is a one-word-at-a-time, searching type of articulation with inappropriate pauses. When speech is impaired in MS, the most apparent problems are with loudness control and articulation. The loudness-control problem is having too soft or too loud speech. The articulation problems usually involve coordination and distinctness of sound production. In addition, patients often display a harsh voice quality, and some have hypernasality. Multiple sclerosis is a dysarthria resulting from damage to multiple systems, depending on which ones are damaged. Actor, director, and talk-show host Montel Williams reportedly has MS.

Amyotrophic lateral sclerosis (ALS) also results in a dysarthria from damage to multiple motor systems. Degeneration of both the upper and lower motor neuron systems characterizes this progressive disorder. As a result, it has symptoms of both flaccid and spastic dysarthria. Typically, this type of dysarthria does not present with equal spastic and flaccid symptoms; one or the other may be prominent at any given time.

The speech of patients with ALS is usually severely impaired. As with Stephen Hawking, speech can deteriorate to the extent that communication can be done only with an assistive device. When there is some oral speech capability, articulation is severely impaired, and there is hypernasality and nasal emission. When there is voice, it is often strained-strangled, with a "wet" quality. There are often audible inhalations, sometimes accompanied by voicing sounds.

Several other disorders and diseases result in multiple dysarthrias. Certain types of head traumas that damage more than one area of the brain, multiple strokes, and generalized brain and nervous system diseases can cause multiple types of dysarthria. In addition, certain progressive diseases can cause one system after another to be damaged, thus causing an evolution of dysarthric speech symptoms.

Dysphagia

Some patients who have paralysis or weakness of their speech musculature have **dysphagia,** a swallowing disorder. It is often seen in patients with dysarthria because the same muscles used for speaking are also used for sucking, chewing, and swallowing. Sometimes, however, dysphagia can occur alone and not be accompanied by a speech pathology. Over the years, because of their knowledge and expertise, speech–language pathologists working in medical environments have accepted evaluation and treatment of dysphagia as part of their clinical responsibilities. Their knowledge of the nature and function of the oral, laryngeal, and respiratory structures makes them qualified to deal with dysphagia. Evaluation and treatment of dysphagia is a very important part of patient management because dysphagia can be life threatening.

Before discussing the evaluation and treatment of dysphagia, describing the stages of a normal swallow is necessary. There are three interconnected stages of a swallow: oral, pharyngeal, and esophageal–laryngeal. (In this book, the third stage is called esophageal–laryngeal rather than simply esophageal. This is to show the importance of laryngeal protective actions during the combined stages of the swallow, particularly during the pharyngeal activities.) Perlman and Christensen (1997) suggest the term pharyngealolaryngeal to more accurately include the laryngeal actions. The *oral stage* is when liquid or food is prepared for swallowing. At this stage, liquid is controlled and contained. Food is chewed, or masticated. Mastication involves breaking down the food into small pieces and the creation of a bolus, a ball of food that can easily be moved to the back of the throat. The bolus is lubricated by liquids in the food and by saliva. The second stage of swallowing occurs at the *pharyngeal level* in which the liquid or bolus is positioned for swallowing. At this stage, the velum elevates, closing off the air passageway to the nose, and the larynx elevates. The esophageal–laryngeal stage is the conclusion of the swallow; the airway is protected, and food is propelled into the stomach. Logemann (1998) notes that the esophageal stage of the swallow cannot be modified by therapy. Coordination of the oral, pharyngeal, and esophageal–laryngeal stages is important to protect the airways from getting food or liquid in them. The vocal cords are closed, protecting the air passageways. The epiglottis, a flaplike cartilage structure of the larynx, also snaps over the vocal cords, helping keep food and liquids out of the lungs and the passageways leading to them.

In a normal swallow, food and liquid are naturally and easily moved from the oral cavity to the stomach. However, when there are muscle paralysis, weakness, or sensation problems (numbness) in the mouth or throat, food and liquid are not properly contained and swallowed. Sometimes, choking and coughing accompany these problems, and other times the patient can have silent aspiration. Silent **aspiration** is when food or liquid gets into the lungs or the passageways leading to them, and the patient does not choke or cough. Food and liquid, which have bacteria, can cause pneumonia when aspirated. Aspiration pneumonia can lead to serious medical complications, particularly in feeble and weak patients.

The Swallowing Evaluation

There can be two parts to a swallowing evaluation. The first aspect is the bedside assessment in which the clinician assesses the patient's swallowing ability; the patient can be in bed or sitting up in a chair. During the evaluation the patient is given food and liquid and observed to see how well he can manage them. However, some patients are designated NPO, which means that they are not to be given anything orally, because they may choke or aspirate. When patients are on an NPO status, swallowing is assessed indirectly by determining strength and mobility of the muscles and structures of swallowing.

The bedside evaluation involves assessing several swallowing functions at the oral, pharyngeal, and esophageal–laryngeal stages (Tanner & Culbertson, 1999). At the oral stage, the patient's abilities to accept food and create a bolus, seal the lips, and masticate are assessed. The teeth are observed to see if there are enough of them and whether they are functional for tearing and chewing food. The tendency of some patients to pocket food, leaving the bolus or particles of food in their cheeks after swallowing, is noted. Tongue mobility is evaluated. Does the tongue protrude, retract, elevate, depress, and lateralize normally? The patient's ability to propel the bolus along the palatal vault is determined. A determination is also made as to whether the patient is impulsive with eating. Does he pay attention and think about how fast and how much he is attempting to swallow?

Bedside assessment of the swallow at the pharyngeal level involves noting whether the patient can initiate a swallow and whether he can manage his own saliva while awake and during sleep. Using a penlight and a tongue blade, velopharyngeal closure is observed while the patient says "ah." **Velopharyngeal closure** is the closing off of the nasal passageway with the **soft palate** by contacting the posterior pharyngeal wall. Gently probing both sides of the back of the throat and posterior tongue also assesses the **gag reflex.**

The primary goal of the bedside assessment at the esophageal–laryngeal stage is to see how well the patient can ultimately protect and clear his airway from foreign bodies and propel food to the stomach. Does he have a productive cough, elevate and tip anteriorly the larynx, and close the vocal cords? To see if the vocal cords are capable of completely closing during the swallow, the patient's voice quality is assessed. Does he have a weak, breathy, or absent voice?

Only so much can be learned about a patient's swallow at the bedside. It is particularly difficult to know whether the patient silently aspirates by this assessment. Daniels, McAdam, Brailey, and Foundas (1997) found six critical features indicating severe dysphagia: dysphonia, dysarthria, abnormal volitional cough, abnormal gag reflex, cough after swallow, and voice change after a swallow. The presence of two of the clinical features distinguished patients with moderate to severe dysphagia from patients with a normal swallow or mild dysphagia. When the bedside evaluation shows that the patient is at risk for aspiration, a special type of X-ray procedure is warranted. The second part of the dysphagia evaluation is called a *videofluoroscopic swallow study* (VSS). This test, which is done in the radiology department, is sometimes also called a *modified barium esophagram*, or simply a *barium swallow*.

A VSS is an important test to decide whether a patient is aspirating food or liquid. Barium is a liquid or paste that, when swallowed, shows up on an X-ray procedure. A VSS is a moving X-ray procedure where the movement of the liquid or paste is seen in real time; it can also be taped and studied later. Sometimes, another food item, such as a cookie, is soaked in the barium liquid to show better how well the patient can chew and swallow.

During a VSS, the speech–language pathologist is present. The clinician watches the substance move from the patient's mouth to stomach on a television monitor. During the study, problems with liquid containment, mastication, bolus creation and movement, swallow reflex initiation, and coordination are noted. What is most important is that the clinician note whether liquid or particles of food are aspirated into the air passageways, and whether the patient can remove them with a cough or by throat clearing. Sometimes during the study, the clinician has the patient try to chew and swallow differently to see if there are safer ways to eat.

A common reason why a patient aspirates food and liquid into the air passageways is because of pooling. Liquid and food particles sometimes pool at the base of the tongue at a place called the *vallecula* or in the *pyriform sinuses* at the level of the vocal cords (Figure 7.2). Then, when the patient inspires, or breathes in, the liquid or foodstuffs are sucked into the air passageways. If she cannot feel this happen or does not have enough strength to clear the airway, then foreign bodies get into the lungs. When a sufficient amount of bacteria-laden substances contaminates the lungs, then the patient is at risk for aspiration pneumonia. The occurrence of pneumonia is 7.5 times greater in stroke patients who aspirate than in those who do not (Schmidt, Holas, Halvorson, & Reding, 1994). Pneumonia is a dangerous and life-threatening medical condition with the mortality rate of 43% in hospitalized elderly patients who develop it (Gonzalez & Calia, 1975).

Dysphagia Therapy

Although there are several therapies for patients with dysphagia, the success of these therapies depends on the nature and severity of the disorders. These therapies are commonsense changes in the way that the patient eats, to help him more successfully manage food and reduce the risk of choking and aspiration. Fortunately, with therapy, many patients can learn to meet their nutritional needs orally and again have the pleasure and satisfaction of eating normally.

The patient's attending physician, nurse, nurse's aide, occupational therapist, registered dietitian, and speech–language pathologist work together in dysphagia therapy, which usually has three aspects. First, the texture of the foods and the thickness of the liquids given to the patient may need to be adjusted. As a rule, the thicker the liquid, the easier it is for the patient to control it. Consequently, patients are given naturally thick liquids such as some soups, sauces, and gravies. Sometimes, the clinician will make naturally thin liquids thicker by adding a tasteless, artificial thickener. It can be added to coffee, teas, and thin soups to make them thicker, thus easier for the patient to handle. A registered dietitian oversees the thickness of the food items. Most patients must start with a pureed diet, food that has been chopped and blended to a near-liquid form. Patients with mild dysphagia may be able to tolerate chopped food or soft diets. In therapy the temperature of the food or liquid is used to help the patient track it in her mouth, throat, and stomach. When food or liquid is either hot or cold, rather than tepid, the patient can better monitor it.

The second part of dysphagia therapy involves head and body positioning of the patient. Some patients do better if they are sitting up in a chair or in their bed, whereas others can swallow more efficiently if they are leaning a little forward or backward. The goal is to let gravity help with the swallow. Having the patient turn her head during the swallow is also helpful for some types of dysphagia.

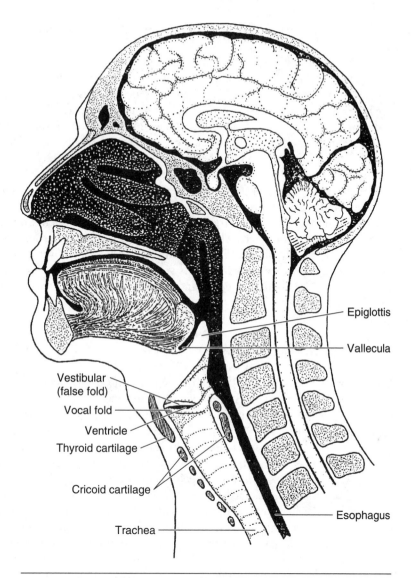

Epiglottis

Vallecula

Vestibular
(false fold)

Vocal fold

Ventricle

Thyroid cartilage

Cricoid cartilage

Esophagus

Trachea

FIGURE 7.2   *The Vallecula and Other Laryngal Structures*

Source: W. Culbertson & D. Tanner, *Introductory Speech and Hearing Anatomy and Physiology Workbook.* Copyright 1997. Reprinted by permission by Allyn & Bacon.

The third aspect to dysphagia therapy involves having the patient time and monitor chewing and swallowing. The patient is taught to carefully chew and contain the food and liquids and to be mindful and prudent when moving them to the back of the throat for swallowing. Many patients find it helpful to take a deep breath before swallowing and to push the air out after the swallow, sometimes while saying a sound such as "ah." They must be careful never to attempt to breathe while the food or liquid is in the throat. Dry swallows are encouraged to help the patient better clear the throat after ingesting food or liquids. *Dry swallows* are the purposeful repeated swallows after the initial one to help clear the air passageway.

For patients with severe dysphagia, sometimes it is necessary that they have an IV, NG, or PEG tube. An IV, or an intravenous line, is a needle inserted into a blood vessel. An NG, a nasogastric tube, goes through the patient's nose to the stomach. A PEG tube is like a nasogastric tube, but it goes directly into the patient's stomach. All are used to supply needed fluids and nutrients. The IV and NG tubes are usually temporary ways of providing fluids and nutrients to the patient. They are sometimes used while the patient is getting dysphagia therapy. The PEG tube is often a permanent way the patient can get fluids and nutrients. It is used for patients who are never able to meet their nutritional needs orally.

Although dysphagia is not a communication disorder, it has become an important clinical responsibility of the profession of speech–language pathology. Clinicians practicing in a medical environment have a large number of dysphagic patients on their caseloads. Even speech–language pathologists who work in educational settings sometimes evaluate and treat children who have dysphagia. Feeding and swallowing objectives can be a part of the treatment of children who have birth defects such as cerebral palsy, muscular dystrophy, cleft lip, and cleft palate. In addition, feeding and swallowing problems are seen in pediatric traumatic brain injuries.

Literature and Media Stereotypes

Patients who have motor speech disorders are not necessarily cognitively impaired. Although motor speech disorders can occur with diseases and disorders that can reduce intellectual functioning, when they occur in pure forms, they are not a result of mental impairments. Therefore, many people with apraxia of speech and the dysarthrias can continue to function in society, albeit with impaired communication. This allows them to be both viable and visible. They can continue to function as scientists, actors, and politicians.

Because people with motor speech disorders can be highly functional even with severe communication disorders, society seems awed by them. As with Stephen Hawking, this can cause dissonance between preconceived notions about people with severe communication disorders and the reality of his mental abilities. The stereotypical view of people confined to a wheelchair and being unable to talk signals severe intellectual incompetence. Conventional wisdom suggests that a person with a severe disability must also be mentally retarded. The reality of Hawking not being mentally deficient and actually intellectually superior to most people is remarkable and awe provoking. He is also highly visible. He appears on television and expresses, through his speech synthesizer, complex and thoughtful ideas. Hawking is a superb example of stereotypical beliefs and attitudes being in direct conflict with reality about some people with severe communication disorders.

Rarely do media and literature distinguish between the language disorder of aphasia and the motor speech impairment of apraxia of speech. Writers and filmmakers tend to lump them together and do not separate "language" disorders from "speech" pathologies. Consequently, many people believe aphasia is when a person "knows what he or she wants to say but cannot say it." Actually, this best describes motor speech disorders, not aphasia. In aphasia the words are not available; aphasics have a language disorder. In pure apraxia of speech, the words are available in internal monologue, but it is the plan of speech that is lost.

Like stuttering and articulation impairments, some motor speech disorders continue to be used by filmmakers for their humor value. In the film *Deuce Bigalow: Male Gigolo*, the hyperkinetic dysarthria associated with Tourette syndrome is used to add bizarre humor to one of the characters. Although the film is a comedy and not intended to be a detailed exploration of human maladies, it does not delve into the character's psychological predicament. There is no attempt to explore Ruth's ways of dealing with the disorder. The film does make a social statement when her coprolalia occurs at a baseball game, suggesting that uncontrolled swearing is sometimes acceptable depending on the situation. Her behaviors at the baseball game were not considered extremely unusual.

Many books and films deal with individuals who must be fed by their loved ones. However, nothing in popular literature and media clearly shows the risks of aspiration pneumonia. Most books and films simply reveal the need of the patient to be fed by a friend or loving family member. The writers do not try to explain the risks of choking and aspiration pneumonia. They have not fully used the educational value of media and literature to give the public more information about choking, silent aspiration, and pneumonia.

Motor speech disorders, particularly the dysarthrias, create dissonance in public perception. Many people with motor speech disorders are highly visible and continue to have productive, successful lives. Their ability to adjust and cope with their communication disorder both intrigues and confuses many people.

Summary

Motor speech disorders impair the motoric aspects of speech communication. There are two categories of motor speech disorders: apraxia of speech and the dysarthrias. Both neurogenic communication disorders affect to various degrees the motor aspects of speech production: respiration, phonation, articulation, resonance, and prosody. In pure motor speech disorders, there are no cognitive, language, or intellectual deficits. Oral and limb apraxia are nonspeech programming disorders that sometimes occur with neurogenic communication disorders. The treatment of apraxia of speech and the dysarthrias depends on the type of motor impairment. Dysphagia often occurs with neurogenic communication disorders, and the evaluation and treatment of it has become a major responsibility of clinicians working in a medical setting. The most common fallacious stereotype about motor speech disorders is that people with them must also be mentally deficient. Cognitive dissonance is experienced by many people when they discover that intellect is not necessarily impaired even in the most severe cases of motor speech disoders.

Study Questions

1. List the five motor speech processes.

2. What are the "big three" neurogenic communication disorders?

3. Provide examples of overshooting and undershooting of the speech articulators.

4. Describe *automatic speech*.

5. List and discuss the apraxias.

6. Describe how antagonist and agonist muscles work.

7. List each of the dysarthrias and describe their symptoms.

8. What is the *acceleration phenomenon*?

9. Describe the three stages of a normal swallow.

10. What is a *video swallow study*?

11. What is an *IV*, an *NG tube*, and a *PEG tube*?

12. What are some common misconceptions about people with motor speech disorders?

Suggested Reading

Duffy, J. (1995). *Motor speech disorders.* St. Louis: Mosby. This text covers the motor speech disorders and provides comprehensive information about them.

Tanner, D. (1999). *The family guide to surviving stroke and communication disorders.* Boston: Allyn & Bacon. This book, written in easily understood language, discusses the "big three" neurogenic communication disorders. There is also a short story about a man who has apraxia of speech, dysarthria, and dysphagia and goes through rehabilitation.

Tanner, D. (2003). *The psychology of neurogenic communication disorders: A primer for health care professionals.* Boston: Allyn & Bacon. This book explores the psychology and coping characteristics of people with motor speech disorders.

8

Aphasia in Adults

Chapter Preview

Aphasia is a language disorder, and it disrupts or eliminates all avenues of communication. In this chapter you will learn about the areas of the brain that are responsible for language expression and understanding. In addition, you will learn the causes of aphasia and related disorders and the ways of classifying them. This chapter discusses specific speaking, reading, writing, mathematical, gestural, and understanding manifestations of the syndrome of aphasia. Also explored are the word-retrieval behaviors employed by people with aphasia and their tendency to be on a concrete level with regard to thinking. You will discover that aphasia can be very frustrating. There are also several psychological components to aphasia: exaggerated emotions, anxiety, depression, grief, and how some patients have difficulty shifting from one thought and behavior to another. Finally, you will examine how the media and literature deal with this major communication disorder.

Aphasia is a loss of language due to stroke, head trauma, or another type of brain damage. It results in partial or complete impairment of all avenues of language expression and reception. Few disorders and disabilities can wreak as much havoc on a person's life as does aphasia. (See Box 8.1.) Aphasia usually comes on suddenly, giving the individual little time to prepare for it. Before aphasia, a person is enjoying the capacity to use language in all its forms. He will be speaking with loved ones, writing notes and letters, reading magazines and books, and understanding the speech of others. Then, in an instant, this marvelous human ability to use and understand language can be taken away. Aphasia can be devastating to the person afflicted by it and to his loved ones.

Language plays a vital role in our day-to-day existence. Modern society revolves around it. Spoken and written language are fundamental to our educational, political, and religious institutions. Language is the foundation of literature, and there would be no media without it. To be deprived of language because of aphasia is to be reduced to near-primitive levels of existence. Aphasia can devastate relationships with family and friends and eliminate one's livelihood. Nevertheless, many people are not victims to this disorder; through rehabilitation, work, and sheer determination, they become victors.

Literature, Media, and Personality Profiles

Patricia Neal

Actor Patricia Neal was born in Knoxville, Tennessee, and after high school she traveled to New York City to pursue an acting career. In 1946 she moved to Hollywood to work for Warner Bros. Studios. Her films include *John Loves Mary* and *The Hasty Heart*, with Ronald Reagan; *The Fountainhead*, with Gary Cooper; and *Operation Pacific*, with John Wayne. She also worked in the United States and England on several stage plays. In 1963, she won an Oscar for Best Actress in her role in the movie *Hud*, with Paul Newman.

When she was 3 months pregnant, Neal suffered a series of strokes that left her paralyzed and aphasic. After years of rehabilitation, she returned to her acting career and won an Oscar nomination for the film *The Subject Was Roses*. Since her strokes she has had several television roles including *The Lou Gehrig Story* and *All's Quiet on the Western Front*. She has appeared on *Little House on the Prairie* and *Murder, She Wrote*. She also appeared in *Cookie's Fortune*, which was released in 1999.

Neal has been very active in advocating for head trauma and stroke survivors. The Patricia Neal Rehabilitation Center in Knoxville—a 72-bed rehabilitation facility for stroke, spinal cord injuries, and traumatic brain injuries—is dedicated to her. Her autobiography, *As I Am*, was published in 1988. Neal continues her acting career and has become a role model for many people with aphasia.

Regarding Henry

Paramount Pictures released *Regarding Henry* in 1991. Directed by Mike Nichols and Jeffrey Abrams, it stars Harrison Ford as Henry Turner, an ambitious, ruthless, and successful New York lawyer. He is shot in the head during a holdup, and the story revolves around his rehabilitation and rebuilding of the relationships with his wife and daughter. Besides several physical and psychological disabilities resulting from the gunshot wound, Henry is initially aphasic. In many ways the head trauma reduces him to a childlike state, and he learns to appreciate the simple aspects of life. Henry becomes more likable as he rediscovers himself, his wife, and his daughter. Ultimately, the head trauma serves to make him a better man.

Wings

In 1978 Arthur Kopit released *Wings*, a Broadway play about aphasia. The play was commissioned by Earplay, the drama project of National Public Radio. Kopit's interest in the subject was prompted by his father having a stroke that rendered him aphasic. While his father was in rehabilitation, Kopit observed several people with aphasia and began pondering what their worlds were like. One female patient was a former "wing-walker," and the title of the play grew from the courage and freedom of that vocation. In the play Mrs. Stilson has a composite of aphasic symptoms; she does not just present with one type of aphasia.

Kopit was drawn to the inner world of aphasia by watching his father and trying to understand what it was like to be deprived of language. Kopit detected an attempt by his father to communicate. Despite the global reduction in his communication abilities, his father tried to escape his prison.

Wings is a monumental work of art about aphasia. The author conducted extensive research into aphasia and then created a play that captures the isolation, desolation, and hope in a way only a skilled playwright can do. In many ways the audience walks away from *Wings* knowing more about this disorder and the people who have it than can be learned by reading textbooks and case studies on the subject.

The New Twilight Zone: *"Word Play"*

The New Twilight Zone was based on the bizarre theme of Rod Serling's 1960s hit television series *The Twilight Zone*. *The New Twilight Zone* episodes, produced by CBS Entertainment Productions, were in color and had more production value. One episode entitled "Word Play" involved a man who gradually loses the semantics of language. Written by Rockne S. O'Bannon, directed by Wes Craven, it stars Robert Klein and Annie Potts.

The semantic nightmare begins when a medical salesperson, Bill Lowerly (Robert Klein), dresses and goes to work. At first, his wife, played by Annie Potts, only occasionally uses a word wrongly. At work a coworker remarks that he and Lowerly have "one thing only time can give you . . . 'mayonnaise.'" On the telephone Lowerly's boss reports that they cannot meet because he and his wife are going to celebrate their 17th "throw rug." In the elevator, a coworker asks Lowerly if he knows a good place to take a date for "dinosaur," and at home his wife remarks that his son was too sick to touch his "dinosaur." At this point Lowerly panics and demands to know if "dinosaur" is a new expression for lunch. He finds that the word *lunch* now means a "reddish" color. As time progresses, all the meanings of words he once shared with the community are lost. This is true for written words as well; a sign in his car reminds him to fasten his "Step Dad." During a medical crisis a hospital, Lowerly is completely unable to communicate with his wife and the medical staff. While evaluating his son, a nurse remarks, "One mental eight been cattle renting Jupiter."

Although the main character in this episode apparently does not suffer a stroke or other brain injury, the television show portrays the mulitmodality loss of language experienced by many aphasic persons. It vividly shows the isolation, separation, and panic felt by a person who has lost the ability to communicate. Even while praying, Lowerly wonders if God can understand him. At the conclusion of the show, he is shown trying to learn the words and their meanings in much the same way as aphasic persons do. Lowerly is staring at a picture of a dog and learning to call it "Wednesday."

Legends of the Fall

Released by TriStar, *Legends of the Fall* was nominated for four Golden Globe Awards and won the 1994 Academy Award for Best Cinematography. The story is about a retired colonel and his three sons in Montana during the early 1900s. It is a love story about the three sons and the woman they loved. Toward the end of the movie, Colonel Ludlow, played by Anthony Hopkins, suffers a stroke and is aphasic and dysarthric. Initially, he communicates by writing on a slate, which hangs around his neck. Based on the novella by Jim Harrison, it was directed by Edward Zwick and stars Brad Pitt, Aidan Quinn, Julia Ormond, and Henry Thomas.

Language and the Brain

The brain is divided into two halves, or hemispheres. These two sides are almost identical in appearance, but they are not identical in function. The right side of the brain controls the left side of the body, and vice versa. Consequently, a person who has damage on the left side of the brain often has paralysis or weakness on the right side of the body. In most people the left hemisphere is dominant for most language functions. The right hemisphere is sometimes

BOX 8.1 • *Understanding Aphasia*

Understanding what it is like to have aphasia is difficult because language is second nature. One way of understanding aphasia is to compare it to being in a foreign country and not being able to speak the language. Suppose you were transported to this new country and found yourself in a college classroom. As you sit in the classroom, you can hear and see the professor speak, but you do not understand one word that is being said. You also hear other students in the classroom talk among themselves, but you do not understand them, either. The professor writes on the blackboard, and the marks appear as random scribbles. When you ask for information or direction, the people in the classroom look at you with confusion because your speech is strange and bewildering to them. In aphasia your inner speech may also be disrupted. When you think to yourself, your words do not make sense or they are unavailable. Your experience in this classroom is similar to what it is like to have aphasia.

wrongly called the "silent" hemisphere, but it is not completely silent and is certainly *not* inactive. Basic, noncomplex speech and language functions are located in the right hemisphere in most left hemisphere–dominant people. In a small percentage of left-handed people, the right hemisphere is dominant for language.

The right hemisphere is involved in spatial–temporal planning and execution. *Spatial–temporal functions* concern planning and executing movements over space and time. The right hemisphere is also more intuitive, artistic, and creative. When there is damage to the right hemisphere of the brain in a left-dominant individual, the person may have trouble grasping the totality of an idea and completing a job that requires a series of small steps. Sometimes people with right-hemisphere damage have denial of their disabilities and show "la belle indifference," or lack of concern about them.

The left hemisphere is considered the logical and rational side of the brain. It is also where complex language processing occurs in most people. When discussing language processing, dividing this hemisphere into two sections is convenient. The dividing line, a fissure that separates the frontal lobe from the parietal lobe, is the **central sulcus,** or the fissure of Rolando. Although certain functions can be attributed to particular lobes, they get their names from the bones of the skull. The lobes of the brain are not functional designations, they are anatomical ones.

The area in the front of the central sulcus, the area anterior to it, is important in motor movements. This area contains the **motor strip,** which is involved in causing movements. It also contains **Broca's area**—named after an early neurologist, Paul Broca, who identified the area of the brain in the frontal lobe that is responsible for combining the movements of the articulatory structures into words (see Chapter 7). He discovered this area by doing postmortem examinations on patients who had been under his care during the final months of their lives and who had problems expressing themselves. Their speech problems were not due to tongue paralysis. In 1865 Broca uttered this famous statement: "We speak with the left hemisphere."

When a person has damage to this area of the brain, she has Broca's aphasia. A person with Broca's aphasia has choppy and nonfluent speech with pauses, fillers, and struggled attempts to speak. It is primarily an expressive communication disorder, meaning that comprehension is usually near normal. Often, there are also word-finding deficits and expressive grammatical problems. Depending on the nature and degree of the damage to the anterior parts of the left hemisphere, patients also may have problems writing and using complicated gestures.

Wernicke's area is primarily in the temporal lobe. It is named after the nineteenth-century neurologist Karl Wernicke who discovered the area of the brain where reception and understanding of speech occur. It is posterior and inferior, or behind and below, the central sulcus. When a person has damage to Wernicke's area, it is called Wernicke's aphasia.

Wernicke's aphasia causes difficulty comprehending the language of others. Most of the time, damage to this area does not result in the patient having problems initiating and planning speech. Whereas patients with Broca's aphasia have trouble with the expressive aspects of communication and are nonfluent, patients with Wernicke's aphasia have problems comprehending language, and their speech tends to be **fluent.** Fluent speech that is empty of meaning is called **jargon.** These expressive and receptive disorders are discussed in detail later. Figure 8.1 identifies Broca's and Wernicke's areas of the brain.

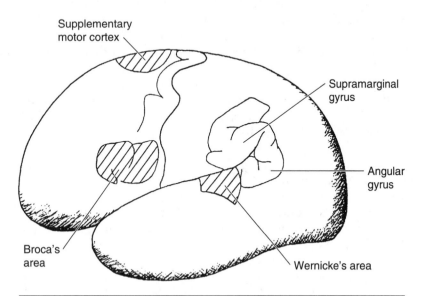

FIGURE 8.1   *Broca's and Wernicke's Areas of the Human Brain*

Source: W. Perkins & R. Kent, *Functional Anatomy of Speech, Language, and Hearing.* Copyright 1986. Reprinted by permission by Allyn & Bacon.

Etiology of Aphasia and Related Disorders

One of the leading causes of aphasia and other neuropathologies of speech and language is stroke. A **stroke** occurs when the blood supply to the brain is interrupted. There are two categories of strokes: hemorrhagic and occlusive.

A *hemorrhagic stroke* happens when there is a "blowout" of a blood vessel. Usually because of high blood pressure, an area in the vascular system bursts. Sometimes this burst is preceded by an **aneurysm,** a swollen part of an artery. When the burst is in the brain, a stroke occurs. Consequently, blood cannot flow to areas that need it. In addition, blood spills into other areas of the brain, increasing the pressure inside the skull. An *occlusive stroke* occurs when there is a blockage, or "plug," in an **artery.** The blockage can be a blood clot or other type of obstruction. When the plug originates elsewhere in the body and finally lodges in the brain, it is called a cerebral **embolism.** When the blockage originates in the brain, it is called a cerebral **thrombosis.**

The severity of aphasia is related to the site and size of the brain damage. As a rule, larger brain damage results in more severe aphasia. However, when small areas of the brain that are important to language are damaged, severe aphasia can result. Even small strokes can result in severe communication disorders. Sometimes, the blood flow to the brain is only temporally interrupted. When the blood flow to the brain is interrupted for less than 24 hours and the person's symptoms are temporary, it is called a **transient ischemic attack** (TIA). When these events result in communication disorders, they are only temporary.

Many diseases that affect the brain can cause aphasia; the most severe is cancer. When the brain tumor affects the speech and language centers, or the tracts leading to or from them, aphasia can result. In addition, chemotherapy, radiation treatments, and surgeries to remove or destroy cancer can also damage areas of the brain that are responsible for speech and language functioning. Infections of the brain, chronic alcoholism, and degenerative diseases can also cause aphasia.

Automobile accidents, gunshot wounds, falls, shrapnel, and blows to the head—to name only a few—can cause head trauma. When head trauma damages the areas of the brain responsible for speech and language functioning, aphasia can result. (Head traumas are discussed in detail in Chapter 10.)

The Syndrome of Aphasia

Aphasia is a **syndrome,** a combination or cluster of symptoms that usually occur together. There are many ways of classifying aphasia and related disorders. Some classification systems have historical importance. Wernicke, for example, was first to classify and describe the various types of aphasia. Other classification systems are of interest to specialists. Physicians, scientists, and speech–language pathologists often have different reasons for labeling and classifying aphasia.

Because the human ability to use and understand language is complicated, classifying language disorders is also complicated. Although there are variations in the different types of aphasia, it is convenient to classify them simply as either predominantly **expressive** or **receptive language** disorders. The expressive disorders go by several names, and aphasiologists are not consistent in their usage. Damage to Broca's and adjacent areas causes expressive problems, and they are sometimes called Broca's aphasia (includes apraxia of speech), telegraphic speech, nonfluent aphasia, predominantly expressive aphasia, motor aphasia, and anterior aphasia. Damage to Wernicke's and adjacent areas causes receptive problems, and they are sometimes called Wernicke's aphasia, jargon aphasia, fluent aphasia, predominantly receptive aphasia, sensory aphasia, and posterior aphasia. Severe or complete damage to both areas of the brain is called global aphasia, irreversible aphasia syndrome, and severe, profound, or complete aphasia. Table 8.1 shows these expressive and receptive categories.

Aphasia: A Multimodality Disorder

Aphasia is not just a problem with talking, and it is not a "speech" disorder (Darley, 1982). It is a language disorder that usually disrupts all modalities, or avenues, of communication. The expressive **modalities** of communication are verbal expression, writing, and expressive gestures. The receptive avenues are auditory comprehension, reading, and receptive gestures. Most aphasic patients also have problems doing simple arithmetic because mathematics is a language unto itself.

Reading and writing are called *graphic modalities*. When reading and writing are disturbed in aphasia, it is not because of vision acuity deficits or hand paralysis. Graphic disturbances in aphasia are a result of central language deficiencies; reading and writing as a linguistic form of communication is impaired. Graphic disturbances are different from other types of communication deficiencies in aphasia because reading and writing are the products of formal education. Unlike speaking and auditory comprehension, which all normal children naturally learn, reading and writing must be taught.

Alexia

Alexia is the complete inability to read and is sometimes called *word blindness*. (**Dyslexia** refers to partial reading deficits, a less severe form of alexia.) Word blindness is an inaccurate

TABLE 8.1 *Expressive and Receptive Language Disorders of Aphasia*

Expressive Language Disorders	Receptive Language Disorders	Expressive and Receptive Language Disorders
Broca's aphasia (includes apraxia of speech)	Wernicke's aphasia	Complete aphasia
Anterior aphasia	Fluent aphasia	Global aphasia
Motor aphasia	Jargon aphasia	Irreversible aphasia syndrome
Nonfluent aphasia	Predominantly receptive aphasia	Severe aphasia
Predominantly expressive aphasia	Posterior aphasia	Profound aphasia
Telegraphic speech	Sensory aphasia	

way of describing reading disturbances because it suggests that the problem is with the patient's eyes. Although strokes, head traumas, and diseases can result in blindness and visual field cuts, the alexia seen in aphasia is not because the patient has difficulty seeing the printed page but is a result of deficiencies in perceiving and processing printed, written, or drawn symbols.

There are several different types of alexia. Sometimes, patients cannot read because they no longer recognize letters and other written symbols. At the perceptual level, patients cannot decipher them. Typically, patients with this type of alexia cannot read words, but when they are traced on their hands or spelled aloud, words can be understood. Some patients cannot read what they have just written; this is called *alexia without agraphia*, reading problems without accompanying writing difficulties.

Alexia can also result from loss of meanings of written words. In this type of alexia, patients can read the word, but they have forgotten what it means. For example, if a written command says "Point to the pen," patients cannot respond correctly because they have forgotten the meaning of the word *point* or *pen*. In *Word Play*, Lowerly experiences alexia when the "Fasten Seat Belt" sign reads "Fasten Step Dad." Alexia also can be caused by poor attention, confusion with the meanings of similar words, and not being able to grasp the entire idea of the text.

The type of alexia seen in aphasia depends on the site and size of the damage in the brain. Often, patients with aphasia and alexia have a combination of reading problems. They have forgotten some of the meanings of written words, are confused about letters, have poor attention, and have difficulties grasping a written idea. The way a patient has been taught to read is an important consideration. Some patients have been taught to "sound out" words, whereas others have been taught to read by learning "sight" words. Some schools teach a combination of methods. It is important to remember that alexia is *not* a result of the patient never being taught to read or to being a poor reader before the brain injury.

Deciding why the patient cannot read is necessary so that appropriate therapies can be provided. Therapy for alexia begins at the lowest level where successful performance can be obtained. Patients may have to relearn letters, small words, or how to keep their attention on the reading task to improve comprehension.

Agraphia

The **agraphia** seen with aphasia is the inability to express oneself in writing, *not* due to paralysis. Some patients have a weak or paralyzed arm, particularly those with Broca's aphasia, and consequently they have trouble writing. However, the writing problems in aphasia are not limited to this motor problem. Patients with agraphia resulting from aphasia cannot write even when they hold the pen or pencil in their left hand. Certainly, when patients who are right-handed try to write with their left hands, it is usually done less legibly, but the thoughts can be expressed nonetheless.

With few exceptions, aphasic patients write like they speak. The writing of fluent jargon by aphasic patients tends to be like their speech—meaningless. It is filled with words that do not make sense in a sentence, letters put together that do not make identifiable words, or unintelligible, random scribbles. Nonfluent aphasic patients write haltingly, much like they speak. The writing of the nonfluent aphasic person is filled with many errors. Letters are created clumsily, and words are misspelled. The patient appears perplexed at the task of writing. In the movie *Legends of the Fall*, Colonel Ludlow suffers a stroke and initially appears to have Broca's aphasia and dysarthria. However, early post-onset, when he writes, his writing is done legibly and with proper grammar and syntax. His writing contrasts with his verbal output, which is typical of severe Broca's aphasia and dysarthria. Although this type of discrepancy between verbal and graphic output can occur, it is not typical of Broca's aphasia.

Patients with severe writing problems may have problems copying geometric forms. For example, if a square is drawn on a sheet of paper, the patient cannot draw it. In higher-level writing deficits, the patient will have trouble writing while someone dictates the sentences.

Not only do patients typically write like they speak, but they often have a concurrent problem with reading. However, there is a rare form of agraphia called *pure dysgraphia*, or *agraphia without alexia*, in which the patient's writing and spelling are impaired, but reading is only slightly affected, if at all.

Therapy for agraphia involves learning to control the pen or pencil, copy geometric forms, make letters, and write names. Writing words of increasing length, sentences, and short paragraphs are also goals of therapy. Writing to dictation is one of the highest goals of therapy. Some treatment models of aphasia suggest that the patient be taught to write with his nondominant hand regardless of whether he has control problems. For example, although a patient is right-handed but still can grasp and control the pen or pencil, it is suggested that he use the nondominant hand so that the nondamaged hemisphere is used. (Recall that the left hemisphere controls the right side of the body, and vice versa.)

Acalculia

Acalculia is the inability to do and understand simple mathematics due to brain damage. **Dyscalculia** refers to partial deficits doing simple math problems, a less severe form of acalculia. It is important to understand that acalculia is for "simple" mathematics. It is not restricted to complex formulas and difficulty doing calculus, algebra, statistics, and geometry. Acalculia is the inability to do simple and common mathematical problems such as counting and knowing that $2 + 2 = 4$ and $5 - 3 = 2$. Making change is one of the most important and practical problems experienced by the aphasic person. A patient with acalculia would not know how much money she should get back from a $10 bill if something cost $6.50. She would also have problems giving a customer the correct change.

There are two reasons why aphasic patients have problems doing simple mathematical problems:

1. Doing mathematical problems involves speaking, reading, and writing. When a person does a math problem on paper, he must write it down and read what has been written. When the math problem is done orally, he must say words and numbers and understand what is spoken to him. Whatever problems an aphasic patient has with these avenues of communication will contribute to the acalculia.
2. Math, too, is a language. Written signs—such as equal, multiply, divide, sum, and percent—have symbolic meaning, the same as typical words do. Math problems have a

grammar and syntax to the expressions. When aphasia disrupts the fabric of language, the deficiencies also extend to the language of math.

The procedures for treating acalculia are similar to those for alexia and agraphia. The goal is to start at the lowest level where successful performance can be obtained and then proceed, in gradual steps, to higher-level performance. With patients with severe reductions in the ability to do math, therapy may require starting with very simple problems such as multiplying or adding single digits. Many patients must relearn the meanings of coins and paper money. Higher-level activities include doing more complex math problems, making change, and doing practical budgeting activities. Fundamental to this therapy is that the patients learn to check their figures for accuracy.

Gestural Problems

Aphasia often disrupts the ability to use and understand complicated **gestures.** This is particularly true of severe aphasia. However, most aphasic patients retain the ability to communicate with simple gestures. Many aphasic patients can understand the meaning of a pat on the back, handshake, or the thumbs-up gesture. They can usually point to something they want or shake their heads no if they want you to stop doing something. This is not to say that in some aphasic patients the ability to use and understand simple gestures is not impaired.

For most aphasic patients, expressing themselves with complicated gestures is impaired. Because of the aphasia, the patient cannot point to several objects in a room to communicate an idea. For example, a patient with severe aphasia would have difficulty indicating to a nursing aide to have a bathrobe brought from the closet so that she can get out of bed and walk to the toilet. The same difficulties would be experienced for the patient when she tries to understand complicated finger and hand gestures.

Sometimes, family and friends ask the speech–language pathologist to teach the patient sign language. The idea behind this request is that the patient can bypass the aphasia by learning to communicate with signs. At first glance, this seems to be a viable option. Unfortunately for aphasic patients, learning sign language is not a productive therapy. Signing is a language just like any other language—for example, English, Hopi, Navajo, or Italian. To teach sign language to bypass aphasia is futile because the language centers of the brain are damaged. The problem with communicating is not with the function of the breathing mechanism, larynx, or articulators; it is the use and understanding of symbols that is lost. In addition, teaching sign language is not practical because most people do not use or understand it. For sign language to be a viable option, everyone who tries to communicate with the aphasic patient would have to learn it. Sometimes a speech–language pathologist will teach an aphasic patient hand gestures as part of therapy. However, the goal is to help the patient retrieve words and to facilitate expressions, *not* to use gestures as an alternative to speech communication.

Sign language can be a viable option for some patients with motor speech disorders. For patients who have not had their language centers damaged by a stroke, head trauma, or disease but who have problems with breath support, voicing, and articulation, sign language can be an alternative communication system. However, even in these cases, often better alternatives—such as speech synthesizers, communication boards, and computers—are preferred. Practical gestures, such as pointing to a picture and being able accurately to nod yes/no, can be taught to many aphasic patients, to help them learn **functional communication.**

Predominantly Expressive, Nonfluent Aphasia

In expressive aphasia, patients have trouble writing and using complicated gestures to express themselves. These are expressive components of the syndrome of aphasia. However, most people use speech as the primary way of expressing their thoughts and feelings on a day-to-day basis. Professionals and laypersons often label the speech of expressive aphasic patients as Broca's aphasia. (Recall, Broca's area is in the frontal lobe of the left hemisphere of the brain.) Broca's and adjacent areas of the brain—and the tracts leading to and from them—are responsible for expressive speech and language in most people.

There are four components to the speech of a person with expressive aphasia (Table 8.2). The first aspect is motor speech programming (see Chapters 4 and 7). The motor-programming disorder in which the person has trouble planning, sequencing, and executing the actions necessary to make speech sounds is called **apraxia of speech.** For example, when a patient wants to say a word, he must create and execute the speech plan necessary to get the respiratory, phonatory, articulatory, and resonance processes to do it. The respiratory system must take in the correct amount of air and compress it to the degree necessary to get the vocal cords and articulators to shape and valve it into speech. The velum must elevate and lower at just the right times and for the correct duration, to create proper nasalization. Pitch has to be adjusted correctly by the muscles in the larynx and appropriate loudness levels maintained. There also has to be the correct rhythm, speed, cadence, and melody to the expression. All these movements must be planned and executed properly for the word to be said normally. Damage to Broca's area—and the tracts leading to and from it and other areas of the brain—can cause this process to break down. The result is apraxia of speech, and there are struggled, nonfluent attempts to speak because the articulators overshoot, undershoot, or miss completely their targets. Mild levels of apraxia of speech often resemble stuttering, although they are two distinctly different disorders (see Chapter 2). Severe apraxia of speech can render a patient mute.

The second aspect to expressive aphasia is a word-finding problem sometimes called **anomia.** The patient has trouble recalling and saying the correct words for expression. For

TABLE 8.2 *The Factors Associated with Broca's Aphasia*

Factor	Manifestation
Motor speech programming (apraxia of speech)	Person has trouble planning, sequencing, and executing the actions necessary to make speech sounds.
Word-finding problem (anomia)	Person has trouble recalling and retrieving the correct words for expression.
Telegraphic speech (agrammatism)	Person omits function words and uses only content words.
Automatic speech (subcortical speech)	Person has difficulty with purposeful speech but has little problem fluently and clearly saying some words with little forethought.

example, if a patient is asked to name parts of her body, she might correctly say, "nose," when it is pointed to. However, when the examiner points to an ear and says, "What is this called?" the patient might say, "chin" or nothing at all. Further, when the examiner gives the patient several possible names from which to choose, often the patient can recognize the correct one and then say, "ear." These expressive word-finding problems can occur during confrontational naming tasks, like in the above example, or they can occur during spontaneous speech. Severe anomia can render a patient mute, whereas mild word-finding problems can simply be a nuisance.

The third aspect to expressive aphasia is **telegraphic speech:** Function words are omitted, and the patient uses only content words. This type of speech resembles a telegram. When telegrams were used to communicate over long distances, the companies charged by the word. Naturally, the sender would omit **function words,** such as articles and conjunctions, that were not necessary to express the idea. What remained were **content words** such as nouns and verbs. Aphasic patients with telegraphic speech "telegraph" their ideas in a similar way. Instead of saying "I want to go to the bathroom and brush my teeth," the patient would condense it into "I go bathroom, brush teeth."

Telegraphic speech is sometimes called **agrammatism,** an impairment in the ability to use words in their proper sequence or according to their grammatical functions. It is a breakdown of grammar and syntax. This is a controversial area of aphasia. Some authorities believe that the telegraphic speech is a result of damage to the grammatical and syntactical centers of the brain; that is, telegraphic speech occurs because of a disruption of grammatical and syntactical functions of language. Other aphasiologists believe that telegraphic speech is a result of a general loss of words. Because there is an across-the-board loss of vocabulary and there are more content than function words, telegraphic speech occurs. It is likely that telegraphic speech is a result of both factors.

The fourth aspect of expressive aphasia is **automatic speech** (see Chapter 7), which is sometimes called **subcortical** speech because it is nonpurposeful and nonvolitional. It is the ability to automatically say a sound, word, or phrase when little thought is given to it. It is often present on swear words. A patient with automatic speech may have difficulty with purposeful speech but have little problem fluently and clearly saying swear words. Automatic speech is also present on overlearned and frequently rehearsed utterances such as poems, songs, and memorized phrases.

The following is typical of expressive aphasia. Describing a picture of people on a picnic, the patient displays all four aspects of this communication disorder:

> Ita . . . ita . . . pecture, picture of farge, arge, . . . large, famirly on a sickpic, picnic. The boy Frisbee dog. Table is deeeing, seeing, tet, ah, uh, tet, uh, set. In the tree, a, . . . , a, . . . , In the tree, . . . Everyone, uh, stappy, uh, . . . mappy, . . . Damn it, anyway! Sicknic, picnic happy time.

The motor speech–programming deficit of apraxia of speech is present when the patient tries to say the word *large*. Because the speech act is disrupted at the planning, or execution, level, he overshoots and undershoots the articulation targets. The same types of errors are present on *picnic, being, set,* and *happy*. The patient also cannot remember the word *bird*, which is perched in a tree. This is an example of a word-finding problem, or anomia. It is often difficult to clearly separate an apraxia of speech error from a word-finding one because of their close relationship. Telegraphic speech is present when the patient says, "The boy Frisbee dog." This is a telegrammed statement for "In the picture, the boy is playing Frisbee with his yellow dog." Automatic speech occurs when the patient, in frustration, clearly, fluently, and articulately says, "Damn it, anyway!"

Therapy for predominantly expressive, nonfluent aphasia involves helping the patient retrieve and program words and expand utterances. The grammatical and syntactical structure of expressive utterances are also taught. The goal is to use expressive words and utterances to create the most functional communication system for the patient.

Predominantly Receptive, Fluent Aphasia

The communication disorder of a patient with a predominantly receptive language disturbance is often labeled Wernicke's aphasia. The primary area of damage is Wernicke's area, which is in the temporal lobe; it is the center for understanding oral language. The receptive language centers also extend into the parietal lobe in most people. Understanding what others have spoken is impaired in Wernicke's aphasia. The degree of impaired understanding can range from several words to a complete loss of verbal understanding. Sometimes, jargon speech is also present. There are two types of jargon. Patients with receptive aphasia sometimes make up words called **neologisms.** Of course, all words are made-up, but a neologism is one that cannot be identified as part of the patient's or society's language structure. This type of jargon would sound like this: "The tula er est et tula tula." In the second type of jargon, the patient uses established words but in sentences that do not make sense. An example of it is in "Word Play" when the nurse was reporting on the medical condition of Lowerly's son and said, "One mental eight been cattle renting Jupiter." Many receptive aphasic patients engage in combinations of the two types of jargon.

Why do many receptive aphasic patients speak in jargon? This question arises because, in receptive aphasia, there is little if any damage to the expressive language centers. There is no general agreement among aphasiologists about why patients with this type of aphasia speak in jargon, but there are several possibilities. First, it should be remembered that during communication the brain operates as a whole; that is, no one area operates completely independent of another. Damage to one area often directly or indirectly affects another. Second, jargon speech may result from the patient being unable to monitor her verbal output. Because the patient has trouble understanding, she does not know when nonsense is uttered. Third, the occurrence of jargon speech results from disrupted vocabulary and verbal thinking. Words and their meanings have been disrupted, and the aphasic patient is simply expressing these mixed-up ideas.

The fourth reason why patients speak jargon is psychological. Many receptive aphasic patients continue to attempt to communicate, despite the fact that it has been consistently futile. Why would a person continue to persist in jargon speech when no one apparently understands? In "Word Play" Lowerly finally gives up and simply stops attempting to communicate; he becomes aware that it is pointless. Some patients with jargon aphasia do not give up and stop talking because of the psychological defense of **denial:** They deny there is something wrong with their speech even when it is evident that no one understands them. Some also project their inability to understand on others. The psychological defense of **projection** is the attributing of one's own wishes, thoughts, motivations, and feelings to another person. The patient believes that if the listener would try harder, he would be able to understand. In an interesting study conduced by Lazar, Marshall, Prell, and Pile-Spellman (2000), the authors induced temporary Wernicke's aphasia in a patient. After the patient returned to normal, he was able to recall his attempts to communicate. The study found that there were several independent aspects of Wernicke's aphasia supporting the view that more than one factor accounts for jargon speech.

Although receptive aphasia results in problems understanding the speech of others, it is not the only reason a patient may have trouble correctly answering questions or following instructions. To test comprehension, patients are asked to perform a series of tasks or to answer questions. The degree of auditory comprehension problems is reflected in how well they follow simple and complex verbal instructions and how correctly they respond to the questions. A patient may not be able to follow complex instructions and answer questions correctly because of several reasons.

Factors in Following Complex Verbal Instructions

If a patient is asked to complete a task that requires several steps such as "Please pass the salt, pepper, and sugar," her success indicates more than just intact auditory comprehension. In addition, the type of failure suggests the nature and degree of problems she may be having. A review of how a patient responds to a simple request at the dinner table illustrates the type and nature of potential deficiencies.

The first and most obvious reason the patient may not be able to perform the task may be because her arm is paralyzed or because of limb apraxia (see Chapter 7). In the first instance, the patient understands and knows what to do, but she cannot because of paralysis. In the second instance, the patient may have limb (body) apraxia, and although her arm is not paralyzed, she cannot get it to do what is wanted. For purposeful acts, the patient cannot "will" her arm to do the movements necessary to grasp the salt, pepper, and sugar.

The second reason the patient may not be able to follow the command is because of hearing loss or deafness (see Chapter 6), thus not hearing what you are saying. Most deaf people, however, can understand gestures or sign language or can read your lips to understand the request.

Lack of attention is the third reason the patient may not be able to pass the salt, pepper, and sugar. Her attention may be directed elsewhere. The patient may also be engaging in a psychological defense called *fantasy escape*, where she fantasizes about something pleasurable rather than confront the disability (Tanner, 2003). Partial completion of the task indicates two types of attention deficits: slow rise time and auditory fade.

Slow rise time is when the patient has trouble attending to and comprehending the initial part of the request. To the patient your request may sound like this: ". . . . . . pass . . . the sugar." Consequently, you are likely to get only the sugar, and the salt and pepper will remain on the other side of the table. Auditory fade is the opposite of slow rise time. In *auditory fade* the patient attends to and comprehends the initial aspects of the input, but the final parts are ignored. To the patient your request may sound like this: "Please pass the salt, . . . , . . . , ..." The salt will be given to you, but you must ask again or reach to get the pepper and sugar.

The fourth reason for the patient not to complete successfully the verbal request may be because of agnosia. **Agnosia** is a perceptual disorder in which the patient has trouble attaching meaning to sensory information (see Chapter 4). Agnosia can occur in all the senses. **Auditory agnosia** is a deficit in which the patient has problems with the **perception** of all auditory input. It includes language and nonlanguage signals. With regard to nonlanguage signals, the patient may not appreciate the significance of common environmental sounds such as the ringing or pulsing of a telephone, a knock on a door, or the sound of a smoke alarm. A person with this type of agnosia might answer the door when the telephone rings or do nothing when the fire alarm goes off. **Acoustic agnosia** is a specific type of auditory agnosia in which the patient has trouble distinguishing speech sounds, especially similar ones. To the patient with acoustic agnosia, the individual sounds in your request to pass the salt, pepper, and sugar may seem foreign and unrecognizable.

Salt, pepper, and sugar may not be passed to you because the words have lost their meanings to the patient. This is the fifth reason why she may not be able to follow complex commands. Brain damage may have caused problems with semantic associations. Because of brain injury, the patient may think that "pass" means "point," or she has forgotten altogether what the word means. The patient might give you a spoon rather than the salt or coffee creamer rather than the sugar.

The final reason the patient may be unable to follow your request may be because of cognitive and intellectual deterioration (see Chapter 9). Perhaps, because of cognitive and intellectual deficiency, the patient does not realize that she is in a restaurant or that it is dinnertime. The patient may have difficulty appreciating the situation and what she is supposed to do. Table 8.3 lists the reasons why patients may not follow directional commands.

As you can see, there are a myriad of reasons for patients to be unable to perform complex requests, and they are not necessarily limited to auditory comprehension problems. Many patients with receptive language problems have one or more of the preceding reasons for not following commands or answering questions correctly.

Family members and friends of the patient are often frustrated at being unable to communicate with the aphasic person. Typically, when they find that the patient does not follow requests or answer questions appropriately, they speak louder or even shout. This is a natural thing to do, but it is often confusing for the patient. In the play *Wings*, shouting confuses and angers Mrs. Stilson. Shouting is not helpful in getting the aphasic patient to understand, and it often causes confusion and anger. Therapy involves learning to recognize and understand

---

TABLE 8.3 *Why Patients Might Not Follow Directional Commands*

May not be able to perform the task because of limb paralysis or limb apraxia.

May not be able to follow the commands because of hearing loss and/or deafness.

May have attention directed elsewhere (slow rise time; auditory fade; fantasy escape).

May have trouble attaching meaning to sensory information (agnosia).

May not be able to remember meanings of words.

May have cognitive and intellectual deterioration.

simple, short words and gradually improving the patient's ability to understand the speech of others. Reduction in jargon speech usually happens as auditory comprehension improves.

Loss of the Abstract Attitude

Aphasia, a language disorder, is a form of amnesia; specifically, it is amnesia for words. The person with aphasia has trouble remembering the names of people, places, colors, objects, and so on. There is more to aphasia than just amnesia for words, but loss of the semantics of language is a major aspect of it. Early in the study of aphasia, it was found that this language disorder is associated with an abstract–concrete imbalance in many patients. Aphasic patients, as a group, tend to be on a concrete level for both verbal and nonverbal cognitive tasks. People with aphasia do not do as well as nonaphasic persons with solving higher-level abstract problems, putting things into categories, interpreting proverbs, and the like. This loss of an **abstract attitude** is thought to be a result of impaired language and the resulting inability to bring order to the world.

You would expect there to be difficulty with higher-level cognitive activities on verbal tasks because of the impaired language. However, it has been found that aphasic patients, as a group, also have problems with abstraction on nonverbal tasks such as sorting by color, shape, and size. Although several reasons could account for the loss of abstract attitude for nonverbal tasks, it is possible that this concrete behavior is because of the disruption of language. When a person sorts, categorizes, and sequences objects, and engages in other nonverbal behaviors, language facilitates the process. Words are used to label and generalize and are important parts of abstract cognitive behaviors.

Does an impairment with the ability to abstract mean that aphasic people are mentally retarded? No. Obviously, aphasia results in a cognitive impairment because language is an important part of normal thinking. Nevertheless, aphasia, even severe global aphasia, does not return an individual to a childlike state. Sometimes, literature and media portray an individual with aphasia as being returned to the thinking patterns of a child, such as Henry Turner in the film *Regarding Henry*. Certainly, there are brain injuries, such as bilateral damage to the frontal lobes and diffuse brain damage, that can result in a person regressing to the developmental levels of a child. However, the syndrome of aphasia does not make an individual mentally retarded. An aphasic person may read, write, talk, and even understand the speech of others at reduced levels, but he has *not* been returned to the psychological and cognitive plane of a child. Most patients still retain the memories, visual associations, beliefs, and emotional maturity they possessed before the aphasia. They do not look at the world through the eyes of a child, even though their communication abilities make them appear childlike.

Word-Retrieval Behaviors: Rhyme or Reason

When an aphasic person has problems remembering words, researchers have discovered that there are several retrieval behaviors that can be employed. A good way of exploring their word-retrieval behaviors is to examine what normal people do when they try to remember a person's name. Take, for example, what you do when trying to remember the name of an acquaintance.

Suppose you meet an acquaintance on the street and greet one another. You recognize the person's face and are familiar with her. However, you cannot remember her name. There are several behaviors in which you can engage when trying to place a name with the face. These word-retrieval behaviors are similar to those employed by an aphasic person trying to remember the name of an object, concept, color, animal, and so on.

The first behavior in which you can engage is to search your memory for words that rhyme with it. For example, if the acquaintance's name if "Mary," you might find yourself recalling names like "Sherry," "Terri," and "Carrie." When aphasic patients try to retrieve names of common everyday things, they also may say words that sound like the desired ones. For example, if an aphasic person is trying to say the name of the eating utensil *fork*, he or she might say, "pork," "stork," and "cork," while searching for the correct word. These types of word-retrieval behaviors go by several names including *phonemic paraphasias*, *literal paraphasias*, and *approximation errors*.

The second strategy you might use is to search your memory for the context or situation in which you know her. For example, you might try to remember if the acquaintance is a fellow student, professor, coworker, or member of your church. How are you associated with her? Aphasic patients also look for **associations** when trying to retrieve words. In the example of the patient trying to retrieve the word *fork*, he might say words that have a relationship in meanings. The patient may say, "knife," "spoon," or "plate." Sometimes, these errors of association can be embarrassing to the patient and cause family and friends to suspect that the patient is disorientated. A patient may accidentally call his wife his "mother" or call a current mate by a previous mate's name. *Semantic paraphasias*, *verbal paraphasias*, and *association errors* are words used to describe this type of word-retrieval behavior in aphasic patients.

Suppose you are discussing the acquaintance with some of your friends. You see the person in your mind's eye, but cannot remember her name. To retrieve the word, you might engage in a description of the acquaintance's face, hair, and typical clothing she wears. This is the third type of word-retrieval behavior, called description. Similarly, the aphasic patient, when trying to remember the word *fork* might describe its features, form, or function. The patient might say, "It has prongs and you eat with it." *Description* is a strategy to remember the word or to have someone supply it.

Aphasiologists call a naming error that is neither an association, a description, nor an approximation of the desired word a *random error*. A random-naming error is one in which the listener cannot detect the rhyme or reason for it. An example of a random error when trying to retrieve the word *fork* would be to call it a "banana" or "window." These words are neither associations, descriptions, nor approximations of the desired word. Although aphasic patients, and normal speakers as well, sometimes say words that are random-naming errors, often an association is not readily apparent. Maybe, the patient was thinking of a banana or looking out of a window while trying to search for the word.

Tip-of-the-Tongue Phenomenon

Most people have experienced a situation where they know the name of something, but they cannot retrieve it. They are close to saying it, the word seems on the surface of their memory, but it lacks a trigger to be able to recall it. In aphasia this is called the *tip-of-the-tongue phenomenon;* it is one of the most frustrating aspects of aphasia.

Two clinical behaviors are important when discussing the tip-of-the-tongue phenomenon: awareness of errors and the ability to self-correct. A patient who has awareness of errors knows when he or she makes a naming mistake. For example, the patient knows a mistake has been made when she says, "Please pass the sugar," when in fact the salt was wanted. There is an awareness that the wrong word has been spoken. The ability to self-correct is apparent when the individual, without cues or assistance, corrects the mistake and says, "Not sugar . . . salt." As a rule, aphasic patients who are aware of their errors and can self-correct have a better prognosis for recovering the maximum amount of language possible. They can work independently on their naming problems because they are both aware of errors and can self-correct. Self-therapy occurs every time the patient talks. When she makes a mistake, it is recognized and corrected. A therapist is not needed to show when there is an error and how to correct it.

The tip-of-the-tongue phenomenon is present if the patient has problems self-correcting because he cannot remember the word, but it is close to being recalled. Often, all a patient needs is a cue or to have someone provide several options. The patient can usually recognize the correct word from several possibilities. Recognition of a correct response is usually easier than recalling it.

The Psychology of Aphasia

Aphasia can be a devastating disorder. Even mild aphasia can cause a patient to be frustrated, depressed, angry, and frightened. Severe aphasia can eliminate functional communication between a patient and her family and friends and disrupts their lives. When loss of language severs the ability to communicate, it can leave a patient isolated from loved ones and clinically depressed; loss of language can also cause a host of other psychological reactions. Often, the road to recovery is uphill and slippery. The recovery process for survivors of brain injury who have aphasia is more than relearning language; it is also learning to cope with and adjust to the major unwanted life changes wrought by the disorder. In December 2000 the Public Broadcasting System's *ExxonMobil Masterpiece Theatre* broadcast an exploration into many of the psychological issues associated with stroke. Entitled "Lost for Words," it is about an old woman who tries to remain independent despite a series of strokes. In many ways, for both clinicians and patients, the psychology of aphasia is as important as its neurology. Code, Hemsley, and Herrmann (1999) found that the emotional aspects of aphasia can have a marked negative impact on recovery, response to rehabilitation, and psychosocial adjustment.

What is it like to have language suddenly removed from your life? What psychological toll does the loss of the ability to speak, read, and write and to understand spoken words demand? This question prompted Arthur Kopit to write the play *Wings*, and it was the theme of *The New Twilight Zone* episode "Word Play." Loss of language is so unusual to our lives, so bizarre, that many people cannot fathom the implications. Aphasia is a powerful and life-shattering communication disorder.

During the early years of aphasiology, little attention was given to the psychology of aphasia (Tanner, 2003). Patients suffering from aphasia were studied as medical oddities, and little attention was given to their recovery or adjustment. In recent years, aphasiologists have begun to explore the social, emotional, and psychological issues related to it. Currently, a patient's **quality of life** following a brain injury is being addressed. As more patients survive a stroke, head trauma, or brain disease and live longer lives, their quality of life has become a concern. Clinicians are concerned about the patients' happiness and satisfaction with life. Although there is little that can be done to change the neurology of aphasia, there is much that can be done in the psychological realm.

The Five Major Psychological Concomitants of Aphasia

Over the years, aphasiologists have discovered five frequently occurring major psychological aspects of aphasia. Psychological adjustment factors are so prominent in aphasia that they can be considered part of the syndrome of this communication disorder. Not all patients experience all five of them, but psychological adjustment factors are as much a part of aphasia as are the reading, writing, and speaking problems. Few aphasic patients are spared one or more of the psychological concomitants. Identifying the neurological substrates of these co-occurring reactions to brain injury is difficult, but they are either completely or partially psychological reactions to unwanted life changes and to the stress associated with them. The five psychological concomitants are emotional lability, catastrophic reactions, perseveration, organic depression, and the grief response (Table 8.4).

Emotional Lability

You would expect that when a person suffers a major brain injury and resulting neuropathology of speech and language, it would be considered a negative, sad event. Crying, a natural reaction to sadness, would be expected. In aphasia, there is much to cry about. However, some patients have exaggerated emotional reactions, which is called emotional lability,

TABLE 8.4 *Psychological Concomitants of Aphasia and Related Disorders*

Psychological Concomitant	*Reaction*
Emotional liability	Exaggerated emotions
Catastrophic reactions	Panic attacks and the need to flee or fight
Perseveration	Tendency for a thought or motor act to persist
Organic depression	Chronic severe negative emotions as a result of a chemical imbalance
Grief response	Moving through predictable stages of adjustment to unwanted changes

following brain injury. This exaggerated emotional reaction is sometimes called *pseudobulbar emotional lability* because it is associated with damage to the upper **motor neurons** in the brain. It is more common in patients who have spastic dysarthria, a common motor speech disorder (see Chapter 7), which often co-occurs with aphasia. This psychological concomitant to aphasia causes patients to lose their emotional inhibitions. They laugh and cry too easily, too much, and too long. But because there is more to cry about, it usually involves crying.

The distinction between *exaggerated* and *inappropriate* emotional responses is important. Early in the study of aphasia, emotional lability was considered an inappropriate response. Patients who cried were thought to be acting in an inappropriate way. Their emotional reactions to the brain injury were out of context. Later, aphasiologists realized that the patients' emotions were not out of context but were exaggerated. Patients had reasons for crying or laughing, but they did it too long or too often.

Today, emotional lability is considered the result of a lowered emotional threshold. The trigger point that sets off an emotional response is lowered, consequently, patients' emotions are closer to the surface. There is an aberrant duration and spread of emotions. It is also important to recognize that not all emotional responses are a result of emotional lability. Aphasia is a powerful, emotional event in a person's life, and considering all emotions as symptoms of emotional lability does a great disservice to the patient by denying him normal and natural psychological reactions.

Some aphasiologists believe that emotional lability consists of just the motor behaviors of crying (or laughing), without the feelings typically associated with them; that is, crying is only the motor behaviors. The sobbing, tears, and sad face are devoid of feeling. This may be true in some individuals, but in the majority of patients with emotional lability, their feelings are real, albeit exaggerated. Further, emotional lability is a psychological reaction. It should always be remembered that "people" have brain injuries that lead to aphasia. People have aphasia; it is not simply a symptom of damaged areas of the brain. In aware patients there is a human, psychological reaction to all brain injuries that impair functioning (Tanner, 2003).

Typically, three factors can trigger a bout of emotional lability: words and thoughts, people, and situations (Tanner, 1999a). Certain words and thoughts can cause a bout of crying. Some words carry more emotional content and can set off negative thoughts. In some patients, simply saying words like *nursing home* or *stroke* can cause negative thoughts that trigger emotional reactions, resulting in exaggerated crying. Certain people can be the trigger of labile crying. Simply mentioning the names of family members or showing pictures of children or grandchildren can cause crying. Situations—such as going to church, visiting home on a day pass, or being transported to the physical therapy gym—are the third trigger. These triggers cause patients to be aware of their negative predicaments, and can cause the emotional reactions associated with them.

Besides being distressing to the patient and her family, severe emotional lability can interfere with rehabilitation. Emotional lability can be treated though behavior modification or with medications. Behaviorally, a patient is taught to reduce the occurrences of emotional lability by ignoring the stimuli that cause them. The idea is to desensitize the patient to them. Once the emotional behaviors have begun, decreasing the duration of them is helped by focusing on positive stimuli or encouraging distraction. Antidepressants are also successful in helping some patients control their exaggerated emotional reactions.

Catastrophic Reactions

When an aphasic person is overwhelmed with anxiety and there is the need to flee or fight, a catastrophic reaction can occur. A patient experiencing a catastrophic reaction can become irritable, angry, or withdrawn. Lack of eye contact, sweating, and trembling are also symptoms of a catastrophic reaction or an impending one. Patients may verbally report the need to escape and have a feeling of impending doom. In some patients, striking out or a loss of consciousness can occur. Catastrophic reactions are more common in expressive rather than receptive aphasia. Because expressive, nonfluent aphasia is more common in women than men, women tend to suffer this anxiety-based disorder more often. A **catastrophic reaction** is both a psychological and physiological breakdown.

Psychologically, a catastrophic reaction occurs when a patient is given too many demands that have a *temporal urgency:* Several tasks are to be completed in a short period of time. It is no wonder that patients with predominantly expressive, nonfluent aphasia are more prone to them. Expressive nonfluent aphasia can be very frustrating. Patients effortfully search for words and how to say them, only occasionally being able to talk normally. Noise often precipitates catastrophic reactions. Patients feel overwhelmed by too many demands, too little time to complete them, and too much competing noise. And given that language helps bring order to reality, aphasia is a two-edged sword. It causes tension, anxiety, and frustration and eliminates or reduces the ability of language to comfort and bring order to the world.

Physiologically, a catastrophic reaction prompts the *flight-or-fight response.* This is a primal response to threatening situations, a remnant of earlier evolution. The human brain has retained the ability to mobilize the body's physiological abilities to run from or fight a potential dangerous threat. In primitive times these threats were usually physical, life-threatening situations, people, or animals. When confronted with the threat, the person mobilized the biological functions to flee or fight. This natural defense is activated in some aphasic persons when confronted with threats to their psychological integrity. They feel threatened and the biological reaction to flee or fight arises. But there is nowhere to run, no one to fight, no place to hide.

It is thought that catastrophic reactions occur in a small number of patients; they are not a common psychological concomitant to aphasia. However, they may be more common than traditionally thought. First, there are degrees of catastrophic reactions. Not all are dramatic, psychological, and physiological breakdowns. Second, not all catastrophic reactions are observable. Even predominantly receptive, fluent aphasic patients may have them, but they do not have observable symptoms. The symptoms are not readily apparent, or they are masked by other behaviors such as walking away, blanking out, or humor.

Stopping a catastrophic reaction once it occurs is difficult. Immediately reducing stress and providing the patient with an avenue of escape is helpful. Calming the patient with comforting and supporting statements can also reduce the extent and duration of a catastrophic reaction once it has begun. However, prevention is the best medicine. Aphasic patients prone to catastrophic reactions should be seen in comfortable, calm settings. Demands, especially those related to communication, should be kept to a minimum and gradually increased as the patient's speech and psychological abilities permit. For patients who frequently have catastrophic reactions and do not respond to behavioral prevention strategies, medication can help. Physicians can prescribe antidepressants and antianxiety medications to help prevent or minimize the occurrence of catastrophic reactions.

Arthur Kopit (1978), in the prelude to *Wings*, describes the seeds of a catastrophic reaction in Mrs. Stilson's new world:

> In this new world, she moves from one space or thought or concept to another without willing or sometimes even knowing it. Indeed, when she moves in this maze-like place, it is as if the world around her and not she were doing all the moving. To her, there is nothing any more that is commonplace or predictable. Nothing is as it was. Everything comes as a surprise. Something has relieved her of command. Something beyond her comprehension has her in its grip.
>
>   In the staging of this play, the sense should therefore be conveyed of physical and emotional separation (by the use, for example, of the dark transparent screens through which her surrounding world can be only dimly and partly seen, or by alteration of external sound) and of total immersion in strangeness. (p. 10)
>   Kopit, A. (1978). *Wings:* A Play, (p. 10). New York: Hill & Wang.

Perseveration

Perseveration is the tendency for a sensory or motor act to persist for a longer duration than would be warranted by the intensity and significance of the stimuli. Once a behavior has begun, the aphasic patient with perseveration is unable to stop or modify it, even though he may know it is inappropriate. The two perseveratory behaviors seen in some aphasic patients are during speaking and writing. During speaking, the aphasic patient with perseveration tends to utter the same word repeatedly. This behavior is apparent during sentence completion activities. When the patient is asked to complete this phrase, "I want a drink of _____," he may answer it appropriately by saying "water." When asked to complete the next phrase, "Knife, fork, and _____," the patient may again say, "water." The tendency to perseverate is apparent when the patient says, "water," to complete the phrase, "The United States of _____."

Severe perseveration, which can significantly interfere with communication and reduce the benefit the patient can obtain from therapies, has been likened to a "song going over and over in the mind." A patient with sensory perseveration may have a word or thought that continues in her inner speech. She cannot shift to another train of thought, and the flexibility of thinking is reduced.

Sensory perseveration is also manifested as **echolalia,** the tendency to repeat words or phrases that are spoken. The word *echolalia* comes from the patient "echoing" what has been said. When a person greets an aphasic who has echolalia and says, "Good morning, how are you today?" the patient might respond by saying "Today." Similarly, when the patient is asked what he wants for breakfast, the patient may respond with "For breakfast." It is as though the patient's thoughts are contaminated with the last thing heard.

Not all echolalia is a symptom of brain injury. Children go though a stage where they echo what their parents say; it is a normal stage of language acquisition. Adults also echo what has been spoken when bidding for time. For example, when someone asks, "Do you have the book?" an automatic reply, while trying to process the request, might be, "The book?" Aphasic patients may echo what has been spoken when bidding for time and also have the abnormal tendency for echolalia.

An aphasic patient with writing perseveration often has difficultly shifting from one letter to the next. For example, when writing her name, the patient may continue writing one of the letters repeatedly until it trails off into an unrecognizable scribble. These behaviors may also be present during other graphic behaviors such as drawing or copying.

Kreisler et al. (2000) found that an area in the brain known as the caudate nucleus is a likely area of damage in perseveration. Psychologically, perseveration resembles **obsessive–compulsive disorders** (OCDs). Obsession is the inability to stop thinking about something. When a person does an activity repeatedly and cannot stop, he is engaged in a compulsive behavior. These two disorders often occur together. A person is obsessed with a thought and engages repeatedly in a response to it. For example, the late billionaire and aviator Howard Hughes was said to be obsessed with the thought of germs and compulsively washed his hands and did other things in response to this fear.

Perseveration can be treated with both behavioral therapies and medications. Patients can be taught to shift mental sets and behaviors by rewarding desirable thoughts and actions and discouraging perseveration. Some patients may benefit from medications used to treat psychiatric disorders. Although perseveration is a negative prognostic indicator, a combination of behavioral therapy and medications can help patients respond to aphasia rehabilitation.

Organic Depression

There are two primary causes for depression in aphasic patients (Tanner, 2003). First, depression is a natural occurrence in aware patients because of the losses they experience and the stresses associated with them. It is one of the stages of the grieving process and will be discussed in the next section, The Grief Response. The second cause of depression in patients with neuropathologies of speech and language is organic. **Organic depression** occurs because of brain injury and the disruption of chemicals that control and regulate moods. It is, at least in part, a result of brain chemicals gone awry.

Depression is called the "common cold" of mental illness. Depression is qualitatively and quantitatively different from sadness. Most people have experienced sadness at some point in their lives. Sometimes, sadness results from disappointment over a relationship gone sour, fatigue, hunger, sleep disruption, or follows a period of high activity. Sadness is a natural mood swing that is appropriate in degree to the circumstances that cause it.

Clinical depression is much more than sadness. It can also result from environmental factors, but it is too extreme or lasts too long. Clinical depression is often caused by no apparent reason; a person just becomes depressed. Clinical depression is a prolonged, severe bout of negative emotions. The clinically depressed person may cry frequently, lack concern for others, avoid family and friends, and lose interest in pleasurable activities. Anxiety is also a frequent symptom of clinical depression. Some depressed people become agitated, irritable, frightened, or angry. A clinically depressed person may become suicidal. Their thoughts become saturated with death and dying.

Strokes, head traumas, and neurological diseases can cause clinical depression, and it is common in patients with neuropathologies of speech and language. As was previously noted, patients with injury in the anterior part of the brain, those with nonfluent, predominantly expressive aphasia, are more likely to suffer from depression. Often, patients with communication disorders lose the ability to benefit from psychological therapies to address the depression. Because of their communication disorders, they cannot benefit from the "talking" cures. They have trouble understanding the therapist and talking through their depressive thoughts.

In aware patients the knowledge that they have suffered a brain injury results in reduced self-esteem. There is an altered **self-concept.** There are often feelings of inadequacy. Guilt is also present; patients may feel guilty for being depressed or feel that they could have done something to have prevented the brain injury and communication disorder. These feelings may not be realistic. In reality, perhaps nothing could have been done to prevent the injury. Severe depression can be psychotic in nature; that is, the person can lose touch with reality.

Speech and language therapy can be helpful in treating depression in aphasic patients. Besides helping the patient increase her communication abilities, therapy can help the patient improve body image and other aspects of self-concept and provide hope and optimism. The structure and guidance provided by the clinician can also help the patient focus her attention on positive aspects of life. The clinician's support and encouragement provided during therapy can also be helpful. In addition, several antidepressant medications are available to help patients overcome clinical depression following brain injury. These medications have few side effects and can help even severely depressed patients with communication disorders.

The Grief Response

The human response to loss is grief. The **grief response** involves several stages that people go through when learning to accept unwanted changes associated with loss. In aphasia there is much to grieve. Rarely do patients make absolute, complete recovery from neuropathologies of speech and language. Of course, for the response to occur, the patient must have valued that which was lost and be aware of his predicament.

There are three primary dimensions in which loss can occur in aphasia (Tanner & Gerstenberger, 1996). First, because strokes, head traumas, and diseases take away physical and mental abilities, a patient experiences *loss of self.* The aspects of self that can be lost in aphasia include understanding the speech of others, speaking, reading, writing, and doing simple arithmetic. Even the ability to use and understand complex gestures can be lost. Strokes, head traumas, and diseases can also cause paralysis, blindness, hearing loss, and deafness.

The second dimension is *loss of person.* Because communication with friends and loved ones can be devastated by aphasia, there can be a sense of separation. Although friends and loved ones are not physically taken from the patient, they can be lost because aphasia places a wedge between them. They cannot plan, discuss, and share experiences as they once did. This can result in a deep sense of loss that is sometimes compounded by actual physical separation when the patient is sent to a nursing home or extended medical care facility.

Loss of object is the third area that can cause the grief response in aphasic patients. Because of communication disorders, paralysis, and other infirmities, aphasic patients often lose the ability to use valued objects. They cannot use or enjoy a motor home, sewing machine, computer, bicycle, horse, or pet. Some patients cannot garden, play cards, bowl, or dance because of the mental and physical problems associated with a stroke, head trauma, or disease.

Aphasic patients are like everyone else when they are confronted with serious losses; they go through predictable stages that ultimately lead to acceptance. The first and most detailed process was first proposed by Elizabeth Kübler-Ross in her landmark book, *On Death and Dying* (1969). At first the person psychologically tries to overcome the losses; she engages in denial, anger, and bargaining. In these stages the patient is not completely aware of the extent of the losses. Grieving depression occurs when the patient finally becomes aware that she is permanently separated from abilities, people, and things she once valued. At this stage the person becomes fully aware of the value of the losses, and she is no longer trying to overcome them. Normal grieving depression can last from 3 to 12 months, depending on the value of what was lost. The final stage is acceptance, or resolution of the losses. Here the patient is no longer trying to overcome the losses or is no longer depressed by them. She accepts what has happened and feels neither good nor bad about it. Most patients reach an acceptance of the losses associated with aphasia.

Of course, not all patients go through every stage, and their order can fluctuate. Some patients spend little time in one stage, and others can be fixated in other stages. The common thread in the grief response is that patients who are aware of what has happened, and who valued that which was lost, experience the grief response. The focus of rehabilitation goes from trying to overcome the disabilities to reaching an acceptance of them. According to Code, Hemsley, and Herrmann (1999), the grieving model is powerful in its ability to explain some of the emotional and psychosocial effects of aphasia, but more research about loss, grief, and aphasia is necessary.

Aphasia Rehabilitation

Spontaneous recovery of speech and language abilities occurs in the majority of aphasic patient. **Spontaneous recovery** is the period of time post-onset where the brain naturally resolves part or, in rare cases, all the language disturbance. Spontaneous recovery is both a blessing and a curse. It is certainly a blessing that many patients automatically recover some or all of their communication abilities. The curse is felt by researchers. Because patients improve spontaneously and without the benefit of rehabilitation, research into therapies and treatments is more complicated. It is difficult to separate the effects of rehabilitation from naturally occurring spontaneous recovery.

There are several reasons for spontaneous recovery in aphasia. The medical conditions that can cause aphasia sometimes also result in a buildup of pressure in the brain. This pressure can cause some areas in the brain to not work properly. When the pressure reduces, these areas again can function normally. Besides the pressure drop in the brain, spontaneous recovery can be due to improved blood circulation and because other areas of the brain take over functions of the damaged ones. In addition, some brain cells are just "stunned" by a stroke or head trauma, and eventually they return to normal functioning. There are other reasons why spontaneous recovery occurs, but like other parts of the body, the brain tends to heal itself. Spontaneous recovery is more apparent during the first few weeks following a stroke or head trauma. However, some authorities believe it lasts for up to a year.

Research into the value of aphasia therapy is complicated by spontaneous recovery. Early in the study of aphasia, some scientists attributed all improvement of speech and language in aphasic patients to spontaneous recovery. Some questioned whether speech and language therapy had any value. Over the past four decades, many studies have addressed the value of aphasia rehabilitation. With few exceptions, studies have found that patients who have aphasia therapy do better and make greater recovery in their abilities to communicate than do those who do not receive it. Many patients report that the greatest value of therapy is in the psychological realm. Aphasia can be a nightmare psychologically, and the guidance, support, and encouragement from the clinician are helpful. "There are now clear indications that emotional factors must be addressed in rehabilitation and that rehabilitation programs based purely on the medical model are simply not adequate or appropriate" (Code et al., 1999, p. 28). Unfortunately, it appears that patients with global aphasia do not appreciably improve in their speech and language abilities because of therapy. Global aphasia is sometimes called severe expressive–receptive, profound, complete, or irreversible aphasia (see Table 8.1). Although these individuals may benefit psychologically from therapy, there has been too much brain damage for them, as a group, to significantly improve their speech and language abilities.

Aphasia therapies are commonsense instruction, drills, and exercises designed to help patients regain as much of their language abilities as possible, given the extent of the brain damage. After evaluating patients' communication strengths and weakness, clinicians work to improve patients' expressive and receptive language abilities. They start at levels where patients can succeed, and in gradual, systematic steps improve patients' abilities to communicate. This happens in all modalities of communication, including reading, writing, and the use of gestures. Language stimulation, deblocking drills, rapid naming-recall exercises, and cognitive retraining strategies are employed. One therapy is called *melodic intonation therapy* (MIT). Some patients can sing simple songs much better than they can talk. By using the melody and rhythm of songs, they can be taught to have better verbal expression.

Literature and Media Stereotypes

When an actor successfully recovers from aphasia, the courage and determination in overcoming it become part of his or her public persona. Patricia Neal's return to her acting career, and subsequent Oscar nomination for Best Actress in *The Subject Was Roses*, clearly shows that some people can be victorious over aphasia. Although the public recognizes how formidable aphasia can be, people like Neal show that one need not be victimized by it. Additionally, famous actors often use their power, money, and fame to advocate for others with major communication disorders. A good example of this is The Patricia Neal Rehabilitation Center.

Films such as *Regarding Henry* often portray the "silver lining" potential of aphasia. Although these films tend to simplify neuropathologies of speech and language—even mislead the public over their nature, symptoms, and course—they are good at portraying the personal growth many people undergo. A common theme is that the aphasic person returns to basic values. Aphasia is often viewed as a stimulus for regaining innocent, important, and more compassionate values.

The way films can mislead and simplify aphasia is seen in the movie *Legends of the Fall*. Colonel Ludlow's initial symptoms are not typical of aphasia; they more resemble severe dysarthria. If the screenwriter's goal was to portray aphasia, Ludlow's lack of written and verbal grammatical and syntactical deficits are somewhat misleading, but the film does a good job in showing his independence and strong personality. He is portrayed as a victor rather than a victim to aphasia.

It is difficult for aphasiologists, let alone the general public, to understand what it is like to be totally deprived of all avenues of language expression and reception. In many ways, global aphasia is a bizarre disorder. It takes away language, a naturally acquired ability that is taken for granted; to be totally deprived of language is incomprehensible. Some filmmakers and playwrights are gifted in their ability to portray the inner world of aphasia. *The New Twilight Zone* episode, "Word Play," gives a penetrating glance into a chaotic world of a man suddenly separated from loved ones because of language barriers. It is like the biblical "tower of Babel" parable in current times. Fortunately for the protagonist, he still possesses intact inner speech, which helps him navigate through the fog of confusion. Unfortunately, in many aphasic patients, their inner speech is as disrupted as is their "exteriorized" language. Absent inner speech causes aphasia to be even more confusing and life disrupting.

Arthur Kopit tackles aphasia, in all of its complexities, in the play *Wings*. He does a remarkable job of depicting the confusion of Mrs. Stilson's entry into the world of aphasia. In the preface to the play, he readily admits that much of the imagery of the inner world of aphasia is speculation. However, it is clear that he has done his homework; there are few technical errors in either Mrs. Stilson's language patterns or her responses to others. Kopit, like many playwrights before him, uses the stage as a medium to entertain and inform. *Wings* is a truly remarkable window into the inner world of aphasia.

Media and literature are given a "thumbs up" in portraying aphasia. Although literary license is taken in depicting the complexities of this disorder, authors and playwrights have addressed it in its totality. The public figures who have moved from victims to victors over aphasia offer patients and their families a ray of hope and a plethora of possibilities.

Summary

Aphasia, serious and potentially devastating, is a language disorder that destroys or impairs all avenues of communication: speaking, writing, reading, verbal understanding, and gestures. Aphasia is caused by strokes, head traumas, and diseases that affect the speech and language centers of the brain. There are two categories of aphasia: predominantly expressive and predominantly receptive. In predominantly expressive aphasia, patients have difficulty or cannot express themselves through speaking, writing, and the use of expressive gestures. In predominantly receptive aphasia, patients have difficulty or cannot understand the spoken, written, or gestured expressions of others. Some aphasic patients have catastrophic reactions, uncontrolled crying, depression, and difficulty shifting from one task to another. Most aware aphasic patients also grieve over what aphasia has taken from them.

With the exception of global aphasia, most patients benefit from aphasia therapies, especially psychologically. When aphasia is portrayed in media and literature, it is rarely shown as the complex and devastating disorder it can be.

Study Questions

1. Define *aphasia*.

2. Compare and contrast the functions of the right and left hemispheres of the brain.

3. Draw a human brain and designate Broca's and Wernicke's areas of the left hemisphere.

4. What is the difference between an *embolus* and a *thrombosis*?

5. List the synonyms for expressive and receptive aphasia.

6. What is *acalculia*? Give an example.

7. Compare and contrast Broca's and Wernicke's aphasia.

8. What is the *loss of abstract attitude*?

9. List and discuss the five major psychological concomitants of aphasia.

10. What is *spontaneous recovery*?

11. How do literature and media characterize people with aphasia?

Suggested Reading

Darley, F. (1982). *Aphasia*. Philadelphia: Saunders. This classic text clearly defines and describes aphasia as a language disorder distinct from the motor speech impairments.

Lazar, R. M., Marshall, R. S., Prell, G. D., & Pile-Spellman, J. (2000). The experience of Wernicke's aphasia. *Neurology, 55:* 1222–1224. This study is about a patient who has temporary Wernicke's aphasia, and after returning to normal, he recounts his experiences with the disorder.

Tanner, D. (1999). *The family guide to surviving stroke and communication disorders*. Boston: Allyn & Bacon. This book explores the nature and clinical symptoms of neurogenic communication disorders, using nontechnical terminology and a short story.

Tanner, D. (2003). *The psychology of neurogenic communication disorders: A primer for health care professionals*. Boston: Allyn & Bacon. This book explores three aspects to the psychology of neurogenic communication disorders: (1) organic and biochemical alterations, (2) coping styles and psychological defenses, and (3) loss, grief, and adjustment factors.

Communication Disorders Resulting from Dementia

Chapter Preview

This chapter explores the communication disorders seen in dementia. Dementia, one of the most frightening and disabling conditions that can affect people, is progressive deterioration of intellect, memory, personality, and the ability to communicate. Dementia is not a normal part of growing old; it results from pathological aging. There are several causes of dementia, and Alzheimer's disease is the most common. You will examine behaviors, emotions, hallucinations, delusions, and the specific communication problems experienced by people with dementia. There is an example of the progression of dementia and the early signs and symptoms of the loss of mental functions. You will learn about evaluating and treating the communication disorders seen in dementia and about the stereotypes that society has about people with dementia and how literature and media propagate them.

Few diseases and disorders are more frightening than Alzheimer's disease, intellectual deterioration, organic brain syndrome, senility, and organic mental disorder. Diseases and disorders that affect a person's thought processes, intelligence, and memory are frightening to both the patient and his loved ones. Unfortunately, many diseases and disorders can cause mental deterioration. For the most part, they are irreversible and ultimately fatal. For many people the thought of gradual loss of mental functioning is more frightening than is the thought of death itself.

Losing mental functioning is a basic fear and the ultimate psychological threat. Being unable to remember what one was doing a few minutes ago, getting lost in familiar places, or forgetting loved ones can be psychologically devastating. Fear and panic can grip the heart when memory loss and confusion set in. For many patients a gradual loss of mental functioning is like a slow death. There is a slow irreversible loss of self. These people become more and more dependent on others for even the most minor of day-to-day activities. They often do bizarre and uncharacteristic things and can become a danger to themselves and others.

Their memory impairments disrupt relationships where the continuity of past, present, and future is lost to family and friends.

Often, the first signs of **dementia** are noticed during communication. The person may ask strange questions or make comments that show her confusion. Memory is impaired and she may repeatedly ask the same questions or demand that something irrelevant be done. Even simple instructions are not understood or followed. Conversations become shallow and ultimately meaningless. As dementia progresses, speech and language can deteriorate, and even the ability to engage in functional communication can be lost.

Many people believe dementia is a natural consequence of the normal aging process. The healthy, normal process of aging, however, does *not* include dementia. Certainly, people in their later decades of life may not be as mentally sharp as they once were, but the clinical signs of dementia suggest a pathological state. Life's later years can be a rich, rewarding time filled with growth, discovery, and reflection.

For the most part, literature and media portray people with early signs of dementia with benign tolerance. Their foibles are viewed humorously. Of course, people with dementia are delegated to inferior family and vocational positions. This is often necessary and appropriate. No one wants a person with compromised mental functioning in a position of authority or responsibility. People in late stage dementia become burdens on loved ones and society. Those early fears of dependency, voiced by Ronald Reagan, in a letter to the American people (Box 9.1), often become a reality. Early on, many people fight and struggle to maintain mental integrity: "They do not go gently into that good night." Nevertheless, even with the advances currently being made to prevent or find a cure for many dementia-causing disorders and illnesses, they remain incipient and insidious.

Dementia

"Irreversible dementia is characterized by chronic progressive deterioration of intellect, memory, personality and communicative functions" (Bayles, 1994, p. 535). No one is immune to it. This devastating disorder happens to presidents, longshoremen, cranberry silo guards, scientists, teachers, farmers, professors, vagrants, and poets. It happens to people of all races. No country has borders capable of keeping it out. It strikes the relatively young and extremely old. Dementia can creep up slowly or have a rapid onset. Like other age-related disorders, the number of people affected by it is likely to increase. Review of current research shows that dementia touches 1 in 3 families, as many as 50% of people by the age of 85 have some of the symptoms, and by 2050, 14.4 million people in the United States could have it (Ripich & Ziol, 1998). "It is essential that speech-language pathologists (SLPs) and others who work with persons with dementia are prepared to meet the communication needs of both cognitively impaired persons and their care providers" (Ripich & Ziol, 1998, p. 467).

Many diseases, infections, toxins, vascular disturbances, and traumas can cause irreversible dementia. They are discussed in the pages that follow. Several reversible conditions can be disguised as irreversible dementia. Depression and abuse of prescription medications in the elderly can create symptoms of dementia. Unlike true irreversible dementia, when the depression lifts or the patient stops or changes medication, the dementia-like symptoms stop.

BOX 9.1 • *A Letter to the American People*

My Fellow Americans. I have recently been told that I am one of the millions of Americans who will be afflicted with Alzheimer's disease.

Upon learning this news, Nancy and I had to decide whether as private citizens we would keep this a private matter or whether we would make this news known in a public way. In the past, Nancy suffered from breast cancer, and I had my cancer surgeries. We found through our open disclosures we were able to raise public awareness. We were happy that as a result, many more people underwent testing. They were treated in early stages and able to return to normal, healthy lives.

So now we feel it is important to share it with you. In opening our hearts, we hope this might promote greater awareness of this condition. Perhaps it will encourage a clearer understanding of the individuals and families who are affected by it.

At the moment I feel just fine. I intend to live the remainder of the years God gives me on this Earth doing the things I have always done. I will continue to share life's journey with my beloved Nancy and my family. I plan to enjoy the great outdoors and stay in touch with my friends and supporters.

Unfortunately, as Alzheimer's disease progresses, the family often bears a heavy burden. I only wish there was some way I could spare Nancy from this painful experience. When the time comes, I am confident that with your help she will face it with faith and courage.

In closing, let me thank you, the American people, for giving me the great honor of allowing me to serve as your president. When the Lord calls me home, whenever that day may be, I will leave with the greatest love for this country of ours and eternal optimism for its future.

I now begin the journey that will lead me to the sunset of my life. I know that for America there will always be a bright dawn ahead.

Thank you, my friends. May God always bless you.

Sincerely,

Ronald Reagan

Causes of Dementia

Alzheimer's disease is the most common cause of irreversible dementia, accounting for about half the cases (Hopper & Bayles, 2001). Initially, minor and infrequent symptoms of the disease, such as forgetfulness and confusion, appear, but later in the course of the disease, pronounced disorientation, amnesia, and speech and language pathologies emerge. One of the most perplexing aspects of early-onset Alzheimer's disease is that the symptoms can resemble normal forgetfulness and occasional confusion experienced by everyone. For example, forgetting one's keys or not remembering a telephone number can be both a normal occurrence in a busy person's life and a sign of early-onset Alzheimer's disease.

Literature, Media, and Personality Profiles

Ronald Wilson Reagan

Ronald Reagan, the 40th president of the United States, was born February 6, 1911, in Tampico, Illinois. He attended high school in Dixon, Illinois, and then studied economics and sociology at Eureka College. After graduation he became a radio sports announcer. In 1937 Reagan began acting and, during the next 25 years, appeared in more than 50 films. He had two children from his first marriage to actress Jane Wyman. In 1952 he married Nancy Davis and had two children by that marriage. Reagan served as governor of California from 1966 to 1974. He was elected president of the United States in 1980 and served two terms.

Reagan was nicknamed "The Great Communicator." His ability to skillfully deal with Congress and his economic policies, "Reaganomics," led to a renewal of national patriotism that has been called the "Reagan Revolution." His foreign policy was based on "Peace Through Strength," and during his presidency he significantly increased defense spending. Many believe his hard line with the now defunct Soviet Union, which he called, "an evil empire," helped win the cold war. Shortly after completing his second term as president, Reagan was diagnosed with Alzheimer's disease.

Abraham "Grampa" Simpson

Abraham Simpson is a main supporting character on the long-running hit television show *The Simpsons*. Abe Simpson is the father of Homer, the befuddled patriarch of the dysfunctional cartoon family. Now living in a retirement home, Abe sold his house so that Homer and Marge could buy their current one. In a typical show of gratitude, Homer then sent Grandpa to the Springfield Retirement Castle. Before retiring, Abraham was a cranberry silo watchman. He was married to Homer's mother, Penelope, but she left him. She was forced to go underground because of her 1960s antiwar activities. He has had other romantic interests, including one with Marge's mother. Abe is a member of the mysterious "Stonecutters' Club," a thinly disguised reference to the Masons. He won an Emmy for writing an episode of the violent cartoon within a cartoon: "The Itchy and Scratchy Show." His grandchildren, Bart and Lisa, actually wrote the episode. He was once voted the most handsome boy in Albany, New York. His favorite television show is *Matlock*.

Simpson's medication is two red and one yellow pills daily, taken for undisclosed but apparently age-related disorders. He brags that he can still dress himself and regularly falls asleep in an instant, often during midsentence. Clearly suffering from early symptoms of dementia, Abe has uttered some strange statements:

"Dear Mr. President. There are too many states nowadays. Please eliminate three. I am not a crackpot."

"I always get the blame around here! Who threw a cane at the TV? Who fell into the china hutch? Who got their dentures stuck on the toilet?"

"I can still eat corn on the cob if someone cuts if off and smushes it into a fine paste. Now that's good eatin'!!!!"

"My Homer is not a communist. He may be a liar, a pig, an idiot, a communist, but he is not a porn star."

"My car gets forty rods to the hog's head, and that's the way I likes it."

Simpson is not always confused. He was once instrumental in capturing Springfield's worst criminal: the Cat Burglar. It helped that the criminal was his next-door neighbor and left obvious clues. He continues to live, relatively independently, in the retirement home, enjoying his hobby of collecting beef jerky, napping, and occasionally baby-sitting for Homer and Marge.

Nash Bridges

CBS first telecast the police drama *Nash Bridges*, on March 29, 1996. It features Don Johnson, who had starred in the popular television show *Miami Vice* 7 years earlier. It also stars Cheech Marin. The show is about the personal and professional life of Nash Bridges, acting head of the Special Investigations Unit (SIU). The SIU is headquartered on a barge moored at a San Francisco pier. There are frequent undercover assignments involving cases ranging from robbery to murder.

Nash Bridge's father is Nick, played by James Gammon. He is a retired longshoreman and shares Nash's upscale apartment. Nick is a complex and somewhat tragic character in the series. He drinks too much, smokes cigars, and is a womanizer. He is a loving father but has emotional problems and gets involved in risky schemes. He also shows signs of early-onset Alzheimer's disease. Occasionally, he has memory problems and makes strange statements. In one episode he forgot his lines in a play, became disoriented, and did not recognize his daughter. Nick sometimes forgets that his other son was killed during the Vietnam War. He also suffered a stroke and was comatose for a time.

Age Old Friends

Age Old Friends is about two retirement home residents who must deal with age-related physical and mental deterioration. The film, released in 1989, is based on the play *A Month of Sundays,* by Bob Larbey. It stars Hume Cronyn as John Cooper and Vincent Gardenia as Michael Aylott, who are longtime friends. It also stars Michele Scarabelli as a kind and considerate nurse. Produced by Patrick Whitley, it addresses the fear and adjustments associated with growing old. To keep their minds alert, they play a memory game about the 1937 New York Giants. The film shows the power of friendship in helping to accept the changing roles and identity brought on with aging and subsequent physical and mental impairments.

Some people believe an Alzheimer's disease epidemic is looming on the horizon. Neergaard (2000) reports that the cases of Alzheimer's disease double every 5 years of age from 65 to 85. With the rapidly aging baby boomers, the number of people afflicted with this disease could reach epidemic proportions. "Alzheimer's disease has been determined to be the fourth leading cause of death in the United States" (Kennedy, 1999, p. 230).

The cause or causes of Alzheimer's disease are unknown; there are many possible culprits. The hippocampus, located deep within the brain, is considered a likely site of brain damage. It has long been known that this structure is important for memory and learning. Disorders affecting brain chemistry, vascular disturbances, toxins and heavy metals, fever, a history of neurological disorders from disease or head trauma, and genetics may also play a role. According to Ripich and Ziol (1998), at present the only way to confirm a diagnosis of

Alzheimer's disease is during an autopsy. Currently, research into the molecular mechanism of Alzheimer's disease is showing promise for prevention, treatments, and a possible cure to this devastating disorder (Emilien, Maloteaux, Beyreuther, & Masters, 2000).

Vascular dementia is the cognitive and behavioral deterioration caused by multiple strokes or other diseases that can affect the blood supply to the brain. The symptoms of this type of dementia depend on the site and size of the lesions in the brain. To have dementia of this cause, besides the usual signs of cognitive and behavior deterioration, a patient must also have focal neurological symptoms indicative of a vascular disturbance and brain-scan proof of multiple cortical or subcortical lesions (American Psychiatric Association, 1994).

Separating the symptoms seen in Alzheimer's disease from those occurring in vascular dementia is difficult. There are similar aspects to both disorders. Diagnostic criteria significantly influences the incidence and prevalence of vascular dementia (Chui et al., 2000). Men may be more at risk for developing vascular dementia, whereas the risk to women is slightly greater in Alzheimer's disease (Ripich & Ziol, 1998). Because strokes and other vascular disturbance can come on rapidly, the patient may show signs of confusion, memory loss, and behavior problems more abruptly in vascular dementia.

Another cause of dementia is Parkinson's disease. Some patients who have this disorder, which results from a deficiency of the **neurotransmitter** dopamine, display symptoms of dementia (see Chapter 7). Pick's disease also causes a deterioration of the temporal and frontal lobes of the brain (Ripich & Ziol, 1998). People with advanced alcoholism or head trauma also can show signs and symptoms that resemble those seen in irreversible dementia. Heavy-metal poisoning and metabolic disorders have also been linked to dementia. People in the later stages of the sexually transmitted disease syphilis are often demented. It has been reported that Adolf Hitler and the gangster Al Capone, late in their lives, were suffering from syphilis-induced dementia.

Transient ischemic attacks (TIAs), temporary interruptions of blood flow to the brain, may be due to partial occlusion of one or more arteries. They are like strokes but do not result in permanent brain damage. The symptoms presented by the patient when he is experiencing a TIA depend on the degree of the blood-flow interruption. When a TIA happens, the patient can present with many of the symptoms of dementia. Some people have multiple episodes of TIAs, causing frequent cognitive and behavioral patterns typical of Alzheimer's disease or multiple-infarct dementia.

In early-stage dementia, patients may only present with minor and irregular memory, learning, and behavior problems. Later, they may begin to wander aimlessly and have hallucinations and delusions, particularly paranoid and persecutory ones. In the movie *Age Old Friends*, the first signs of dementia were forgetting a handkerchief, turning the wrong way on a walk to a candy store, and forgetting what had been discussed. The confusion and memory problems get progressively worse as the dementia advances. One patient in the nursing home is found bathing in a pond. Many patients lose the ability to recognize family and friends. One reason for the inability to recognize familiar people is a perceptual disorder called *prosopagnosia*, the inability to recognize familiar faces. In dementia there may be bowel and urinary incontinence. Some patients have **dysphagia,** which is a swallowing disorder (see Chapter 7). They require special diets and careful evaluation, treatment, and monitoring by a speech–language pathologist. Vision and hearing disorders may also be part of the symptoms of dementia, and preexisting ones can exacerbate the memory, learning, and behavioral problems.

Disruptive Behaviors

As dementia progresses, several disruptive behavior patterns can be observed. According to Hartke (1991), although these behaviors can result from a variety of causes, four major sources are (1) organic or physically related causes, (2) environmental causes, (3) cognitive causes, and (4) emotional causes. Organic, or physically related, causes of disruptive behaviors include acute confusional states, fatigue, illness, medication reactions, sensory losses, and pain. Environmental causes include changes in caregivers or routine, noise, lack of privacy, and unfamiliar people. These stressors commonly cause free-floating anxiety and can escalate into a **catastrophic reaction.** Cognitive causes include impairments of memory, communication, insight, judgment, and problem solving. Emotional causes include anxiety, depression, lowered self-esteem, attention seeking, fear, and suspiciousness. According to Hartke (1991), pharmacological and behavioral management are applicable for disruptive behaviors across the etiological categories.

Hallucinations and Delusions in Dementia

As noted previously, patients with dementia may hallucinate. She sees objects that are not there and hears sounds or smells odors that do not exist. These are called *visual, auditory,* and *olfactory hallucination,* respectively. **Tactile** hallucinations involve feeling sensations that do not occur. A hallucination can also involve the misinterpretation of a real sensory experience. Hallucinations are similar to illusions, which we have all had. For example, a person might believe that a leaf touching the skin is a spider preparing to bite. An illusion is the misinterpretation or confusion about something that is sensed. Seeing a face in a cloud or believing traffic noise is the sound of the ocean are illusions. Magicians practice the "art of illusion"; they fool the senses.

Brain injury, drugs, diseases, and alcohol intoxication can cause hallucinations; even migraine headaches and seizures can induce them. The nature and chronicity of hallucinations are related to the area of the brain affected. Nonorganic factors can also cause hallucinations. These types of hallucinations are often caused by stress and loneliness and result from excessive daydreaming and fantasizing. Fatigue and isolation also play an important role in them. Initially, the daydreaming and fantasizing help reduce stress, but as time passes, the person gradually loses contact with reality because of the excessive use of fantasy escape.

Delusions and hallucination often go hand-in-hand. Whereas a hallucination primarily involves the senses, a delusion is a thought disturbance. It is a belief that is untrue but rigidly held by the person. The delusional person will not give up the untrue belief, even when provided proof to the contrary. We have all had delusional-like thoughts, especially when we were children. Walking through a cemetery on a windy, dark night can cause thoughts of ghosts stalking the path to home and safety. Being alone, late at night, after watching a scary movie can cause unrealistic and fearful thoughts. Of course, these innocent flights of the imagination are not true delusions. They are short lived, not rigidly held in proof to the contrary, and not a result of a break with reality.

Most psychiatrists believe that delusions, like hallucinations, can be caused by both organic and nonorganic factors. Illegal drugs can cause them. High-potency marijuana, cocaine, ecstasy, and LSD are known to cause delusions. Prescribed drugs can also have delusions as unwanted side effects. Traumatic brain injuries can also cause these rigidly held thought disturbances, especially in people who are predisposed to them (see Chapter 10). Nonorganically caused hallucinations and delusions are thought to result from low self-esteem, projection, and denial. Isolation, fatigue, and loneliness play a role in their development and maintenance.

There are many types of delusions. A *delusion of grandeur* is when a person believes that he is a superior or supernatural savior of the world. The person may also believe that he is called upon by God to perform some important duty. A *delusion of persecution* occurs when a person believes that she is in extreme danger or at the mercy of powerful forces. These people may wear tinfoil or metal "hats" to protect themselves from unwanted alien thoughts. When a person has a *somatic delusion*, he believes there is something terribly wrong with the body, when in fact all is well. Unfortunately, delusional thoughts sometimes cause a person to harm other people.

Of course, not all rigidly held beliefs are psychotic delusions. Some religious beliefs, which are rigidly held in proof to the contrary, are not necessarily delusions; they are simply part of a person's belief system. Many people are firmly convinced that there are government plots to imprison them or steal their property. This type of delusional thinking was portrayed in the film *Conspiracy Theory*. Others are certain they have been abducted by aliens. Sometimes it is hard to know when a rigidly held belief is a delusion, an aspect of faith, an accurate appraisal of reality, or just an incorrect idea. The problems of reality testing with delusions and hallucinations are accurately portrayed in the 2002 film *A Beautiful Mind*.

Communication Disorders in Dementia

Ripich and Ziol (1998) have identified the communication changes seen in patients with Alzheimer's disease. They examined the pragmatic, semantic, syntax, and phonology aspects of communication disorders that occur during the early, middle, and late stages of the disease. As was discussed in Chapter 5, **pragmatics** is the functional use of language, the context and intent in which it is used. **Semantics** concerns the meaning of words in language. **Syntax** refers to the rules and way words and other elements of language are ordered to convey meaning. **Phonology** is the rules governing the way sounds are combined in a language.

Box 9.2 provides an illustration of communication disorders in dementia.

Early Stage

Ripich and Ziol (1998) report that in the pragmatic category, during the early stages of the disorder, the patient is generally aware of the problems with communication. There is some difficulty with storytelling and giving instructions. There are frequent requests for clarification and confirmation of what has been said. Patients in early-stage Alzheimer's disease drift from the topic and tend to be vague during communication. There may be specific difficulties understanding humor, analogies, sarcasm, and abstract expressions. In the semantic category, word fluency is compromised. However, Bayles (1994) reports that patients with

BOX 9.2 • *The Progression of Dementia*

Donald, a semiretired farmer, did not show major signs of early-onset dementia until he was 73 years old. Donald continued to help his son with the large family-owned potato and wheat farm. Before the "truck incident," there were some problems with communication, which his family attributed to the fact that he was getting on in years. For example, in the mornings when Donald and his son would have breakfast and plan the day's activities, he would have trouble communicating a series of farm jobs that needed to be done. His son also noted that, although Donald would agree to do several jobs during the day, only one or two would be done, and the others were apparently forgotten. During the early-morning breakfasts, Donald would often wander from the topic of farming to talk about international politics. Sometimes, it seemed he could not keep focused on farming. Once, when talking about farm subsidies, his son jokingly commented that people "like to eat on a regular basis." Donald took the statement literally and replied, "Heck, son, don't you know that people will die if they don't get enough food!"

The "truck incident" clearly proved that the confusion went beyond normal forgetfulness. To feed the cattle, every day it was necessary that two truckloads of hay be taken from the hay lot to the cattle corrals. Usually, both were loaded and driven to the corrals at the same time, one by Donald and the other by his son. One morning, before loading them, Donald demanded that only one truck be used that day. They would load one, drive it to the corrals, unload it and return to the hay lot. Then, they would repeat the procedure with the second truck. When asked for his reasoning behind this strange and unnecessary change in procedure, Donald replied, "I want to save on gas." When his son questioned why driving one truck rather than the usual two would save gas, Donald was adamant about the change. Perplexed, his son agreed to the change. The next morning, Donald had apparently forgotten the illogical idea, and they returned to the typical feeding of the livestock with two trucks.

Over the next few months, Donald's ability to communicate deteriorated. There were frequent problems remembering words and difficulty keeping his mind on the topic of discussion. His family attributed his frequent requests to repeat statements, failure to follow directions, and confusion about the topic of conversations to a loss of hearing. Even after an audiologist tested him and provided a hearing aid, he still displayed the same types of confused behaviors. He became obsessed with certain obscure governmental policies and took less interest in the day-to-day farming requirements. He also seemed to distance himself from his family. During the late stages of dementia, Donald began making statements that no one could understand. Even his grandchildren commented that he was "talking crazy" and was frequently agitated. Before his family made the hard decision to put Donald in a nearby nursing home, he only spoke occasionally, and when he did, it was often meaningless, an echo of what had been spoken by someone else, or was incomprehensible.

Alzheimer's disease are unlikely to be confused with patients who have nonfluent aphasia because the motor strip is not affected throughout most of the course of the disease. Ripich and Ziol (1998) report no syntax or phonology errors in patients with early-stage Alzheimer's disease.

Middle Stage

According to Ripich and Ziol (1998), patients in middle-stage Alzheimer's disease are less aware and start to have difficulty comprehending complex grammatical structures. Patients have diminished vocabulary and poor word fluency, but there are no phonological errors. The pragmatic category continues to be where most problems with communication are noted. There is poor topic maintenance, frequent requests to repeat statements, and fewer ideas. The patient in the middle stage talks about past events or trivia. "There is rarely correction of mistakes and frequent automatic and stereotypical utterances such as 'I'm fine, dear. How are you? Aren't you sweet!'" (Ripich & Ziol, 1998, p. 476).

Late Stage

According to Ripich and Ziol (1998), during late-stage Alzheimer's disease, the patient is unaware of communication disorders. Pragmatically, there is a lack of coherence, difficulty maintaining eye contact, and poor conversational turn-taking. Verbal expressions may be meaningless or bizarre. Semantic problems include jargon and a poor vocabulary. Grammar is generally preserved, but more phonology errors occur. Comprehension is poor. Some patients become mute in the final stages of Alzheimer's disease. This was the case with nursing home resident George in the film *Age Old Friends*.

The communication disorders seen in other types of dementia depend on the number, site, and size of the **infarcts** to the brain. Whether the damage is cortical or subcortical is an important consideration. According to Bayles (1994), major cortical damage results in amnesia, visuospatial deficits, and aphasia. Subcortical damage is associated with memory impairment and psychomotor retardation.

Other common verbal manifestations of dementia include perseveration, echolalia, logorrhea, circumlocution, confabulation, and tangential speech (Table 9.1). **Perseveration** is

TABLE 9.1 *Verbal Manifestations in Dementia*

Verbal Manifestation	Description
Circumlocution	Saying of an alternate sound, word, or phrase for one that is feared, difficult to produce, or unavailable for recall
Confabulation	Tendency to remark about something without regard to truthfulness or accuracy of the statement
Echolalia	Tendency to repeat the last sound, word, or phrase that was heard
Logorrhea	Continuous production of words that have no apparent semantic connection
Perseveration	Tendency for a motor or mental act to continue for a longer duration than is appropriate
Tangential speech	Lacking continuity and consistency in a train of thought

the tendency for a motor or mental act to continue for a longer duration than is appropriate. It is difficulty shifting from one thought or movement pattern to another. Perseveration involves verbal and written responses. Verbal perseveration is when a patient continually says a word or phrase. For example, if asked what she wants for lunch, the patient may continually answer "salad" even when the question has been changed to "Do you want to go outside?" Graphic perseveration is when the patient repeatedly writes the same letter or word. For example, he may write one letter in his name repeatedly. The tendency to perseverate has not been identified with a specific damaged area of the brain (Swindell, Holland, & Reinmuth, 1998). The more extensive the brain damage, the more likely the patient is to perseverate. Perseveration and echolalia often go hand-in-hand. **Echolalia** is the tendency to repeat the last sound, word, or phrase that was heard. The last word spoken contaminates the patient's train of thought. According to Benson and Ardila (1996), echolalia is a feature of many degenerative brain diseases. (Echolalia and perseveration are discussed in detail in Chapter 8.)

Logorrhea, sometimes seen in patients with dementia, is the continuous production of words that have no apparent semantic connection. The patient engages in nonstop, incoherent speech. Demented patients with logorrhea appear to have a strong need to continuously talk. It seems to satisfy some psychological need to remain verbal, albeit incomprehensible. The patient may also receive an inner reward for hearing her speech. For some patients, logorrhea may provide a cathartic effect.

Circumlocution is the saying of an alternate sound, word, or phrase for one that is feared, difficult to produce, or unavailable for recall. It is a common aspect to stuttering (see Chapter 2). Circumlocution is more likely in early-stage dementia because patients are more aware of their communication problems and attempt to self-correct.

Confabulation is the tendency to remark about something without regard to truthfulness or accuracy of the statement. Demented patients who confabulate appear to make up events and distort real ones. One patient with organic brain syndrome engaged in *morbid confabulation*. She continuously talked about how some animals eat other animals and would make up endings to examples in an attempt to complete an idea. The train of thought got progressively more morbid until she began talking about cannibalism. Finally, she appeared to appreciate the negativity of her thoughts and stopped talking altogether (Tanner, 1977).

Tangential speech is seen when a person lacks continuity and consistency in a train of thought; that is, he mentally wanders. In some patients a word at the end of a statement will set them off on another idea, which they will talk about, and yet another word at the end of that statement will prompt another tangential episode. Tangential speech is an indication of impaired concentration and the inability to focus on the intent and goal of communication.

Evaluating and Treating Communication Disorders in Patients with Dementia

There are three aspects to the management of patients with communication disorders associated with dementia (Table 9.2). First, speech, language, and hearing assessment is necessary to decide the nature and type of the communication disorder. Comprehensive hearing evaluation is important to rule out hearing loss as a possible reason for some of the symptoms of dementia. Problems following commands, completing tasks, and turn-taking during

TABLE 9.2 *Evaluating and Treating Communication Disorders in Dementia*

Intervention	Description
Comprehensive speech, language, and hearing evaluation	• Detailed audiological assessment to rule out hearing deficits and to provide treatment as appropriate • Detailed motor speech assessment to identify speech pathologies and appropriate therapies • Detailed language and cognitive assessment to determine deficiencies and whether patient can benefit from therapy
Direct therapy	• For patients who can benefit from speech language and dysphagia therapies, individual and group therapy • Therapy to include *reminiscence* and *life review* as stimuli for therapeutic activities • Group therapies to improve orientation and memory • Continuous monitoring of treatment objectives and outcomes to determine whether patient can continue to profit from experience
Training and counseling of medical staff and family	• In-service training for hospital, nursing home, and home health care agencies' medical staff, including physicians, nurses, nursing aides, and food service staff • Therapy, training, and counseling to address dysphagia • Ongoing training and counseling of family members and friends of the patient; goals and objectives adjusted to the changing conditions of the patient • Ongoing training and counseling of medical staff, family, and friends to address safety issues

conversations can be related to hearing loss. Hearing loss can also be the reason why patients frequently ask that questions be repeated. Sometimes, a patient may appear to have lost the ability to understand the meanings of words when the problem is in fact hearing them. Surgery and amplification can reduce or eliminate many problems with communication that may have been attributed to dementia. Speech and language evaluation is also necessary to determine which aspects of the communication disorder are likely to benefit from treatment. "Early identification is extremely valuable for patients with reversible dementia, as well as for those with irreversible dementia. Patients with reversible dementia need treatment, and patients with irreversible dementia and their families need information about how to maximize communicative performance" (Bayless, 1994, p. 541).

The second area of intervention involves direct therapy. Although, as a group, patients with communication disorders related to irreversible dementia have not been shown to benefit significantly from speech and language therapy, some individuals may be able to profit from experience and can improve. Some patients' mental functioning deteriorates slowly, and thus individual and group therapies can help stave off communication disorders. Many of the direct therapy approaches used with head trauma patients (see Chapter 10) can be used, including memory drills, reality orientation, and group therapies. Ripich and Ziol (1998) also recommend a unique and innovative approach, called reminiscence and life review, to treat communication disorders associated with dementia. The vocal or silent review of events in one's life is called *reminiscence*. It differs from *life review*, which entails organizing and evaluating the overall picture of one's life. Although little research has been done on the effects of reminiscence and life review, both activities may be helpful in improving behavior, cognition, and self-esteem. Tanner (1977), in a pilot study, found that when cognitively intact volunteer patients in a nursing home engaged in basic reality orientation therapy with patients with mild to moderate dementia, some areas of cognition showed improvement. Both the patients with dementia and the volunteers reported satisfaction with the activities.

The third area of intervention involves training and counseling to the medical staff and the patient's family. Communication problems can interfere with medical management of nondementia illnesses in patients with dementia (Brauner, Muir, & Sachs, 2000). Staff members in long-term facilities and home health agencies are provided with information related to the nature and progression of the communication disorders seen in dementia. This can increase their knowledge, improve communication, and decrease problems related to communication breakdown (Ripich & Ziol, 1998). Family counseling is employed to help them understand the nature of the communication disorders associated with dementia, how to deal with them, and to help prepare for eventualities.

Literature and Media Stereotypes

When important political figures or popular entertainment personalities get a major illness, the public is educated about the cause or causes, nature, and course of the disease or disorder. Both the print and electronic media usually cover the disorder in great detail. Experts about the illness are interviewed, books are written, and television specials are aired about it. When that person is a former president of the United States, such as Ronald Reagan, finding people who are not made more aware of the disease is difficult. The educational value of the president's diseases and disorders was apparent when he had two types of cancer removed and when he was fitted for an all-in-the-ear hearing aid. Even when the spouse of the president has a disease or disorder, there is extensive news coverage and education value. This was true for President Gerald Ford's wife, Betty, and her drug dependency, and with Nancy Reagan and her breast cancer. When famous people openly admit and discuss their illnesses, a consequent reduction occurs in the stigmas and stereotypes associated with them. Alzheimer's disease, hearing loss, cancer, and drug dependency are dealt with in a more factual manner, and the myths and mysteries are often removed from them.

Although Reagan was considered a competent president who helped bring patriotism and economic prosperity back to the United States and who some considered the catalyst for winning the cold war with the Soviet Union, there were early symptoms of Alzheimer's disease during his last term in office. Once, Nancy Reagan finished a speech for him, and there was another instance of him becoming temporarily disoriented. These reports were not widely publicized. The White House, probably with the support of the press core, under-played those and other episodes of confusion and memory lapses.

With his advancing age during his last term, some people questioned his competency, especially in dealing with the deteriorating and volatile Soviet Union. It was hoped that there were checks and balances that would prevent the premature and unnecessary escalation of global conflict due to his, or any president's, mental incompetency. In the United States, however, the president is the commander-in-chief of the armed forces and can give the command to launch thousands of thermonuclear missiles at any country in the world. It is disconcerting to know that a mentally or psychologically incompetent president has this unchecked power. Although removing a president from office for dementia has never been necessary, it would require extensive and time-consuming legal and political processes. Impeaching and removing a mentally compromised president who did not want to leave office would be a difficult task.

Other than with Reagan, the media and literature have not devoted much coverage to people with dementia. The major film studios have not produced a movie specifically addressing this disorder, nor have the major television networks created a prime-time show addressing it. There are two reasons for the lack of film and television coverage about dementia. First, creating such a film would be difficult because as the dementia progresses, the story line and plot would lack consistency. For example, a starring character with dementia would be progressively unable to contribute to the plot or story line as the disease progresses. Second, there may be little entertainment value of watching a movie or television show about dementia. Although the film *Age Old Friends* addressed dementia, it was not received well at the box office.

In the movie *Age Old Friends,* Aylott and Cooper refer to residents of the nursing home who have dementia as "zombies" who live their last days in disorientation and confusion. They also recognize that in some ways becoming a zombie eliminates fear and distress. This lack of awareness of what has happened is a blessing in disguise. The two lifelong friends in the film also view dementia as a "war." Maintaining cognitive integrity is a battle to be fought with slim chances of winning. *Age Old Friends* does an excellent job in showing the fear associated with forgetfulness and disorientation. One of the most poignant observations made in the film is that elderly people often measure the passage of time by what has been lost.

The comedy effect of an older person with early and relatively innocuous symptoms of dementia is used in many movies and television shows. The minor mistakes in judgment, memory problems, and confusion are often used for their humor value. Rarely do they address bowel and urinary incontinence, swallowing disorders, dangerous behaviors, anger, or depression and anxiety associated with it. It is as if dementia is homogenized for public consumption. This comedy-relief value of dementia is seen in the popular and long-running television show *The Simpsons*. Because Abraham Simpson is only a cartoon character, it allows the writers to fully use dementia's entertainment value without having to show the negative emotional effect about his psychological adjustment to it.

Myths and inaccurate stereotypes abound about dementia. Perhaps the worst commonly held myth is that senility is a natural and necessary course of the normal aging process. Some people in their seventh, eighth, and later decades of life do have disorders and diseases that compromise their mental functioning, but many older people continue to be alert, active, and mentally competent. They work well past the typical age of retirement, enjoying their later years and continuing to be viable members of society.

Summary

Dementia can cause several communication disorders, and 50% of people over the age of 85 have some symptoms of it. The most common cause of dementia is Alzheimer's disease, which is the fourth leading cause of death in the United States. Patients with dementia often have disruptive behaviors, hallucinations, delusions, and problems with memory and orientation. In early-stage dementia, most of the communication symptoms are subtle, and the patient is aware of them. In middle-stage dimentia, the patient rarely corrects mistakes and often says automatic and stereotypical statements. In late-stage dementia, coherence is lacking and verbal expressions may be meaningless or bizarre. Although some patients can benefit from speech and language therapies for dementia, as a group, most patients cannot and thus are not candidates for therapy. When dementia is dealt with in literature and media, it is usually in a humorous way and does not depict the panic and fear that many patients experience.

Study Questions

1. Why is an Alzheimer's disease epidemic looming in the future?
2. Compare and contrast the causes of dementia.
3. Define *hallucination* and give two examples.
4. Define *delusion* and give two examples.
5. List and discuss aspects of early-stage dementia.
6. List and discuss aspects of middle-stage dementia.
7. List and discuss aspects of late-stage dementia.
8. What is *confabulation*?
9. What is *tangential speech*?
10. What are the three aspects to treating communication disorders associated with dementia?
11. Do patients with dementia benefit from therapy? Why or why not?
12. How do literature and media portray people with dementia?

Suggested Reading

Kennedy, W. Z. (1999). Delirium, dementia, amnesia, and other cognitive disorders. In P. G. O'Brien, W. Z. Kennedy, and K. A. Ballard (Eds.), *Psychiatric nursing: An integration of theory and practice.* New York: McGraw-Hill. This chapter provides a review of the nature and treatment of cognitive disorders from a nursing perspective.

10

Communication Disorders Resulting from Head and Neck Injuries

Chapter Preview

In this chapter you will learn about communication disorders resulting from injuries to the head and neck. You will learn about the types of head and neck injures and their symptoms. You will explore consciousness and how it is impaired in many patients with serious traumatic brain injuries. Impaired executive functions and disorientation are discussed. Memory problems are examined, including those related to attention, long- and short-term storage, and retrieval. The behavioral problems experienced by some patients with traumatic brain injuries are reviewed, including aggression, disinhibition, and other socially inappropriate actions. There is a section on traumatic brain injury in children; brain damage in children often has different outcomes and prognoses than what is seen in adults. There is a section on audiology and traumatic brain injuries. Rehabilitation of the traumatic brain-injured patient is discussed. Finally, you will learn how literature and media deal with people with head and neck injuries.

It is a sad irony that many people who suffer traumatic head and neck injuries are young, vital, energetic, and athletic. They love the excitement of skiing, the adrenaline rush of bungee cord jumping, and the skilled teamwork of horse and rider clearing an obstacle. The acceleration of a motorcycle smoothly shifting gears onto a freeway ramp is a powerful aphrodisiac to some people. Sadly, the very people who revel in speed, acceleration, and the freedom of mobility sometimes suffer the dire consequences of head and neck injuries and find themselves confined to a wheelchair or bed. Often these people also must suffer the frustration and isolation of communication disorders that frequently occur with serious head and neck injuries.

We also live in an increasingly violent society. It seems that no nightly news telecast would be complete without references to a drive-by shooting, terrorist attack, gang fighting, or a mugging. Purposeful and accidental gunshot wounds to the head are common news items and fuel political debates over gun control legislation. Rarely does a year go by without a media reference to a senseless shooting in a school, replete with the insensitive closeups of the tears and anguish of survivors and families. And, of course, there always seems to be wars. Whether they are little regional conflicts or world wars, some soldiers come home with shrapnel lodged in their brains. As you would expect, head and neck injuries can cause major mental and physical disabilities, including communication disorders.

In the not-too-distant past, not many patients with serious head injuries were on the caseloads of speech–language pathologists and audiologists. They accounted for a small percentage of the patients treated for communication disorders. The reason for this was tragic but simple: Many patients died because of their serious injuries. Improved emergency transportation services and medical advances, however, have dramatically increased the survival rates of people involved in serious automobile accidents, falls, gunshot wounds, and other violent events. Most hospitals are now equipped to treat critically injured patients, and there are many more trauma centers. Additionally, helicopter transportation services are now widely available, enabling emergency medical personnel to rapidly transport patients to hospitals for lifesaving medical care. Rapid transportation to hospitals is important with all serious traumatic injuries, but it is particularly necessary for patients with head injuries. There is a short "window of opportunity" available to neurosurgeons to relieve dangerous pressure within the skull that often happens with serious traumatic brain injuries. "The decrease in mortality and improved outcome for patients with severe traumatic brain injury over the past 25 years can be attributed to the approach of 'squeezing oxygenated blood through a swollen brain'" (Ghajar, 2000, p. 923). Today, many patients are brought to hospitals and trauma centers in time to save their lives. In the United States, the incident of nonfatal traumatic brain injuries (discharge rates from hospitals) ranges from 180 to 220 per 100,000 population each year (Kraus & Sorenson, 1994).

The Head-Injured Person

Who gets a serious head injury? What are the common risk factors? Many studies have addressed the characteristics of high-risk groups, and they have yielded surprisingly similar results. The typical person at risk for a serious **traumatic brain injury** (TBI) is a young male earning a low income, who was under the influence of alcohol at the scene of the accident, and who had probably been admitted to a hospital previously for a head injury.

People between the ages of 15 and 24 years are at the highest risk for TBI (Kraus & Sorenson, 1994). This is because young people tend to be more active and less careful. Bicycle and motorcycle accidents are common among the young, as are climbing and sports injuries. Males engage in more risk-taking activities, especially with automobiles, and tend to work at dangerous occupations. Most studies suggest that males are two to three times more likely to suffer a TBI. According to Gillis (1996), approximately 50% of all injuries are the result of motor vehicle accidents, and alcohol is a significant factor in the cause of them. The research that provides these statistics are often correlational studies. A *correlation* is the way two variables correlate, or are linked. Studies show a positive correlation with low socioeconomic status and TBI; the reason for this positive correlation is unclear. It could be related to the fact that low-income jobs tend to be more dangerous and that younger people,

Literature, Media, and Personality Profiles

James Brady

James Brady was born in Centralia, Illinois, on August 29, 1940. He received a Bachelor of Science degree in Communications and Political Science from the University of Illinois in 1962. From 1973 to 1975, he was the special assistant to the secretary of Housing and Urban Development and later appointed as the special assistant to the director of the Office of Management and Budget. He also served as assistant to the secretary of defense. In 1981 he was appointed White House press secretary. He was shot in the head on March 30, 1981, when John Hinckley, Jr., attempted to assassinate President Ronald Reagan. He spent 9 months in the hospital and underwent two surgeries to remove fluid from his brain. Even though he has a communication disorder resulting from the traumatic brain injury, he is active on the speaking circuit. He is a proponent for gun control legislation and was the driving force behind the 1993 "Brady Bill," which requires instant computerized background checks on buyers of guns.

Christopher Reeve

Christopher Reeve was born in New York City. At a young age, he was attracted to the theater and had several parts in school plays. After graduating from high school, he attended Cornell University where he majored in Music Theory and English. During his final year at Cornell, Reeve and his friend, Robin Williams, were accepted at the Juilliard School of Performing Arts and studied under John Houseman. In 1976 Reeve went to Los Angeles and auditioned for the 1978 movie *Superman*. He also did the time-travel, love story *Somewhere in Time*. He went on to appear in 17 feature films, several TV movies, and over 100 plays. Reeve was a superb athlete who did his own stunts. He was also a pilot, expert scuba diver, and skier. He also loved horses. In May 1995, during a cross-country jumping event, Reeve's thoroughbred balked at a rail jump. Reeve's hands were tangled in the horse's bridle and he landed head first. He was instantly paralyzed from the neck down and unable to breathe. Thanks to prompt medical attention, he survived the broken neck. He spent 6 months in the Kessler Rehabilitation Institute in New Jersey. He operates a wheelchair by sucking or puffing on a straw. Since the accident he has become active in increasing awareness of spinal cord injuries and is involved in fund-raising for research. Reeve continues to make appearances at conventions and on television, but he must be careful about speaking. Sometimes, he cannot speak if his tracheotomy tube is slightly out of position or if his body suddenly spasms and jerks uncontrollably. Since the accident he has regained some sensation in parts of his body. He continues to be very active and has written his autobiography, *Still Me*.

Jan Berry

Jan Berry and Dean Torrence both attended University High School in west Los Angeles, California. They played football together and after practice would harmonize to some of the popular songs of the day. They formed a garage band and began performing as The Barons. The band soon became Jan and Dean. In the early 1960s, Jan and Dean recorded a series of car songs including "Drag City," "Little Old Lady from Pasadena," and "Deadman's Curve," which peaked on the rock charts at numbers 10, 3, and 8, respectively. "Deadman's Curve" was a song about a car accident, which foretold of a serious car crash for Berry. On April 12, 1966, Berry crashed his new Corvette Stingray into the back of a parked truck. The paramedics thought he was dead at the scene. Berry was rushed to UCLA hospital and underwent several brain surgeries. He was in a deep coma for weeks and when he emerged from it, he could not walk or speak. Today, he still has problems speaking, but he is able to sing relatively well. It took 7 years before Jan and Dean could sing together again on stage. In 1977 CBS television made a movie entitled *Deadman's Curve* about Jan and Dean and the accident. Today, they continue to tour and perform nationally and internationally.

Gary Busey

Actor and musician Gary Busey was once nicknamed Gary "Abusey." For decades he has been considered one of the "bad boys" of Hollywood, was heavily involved in drugs, and had several brushes with the law. In 1996 he attended a Promise Keepers rally in Los Angeles and announced that he had found Jesus and freedom from drug addiction.

Busey was born on June 29, 1944, in Goose Creek, Texas. His family were devout Christians. He attended Kansas State University and Oklahoma State University and majored in theater. He moved to Hollywood and appeared in several television shows including *Kung Fu* and *Gunsmoke*. In the 1970s he made several movies, and in 1978 he starred and sang in *The Buddy Holly Story* and was nominated for an Oscar. In 1988 he was involved in a motorcycle accident and was not wearing a helmet at the time; he had been very vocal in his opposition to motorcycle helmet laws. During brain surgery he had a religious experience where God told him to seek spiritual help. His faith in God was further tested in 1997, when he had surgery to remove a cancerous growth from his sinus cavity.

Awakenings

The film *Awakenings* is based on the book by Dr. Oliver Sacks, who was born July 9, 1933, in London and obtained his medical degree from Oxford University. (The book was republished by Vintage Books in September 1999.) The book is an account of several patients who contracted sleeping sickness during the great flu epidemic after World War II. They had been in a comalike state for years when in 1969 Sacks gave them the new anti-Parkinson drug L-dopa. The book explores their lives and the remarkable, temporary recovery caused by the drug.

Directed by Penny Marshall, the film adaptation stars Robin Williams as Dr. Sacks and Robert De Niro as one of the patients. De Niro received an Oscar nomination for Best Actor in his portrayal of Leonard Lowe, who knows he is returning to the comalike state.

Sacks is also the author of the best-selling book *The Man Who Mistook His Wife for a Hat*, a collection of case histories about patients with unusual and interesting neurological disorders.

The Bone Collector

The Bone Collector, released in 1999, is based on Jeffery Deaver's best-selling novel by the same name. Directed by Phillip Noyce, it stars Denzel Washington as Lincoln Rhyme, a criminalist who suffers a spinal injury from a falling metal beam while working at a crime scene. The plot revolves around the attempts of Rhyme, who is confined to bed, to solve several brutal murders. The film also stars Angelina Jolie as Amelia Donaghy, who reluctantly becomes the paralyzed Rhyme's eyes, ears, and legs. At each murder site, the murderer leaves vague clues that only the brilliant Rhyme can decipher. The film poignantly depicts the frustration and despair experienced by Rhyme and the fear that he will suffer a seizure that will result in a permanent vegetative state. The film does an excellent job of showing the technological advances available to paralyzed people, enabling them to be more independent and productive.

(continued)

Literature, Media, and Personality Profiles (continued)

Memento

Memento is the story of a man with short-term memory deficits. The plot revolves around his attempts to take revenge on a man who raped and killed his wife. It is a penetrating view into the confusion caused by this type of memory loss and the strategies used to cope with it. The role memory plays in continuity of life is captured in this quote: "We need memory to remind ourselves who we are." Based on a short story by Jonathan Nolan, *Memento* was directed by Christopher Nolan; stars Guy Pearce, Carrie-Anne Moss, and Joe Pantoliano; and was produced by Suzanne and Jennifer Todd.

who make less money, are employed in them. All published studies show a positive correlation between blood alcohol levels and TBIs. Alcohol also appears to be a negative factor in the patient's rehabilitation and recovery. Some studies also show a high recidivism rate; *recidivism* is the tendency for something to recur. People with TBIs tend to have high recidivism rates because many survivors continue to engage in high-risk activities or dangerous occupations.

The Mechanics of Traumatic Head and Neck Injuries

There are two categories of traumatic head injury: open and closed. **Open-head injury** (OHI) occurs when an object, a missile or projectile, penetrates the head. These kinds of injuries are often seen in combat. Soldiers suffer brain damage because bullets, mine, or bomb fragments enter the head. Open-head injuries also happen to victims of drive-by shootings, rioting, and robberies. Industrial, automotive, and recreational accidents may also cause OHIs. James Brady received an OHI during the assassination attempt on President Reagan. The weapon used was a small-caliber pistol, and the projectile was the lead bullet.

Closed-head injuries (CHI) are more common and are usually the result of motor vehicle accidents or falls. In CHIs, the primary and initial site of the brain damage is the *coup*. It is where the brain is damaged by the force of the impact. In physics we know that for every action there is an opposite and equal reaction, and Newton's law accounts for injury to the brain in other areas besides the primary site of damage. The damage to the brain as a result of the recoil and impact of the brain within the skull is called the *contracoup*. The mechanism of coup and contracoup are also seen in open, penetrating injuries because of the force of the missile or projectile hitting the head.

Both types of head trauma can cause focal and diffuse brain damage. *Focal damage* occurs when the injury is limited to one identifiable site of the brain. *Diffuse damage* involves more than one site. Initially, both OHI and CHI often cause similar symptoms, but as time passes they can diverge in their nature and the way they are presented. Objects that cause penetrating head wounds, particularly small-caliber bullets with hollow and jagged tips, create a tearing and shearing action that damage the brain differently than a blunt blow. Some missile wounds tend to be more specific in the area damaged.

Gillis and Pierce (1996) describe the principal forces that result in brain injury: impact, acceleration, and deceleration. *Impact* occurs when a moving object strikes the head. An impact injury may be caused by a falling tool at a construction site or when a slower moving or stationary object is struck by the head. An *acceleration* injury to the brain can happen when the head is suddenly propelled by an external force such as a club, fist, or bat. A *deceleration* injury occurs when the head abruptly stops when it hits a fixed object such as the pavement or dashboard of a car. Gillis and Pierce (1996) note that the principal type of injury in closed-head trauma is a result of *diffuse axonal injury*, a shearing of the axon during rotational acceleration of the brain.

Neck and spinal injuries are most often classified by the site of the fracture. For example, Christopher Reeve suffered a C1–C2 injury, which is also known as the "hangman fracture" (when people are hanged, the break in the vertebrae is often at the C1–C2 level). A C1–C2 fracture occurs at the junction of the first and second cervical vertebrae. Other ways of classifying spinal cord injuries are by the neurologic level of damage, whether they are complete or incomplete, and by impaired function; there are several spinal cord syndromes (Mackay, Chapman, & Morgan, 1997).

Professional and amateur football players sometimes suffer serious head and neck injuries. Even though these players are provided with state-of-the-art helmets and other protective gear, the forces on the head and neck during a tackle or collision can be enormous. Impact, acceleration, and deceleration injuries can result. Sports announcers often trivialize these injuries by saying that the player has had his "bell rung." The player is taken off the field, often on a stretcher, with serious injuries. Some players continue to play in a dazed state.

Athletic associations have established rules to decrease these dangerous injuries. One such regulation, which has recently been enacted by the National College Athletic Association (NCAA), is the "free blocking zone," or "halo," rule and deals with the kickoff and punt return. The kickoff and punt return are two of the most dangerous plays in football. Often the opposing team members reach the receiver, at full speed, at about the time he is catching the ball. Then he is hit while in a vulnerable standing position by the 200- or 300-pound linemen traveling at maximum speed. The force of the impact during these plays have caused many head and neck injuries. With the free blocking zone rule, the receiver is allowed time to safely catch the ball before attempting the return; that is, a buffer zone is created. This rule should result in fewer football players "having their bells rung" and resulting serious head and neck injuries. The movie *Any Given Sunday* dramatically shows the violence and resulting physical effects associated with repeated football injuries.

Technology has eased some of the frustration for head- and neck-injured people. An example of the revolution in technology for the disabled is seen in the film *The Bone Collector*. Denzel Washington plays the part of Lincoln Rhyme, who has a spinal injury. Left with movement only above his shoulders and in his index finger, he is confined to bed and depends on a nurse, colleagues, and friends for much of his day-to-day care. A sophisticated computer and technology setup at his bed helps him investigate and ultimately solve several murder cases in New York City. He can adjust his bed by using a suck-and-puff device. The computer and other high-tech devices can be activated by minimal movements of his finger. Perhaps the most helpful innovation to the criminalist is the voice-activated technology. By voicing simple commands such as "View," "Scan," and "Search," he can use the computer as easily as a person who can use a keyboard. Rhyme can even play chess with the computer by using voice commands.

Communication Disorders and Impaired Consciousness

Some patients with TBIs and communication disorders are normal with regard to their levels of consciousness; that is, the brain injury does not result in impaired consciousness. The communication disorders experienced by these patients include language disorders in which they have problems remembering words or understanding them when they are spoken by someone else. Expressive and receptive language are disrupted in patients whose TBI is focalized in the speech and language centers. Some patients have difficulty programming and sequencing utterances or problems speaking due to paralyzed speech muscles. (See Chapters 7 and 8 for a discussion of aphasia, apraxia of speech, and the dysarthrias.) However, these patients are not significantly impaired with regard to their awareness of self and the environment. Certainly, because they have experienced these neurogenic communication disorders, they have been affected psychologically. Their sense of self and their psychological integrity have been affected, but their levels of consciousness have not been substantially affected.

The majority of patients with significant OHI and CHI have reduced levels of awareness, as do some patients who have had strokes or diseases of the brain. Patients with TBIs typically experience disorientation, memory deficits, and behavioral problems that are indicative of reduced or impaired consciousness. Some patients are in a deep coma, and others simply experience a slight clouding of consciousness.

Consciousness is an intriguing concept, and a variety of disorders and states can affect it. In the broadest sense of the term, *consciousness* means awareness of self and the environment, but the word means more than awareness. To be conscious implies memory of the past and integration of all aspects of reality into the present. Consciousness is awareness of the past, alertness to the present, and realistic appraisal of the future. Consciousness is the ultimate process of abstraction, and it is impossible to directly measure it; one can only infer it based a person's verbal reports and behaviors. A patient in a deep coma likely has no awareness of self or the environment. At the other end of the consciousness scale, patients suffering from anxiety or depression have altered consciousness; that is, their awareness of self and the environment has been changed and consequently so has their consciousness. However, many patients with TBIs have significantly reduced awareness levels as a result of their injuries, and many are comatose.

Coma

According to Gillis and Pierce (1996), coma is a concept or state without clear definition. In the most basic of terms, *coma* is a state of unconsciousness. A person in a deep coma cannot be aroused with strong prompting and coaxing or even by feeling pain. Also, there is no responsiveness to internal needs. Lesser states of impaired consciousness are called by many terms, including *delirium* and *stupor*. These terms refer to someone who is only partially and inappropriately responsive to her internal needs and external events.

In literature and media, a patient in a coma is sometimes likened to someone who is asleep. Sleep, like coma, has deep and light states. Although similarities exist between sleep and coma, they are vastly different states. Scientists, using instruments that measure brain waves, have found that coma patients go through several states of sleep, as found in normal people. Some patients in a coma do not appear asleep because their eyes are open. This type of impaired consciousness is called an *eye-open vegetative state*—a type of coma in which the patient appears awake because the eyes are reflexively open, but no speech, thought, or purposeful body actions occur. Of course, the main difference between sleep and coma is that the sleeping person can be awakened. In the film *Awakenings*, the patient's reduced levels of consciousness were a result of *encephalitis lethargia*, or swelling of the brain. (It is sometimes called sleeping sickness.)

Several tests are available to measure and evaluate coma. The most widely used test is the Glasgow Coma Scale (Teasdale & Gennett, 1974). This test can be rapidly administered and measures the patient's eye opening, best motor response, and speech. The scoring ranges from 3 to 15. Patients with a score of 8 or less usually have severe head injury, and about half of them die as a result of their injuries. Even patients who score more than 12 on the scale experience problems for several months after the injury. Patients with a score of 13 or higher may not have a loss of consciousness, whereas those with a score of 8 or less usually have a loss of consciousness lasting longer than 24 hours (Gillis & Pierce, 1996; Andrews, 1992).

Another widely used test of cognitive functioning is the Rancho los Amigos Scale (Hagen, 1981). It is a descriptive test, and the patient's scores range from "no response" to "purposeful, appropriate" ones. This test is valuable in providing consistency within the rehabilitation team and can be used to help family understand the process of recovery (Mackay et al., 1997). According to Mackay et al. (1997), Level I (No Response), Level II (Generalized Response), and Level III (Localized Response) are seen most often in intensive care units, and they describe varying levels of coma. Other responses include Confused, Agitated (Level IV); Confused, Inappropriate, Nonagitated (Level V); Confused, Appropriate (Level VI); Automatic, Appropriate (Level VII); and Purposeful, Appropriate (Level VIII).

Communication Disorders and the Site of Traumatic Brain Injuries

When describing the speech and language behaviors of patients with TBI, one quickly becomes aware of terminology confusion. According to Gillis (1996), "One of the greatest problems in terminology within the field of speech–language pathology is the description of neurobehavioral sequelae, in particular the breakdown in communication skills" (p. 90). The problem with terminology is a result of trying to compare the neurogenic communication disorders typically seen in strokes to those seen in patients with TBI. Aphasia, apraxia of speech, and the dysarthrias are presented differently in patients who are lethargic or agitated, disoriented, or who have global memory deficits.

The site, nature, and extent of TBI determines the symptoms presented by the patient. There are three general ways of looking at the speech and language symptoms seen in TBI.

First, a small percentage of patients have only their speech and language centers damaged. Because there is focalized damage to the centers, their primary communication disorders resemble aphasia, apraxia of speech, and/or the dysarthrias, which are seen in many stroke patients. As discussed previously, these patients typically do not have reduced levels of consciousness. Second, some patients have brain damage, but the major speech and language centers are spared. Although these patients may also have problems communicating, the fabric of language and the motor speech processes remain intact. These patients primarily present with arousal, orientation, behavioral, and memory problems. Third, patients can have symptoms of aphasia, apraxia of speech, and the dysarthrias compounded by arousal, orientation, behavioral, and memory problems. The common characteristic that affects communication in most TBIs is reduced or impaired consciousness.

Damage to the right and left hemispheres of the brain causes different symptoms in patients with TBI. The left hemisphere is considered dominant in most people and the side of the brain that is primarily verbal, but the right hemisphere also has verbal functions. According to Mesulam (1985), the right hemisphere is specialized for paralinguistic aspects of communication. The paralinguistic aspects of communication include prosody, attention to and perception of verbal input, organizing and comprehending complex information, and abstraction with regard to language. According to Pimental and Kingsbury (1989), damage to the right hemisphere may seriously impair affective components of prosody, gestures, and facial expressions without disrupting the linguistic features of language. Patients with damage primarily to the right hemisphere may have trouble perceiving and interpreting the emotional content of verbal and nonverbal aspects of language.

Lovell and Franzen (1994) list common sequelae of TBI relative to the lobes of the brain that are damaged. *Diffused damage* often results in information-processing deficits, impairments of attention and memory, decreased motor speed, and reaction times. Damage to the *temporal lobes* causes verbal memory deficits, auditory agnosia, and Wernicke's aphasia. Damage to the *parietal lobes* results in visuospatial impairments. Right–left confusion, acalculia, alexia, apraxia, and denial of illness are also associated with parietal lobe damage. When the occipital lobes are damaged, visual representation is impaired, including reading and writing. Cortical blindness, and **homonymous hemianopsia** (blindness in one-half of the fields of both eyes) is also associated with damage to the occipital lobes. Lovell and Franzen (1994) list other sequelae related to the site of brain damage, but the ones listed above are primarily associated with speaking, reading, writing, and understanding the speech and intent of others.

Frontal lobe syndrome is a common label given to patients who have had TBI. Although the nature of this syndrome is the subject of debate, certain symptoms can be seen in patients who have frontal lobe damage (Stuss & Benson, 1986). Lezak (1982) describes a patient with frontal lobe injuries as having a problem with initiation, inability to shift responses, difficulty monitoring behaviors, and profound concreteness. Loss of self-regulation is an important aspect to frontal lobe syndrome. Patients with frontal lobe damage often lose emotional control and may engage in bizarre behaviors. They lose the ability to understand the appropriateness of actions. There are often delayed response times and memory problems. Expressive aphasia is present when there is damage to Broca's and adjacent areas of the frontal lobes. Of course, the behaviors displayed by a patient depend on the type and severity of damage done to the frontal lobes, his preexisting personality, and the environmental demands. Frontal lobe syndrome is best thought of as being a problem with executive functions.

Executive Functions

Executive functions have been described as the ability to formulate and plan goals and then effectively carry them out (Lezak, 1983). Gillis (1996) notes that the concept is analogous to a business executive or chief executive officer. The top executive at a business is involved in planning, monitoring of progress, and attending to feedback about the course and direction of the company. Loss of or impaired executive functions in a patient is like having absent or disrupted management skills. "Behaviorally these may be observed as inhibition, deliberation, coordination, and self-regulation" (Gillis, 1996, p. 112). Although impairments of executive functioning can be observed in many brain injuries, damage to the frontal lobes plays an important part in patients who are impaired in this high-level ability.

A clinician's primary responsibility is to help people with brain injuries achieve goals and live satisfying lives (Ylvisaker & Feeney, 1998). To help meet that responsibility, Ylvisaker and Feeney (1998, p. 53) have proposed that executive functions be understood as including

1. Self-awareness of strengths and limitations and associated understanding of the difficulty level of tasks.
2. Ability to set reasonable goals.
3. Ability to plan and organize behavior designed to achieve the goals.
4. Ability to initiate behavior toward achieving goals and inhibit behavior incompatible with achieving those goals.
5. Ability to monitor and evaluate performance in relation to the goals.
6. Ability to flexibly revise plans and strategically solve problems in the event of difficulty or failure.

An even broader collection of cognitive skills is **metacognition,** which can be described as "thinking about thinking." The term refers to knowledge about all cognitive processes, their products, and anything related to them:

> It is involved in the monitoring of cognitive processes (input and output). This monitoring includes knowing how and when to attend to and organize information; knowing how, when and what to remember; knowing when a problem exists and which solutions have worked or failed; and knowing the individual strengths and weaknesses of different processes and strategies. (Gillis, 1996, p. 111)

Working with a patient with impaired executive functions and metacognition is a daunting task. It is so encompassing that it is necessary to deal with individual aspects of the processes and specific manifestations of the impairments. Just as a chief executive officer of a company does not solely and completely engage in all activities of management, specific areas of executive functioning and metacognition can be analyzed and treated individually. Some of the more important ones are described next.

Disorientation

One of the most common symptoms of TBI is disorientation. Many patients are confused and disoriented at some time during their recovery. **Disorientation** seen in TBI is classified by time, place, person, and predicament (Table 10.1). Disorientation is strongly related to the memory problems that patients often experience as a result of TBI. Patients are disoriented largely because they cannot remember new and past information.

Sometimes a patient is primarily disoriented to only one aspect of reality. For example, a patient may be confused about time but have better orientation to place, predicament, or person. Most of the time, however, a patient with disorientation is confused in all aspects of reality: time, place, person, and predicament. In the medical world, these patients are said to be disoriented "times four." They consistently report the wrong date, time, place where they reside, and the names of relatives. It is important to remember that these patients are not making errors in naming due to aphasia. They are not **paraphasias** in which the patient simply chooses the wrong word (see Chapter 8). The truly disoriented person is confused and behaves in a disoriented manner (Culbertson, Tanner, Peck, & Hooper, 1998).

Disorientation to time is the most common type of confusion because time is abstract and intangible. Patients who are seriously disoriented to time will be confused about the year, month, or day. For example, a disoriented person might believe it is the month of June when in fact it is December. Patients disoriented to time may think that it is breakfasttime when in fact the meal to be served is dinner. Many patients also have trouble accurately appreciating the passage of time. They believe an hour has passed when in fact only 10 minutes have transpired. According to Pimental and Kingsbury (1989), patients with right-hemisphere damage are likely to be disoriented to time. They consider it striking that even when right brain–injured patients have access to a timepiece, they continue to make errors of time orientation.

TABLE 10.1 *Types of Disorientation*

Type	Description	Example
Time	Confusion about time events and/or the passage of time	Not knowing the season of the year
Place	Confusion about place	Not knowing the city in which one resides
Person	Confusion about familiar people and/or loss of identity	Not recognizing familiar family members or friends
Predicament/situation	Denial, confusion, or lack of awareness about a medical condition	Erroneously believing one is in the hospital for routine tests

Disorientation to place rarely occurs independently of time confusion. Patients who show signs of disorientation to place may not know the city, state, or even the country they are in. Some patients report that they are now in a city and state in which they have never lived. According to Pimental and Kingsbury (1989), sometimes patients with right-hemisphere damage who are disoriented to place engage in a confabulated journey. **Confabulation** is the tendency to remark about events without regard to accuracy or truthfulness of the statements. One patient, a professor who suffered a TBI as a result of an automobile accident, was sure that he was on a train traveling to a convention and the hospital room was a sleeping compartment. The train was in Europe heading for exotic cities. His wife reported that he had never been to Europe and rarely traveled by train. Some patients cannot be convinced that they are in a hospital; they believe they are home or visiting relatives.

Disorientation to person can be most disconcerting to friends and family members of the patient with TBI. The patient may not recognize them or, even worse, call them by the wrong names. Some patients have selective disorientation to friends and relatives; that is, they may only remember certain people. Again, it is important to remember that, in patients with TBI and aphasia, the truly disoriented person is not simply making a mistake with naming. For example, a patient who is making an aphasic naming mistake may call his second wife by his first wife's name; he has made an association-naming error. However, the patient knows the reality of the situation. He knows that he is no longer talking to his first wife and that they are divorced; he knows he is addressing his second wife. Patients who are disoriented to person are confused about past and present relationships; they do not know to whom they are talking. Unlike patients who make an aphasic naming error, patients who are disoriented act confused. Their other behaviors also show the disorientation (Tanner, 1999a).

Some patients are so disoriented to person that they have lost their identities. They are confused about self and may even be confused about gender or about their previous occupations. A male patient who is confused about gender may report that he is a faithful wife. A female patient may comment that she is her father's favorite son. Disoriented patients may erroneously believe that they are adventurers or explorers. Once again, these comments are not aphasic naming errors; they are reports of reality as perceived by the patient.

Disorientation to predicament occurs when the patient is confused about what has happened to her. Some authorities call this confusion *disorientation to situation*. Like other types of disorientation, it may be selective or complete. Some patients disorientated to predicament may report that they are in a hospital for routine tests when in fact they are hospitalized for TBIs due to a motor vehicle accident. Patients who are disoriented to predicament may engage in denial. Even when provided with information showing the reality of their predicament, they refuse to believe it. The denial may be caused by the brain injury, particularly when there is parietal lobe damage. This type of organically based denial is called **anosognosia.** The **denial** may also be a psychological protective mechanism used to buffer the reality of the unwanted changes that have happened to her (Tanner, 2003).

Memory Problems

Many of the cognitive and behavioral problems found in patients with TBIs involve impaired memory. Memory is vital to human functioning. Memory allows us to recall and benefit from past experiences, learn new information, and plan for future events. Memory gives our lives continuity. Without memory a person is bound to the here and now and is less aware of self and the environment. Many parts of the brain are involved in memory, and the **hippocampus** is one of the most important. The hippocampus (from the Greek word for "seahorse" because it is shaped like this sea creature) is located deep within the brain (see Chapter 9).

Loss of memory is called **amnesia.** There are two ways of looking at the memory loss experienced by patients with TBI. First, some patients have **retrograde amnesia,** the loss of the ability to remember events that happened before the occurrence of the brain injury. Large blocks of memories can be taken by the TBI. One patient with retrograde amnesia had lost his beloved brother a decade before his brain injury. During his hospital stay, the patient kept asking why his brother had not visited him. When told that his brother had died 10 years ago, the patient began to cry as though he had just lost him. For the patient, he had just lost his brother, and his grief was normal, given his retrograde amnesia. Another couple was on their honeymoon and were involved in a serious automobile accident. Because of retrograde amnesia, the husband did not remember the marriage ceremony nor the fact that they were on their honeymoon. Sometimes in retrograde amnesia, the patient can lose all recollection of events that occurred over months, even years. (Retrograde amnesia is the theme of the 2001 film *Majestic,* starring Jim Carrey, and in the 2002 blockbuster *The Bourne Identity.*)

Anterograde amnesia is failure to recall events that have happened since the brain injury. For example, a patient may not remember days or even weeks since a fall from a cliff. Many patients cannot remember the event that caused the injury. However, not remembering a traumatic event does not preclude experiencing posttraumatic stresses (Herman, 2000). According to Harvey and Bryant (2000), 14% of subjects with mild TBI experienced acute stress disorder, and 24% of the patients at 6 months and 22% at 2 years experienced posttraumatic stress disorder. There are several organic and psychological reasons for this type of amnesia. Damage to certain areas of the brain can cause this selective amnesia, as can *repression* (Tanner, 2003). It is a common defense mechanism in which threatening or painful thoughts are excluded from consciousness.

The Three Components of Memory

It is convenient to look at the process of memory as having three components: attention, storage, and recall. A breakdown of any one them can cause confusion, disorientation, and behavioral problems. Normal memory is also the foundation to learning. Learning new information—whether it is about time, place, person, and predicament or the correct names of body parts, clothing, or furniture—requires functional memory. In patients with TBI, discovering where their memory is impeded is essential. Once the weak link in the chain of memory has been found, therapies can be designed to help patients overcome the deficiencies.

Attention

The first component of memory is alertness to the world and knowledge of what is going on. For normal memory to properly occur, a person must be aware of the environment and be able to attend to important aspects of it. A functional level of attention must be present for a patient to have unimpaired memory. This is one of the reasons why patients in deep comas cannot benefit from therapy; they are oblivious to the environment and thus cannot benefit from the stimulation or profit from experience. Attentional processes are often disrupted in patients with TBI and contribute to difficulties in remembering new information (Lovell & Franzen, 1994). One aspect of attention is arousal. According to Gillis (1996), *arousal* is a general state of readiness to process sensory input, and it is the initial stage of attentional processing.

For normal memory to occur, the patient must not only be generally aware of the environment but also be able to concentrate on the important aspects of it and ignore the rest. This is called *selective attention*. For some patients coming out of a coma, their confusion and disorientation are related to problems with selective attention. They cannot shut out distractions and are bothered by noise. For example, in some medical facilities, the television in the patient's room is continuously left on. The idea behind this practice is that the picture and sound provides needed stimulation for the head-trauma patient. Unfortunately, for many patients, the images and sounds coming from the television are confusing. They have problems separating the television noise from what a doctor or nurse might be saying to them. The images and sounds emanating from the television, which often consists of artificial dialogues and canned laugh tracks, interfere with their ability to attend to visitors. In some patients the television sound desensitizes them to normal conversational speech. Problems separating important sounds from unwanted ones can be considered a perceptual figure–ground problem.

Figure–ground problems occur in both the visual and auditory modes of many head-trauma patients. The *figure* is that which is important—that is, the stimulus that should be attended to. The *ground* is the irrelevant or unimportant information. Patients with TBI may be impaired in their abilities to selectively attend, and their memories will suffer. (See Box 10.1.)

For patients who are in deep comas, very little can be said or done to make them more responsive. Therapies must wait until patients are ready. Some medications can improve arousal levels, and others—especially those used to control seizures—impair it. In the film *Awakenings*, the anti-Parkinson medication L-dopa had a dramatic but short-lived effect. Although the book and film were based in fact, this was an isolated occurrence based on a specific and unusual type of illness. At present no medications can cause that degree of improved arousal and alertness in the majority of patients with severe TBIs.

BOX 10.1 • *Study Habits and the Figure–Ground Problem*

A good example of the figure–ground distinction is the study habits of some people. Some students can watch television while doing their homework. They are not distracted by the noise or images coming from the TV set and can shift attention back and forth from the television to their homework. For other students, it is impossible to study efficiently when there are competing images and noises because they cannot control their attention to study.

Storage

Storage of information is the second component of memory. There are two types of storage: short term and long term. The concept of short- and long-term memory has been around for decades. Since the advent of the computer, some people liken short-term memory to the computer's operating capacity and long-term memory to its ability to save documents in long-term storage.

When it comes to human learning, **short-term memory,** or working memory, is the ability to retain information for as long as the mind is actively focused on the task. An example of auditory short-term memory is trying to remember a telephone number once you have looked it up in the phone directory. We have all had the experience of looking up a number and while putting up the phone book or attempting to dial the number, we are interrupted or distracted. As long as we were able to rehearse the number, to say it over and over aloud or in our internal monologues, the number is remembered. However, because of the interruption or distraction, we can no longer rehearse the number, and it is forgotten. Then, in frustration, we must again look up the number because it was only held in short-term storage and was lost when we could not continue rehearsing it.

Remembering a telephone number also provides an example of the duration of short-term memory, which is difficult to measure. The normal length of this type of memory is controversial. One way of measuring short-term memory is to determine how many objects, figures, or numbers that a person can hold in his mind while rehearsing them. For example, when assessing short-term auditory memory, an examiner will have a patient try to remember numbers after they are spoken. Normal people have a short-term memory of *seven plus or minus two*. This means that a normal short-term memory for digits averages seven, with five to nine being the normal range. It is no coincidence that the number of digits in a local telephone number is seven. The seven plus or minus two rule is a gross estimate of short-term auditory memory. When testing short-term auditory memory, it is important that the examiner say the test items in a controlled and consistent rate. Presenting them either too fast or too slow will cause unreliable scores, because people "chunk" auditory input. *Chunking* is remembering a series of numbers rather than individual ones. Chunking is easy when the stimuli are associated or said rapidly.

When information goes from short-term to long-term storage, different processes and parts of the brain are involved. Short-term memory is thought to involve continuous nerve energy in the brain. When information is stored in **long-term memory,** an actual change occurs in the chemistry of the brain cells. As always, it is difficult to compare the goings on in the brain to what occurs in a particular person's mind. However, it is generally accepted that when a person stores information in the long term, it has been *internalized*: The person has associated it with information already stored in long-term memory.

To continue the example of trying to remember a telephone number, it is only remembered in the short term as long as the person rehearses it. To remember the number in the long term, the person can either visually or auditorily associate it with existing information in long-term memory. For example, if the numbers to be remembered are 5487, a visual association would involve remembering how they look on the dialing pad of the telephone. The numbers 5, 4, 8, and 7 are next to each other and in descending order. An auditory association would be to remember that the numbers 54 or 487 are related to other numbers in memory. Perhaps, the person trying to remember them is 54 years old, or the numbers 487 is a street address of a friend.

There are purposeful and incidental storage of information. *Purposeful storage* involves designing a strategy with which to remember something, like the examples just given. *Incidental storage* occurs when information simply enters memory with no conscious attention given to remembering it. Some memory is stored because it is related to *peak memory experiences*, which are dramatic, unusual, and important occurrences (see Box 10.2).

Two principles are important when working with TBI patients who have memory-storage problems. First, everyone on the rehabilitation team must be consistent in providing information for storage. The information should be practical, and all team members should work on the same stimuli. Second, the information to be stored should be personally relevant to the patient. For example, if a patient is being taught the days of the week, then each day to be remembered should be made personally relevant. If the patient enjoys going to church on Sunday, then that day of the week should be integrated into her existing memory. Sunday should be taught as the day that she goes to church, and she should associate the day with her particular church and past routines. Targeting the memory of obscure holidays and other

BOX 10.2 • *Peak Memory Experiences*

Peak memory experiences are those in which you clearly remember what you were doing, where you were, what you were feeling, and many other details when you learned of a major life event. Do any of these events qualify as peak memory experience?

The tragedy of the World Trade Towers

The car chase and arrest of O. J. Simpson

The tearing down of the Berlin Wall

The collapse of the Soviet Union

The death of Princess Diana

Your first kiss

The Waco, Texas, tragedy

Your parents announcing an impending divorce

The space shuttle *Challenger* explosion

The bombing of the Federal Building in Oklahoma

The suicide of Kurt Cobain

The mass killings at Columbine High School in Colorado

A marriage proposal

The announcement of the death of a loved one

events that are not important to the patient should be set aside until her storage abilities have improved.

Recall

The process of remembering information is complete when the stimulus that was attended to and stored is recalled. Several factors affect recall, and the individual cannot control many of them. Overall alertness, distractions, anxiety, and psychological defenses all affect the process of recall. Recall also depends on the clarity and strength of what was stored.

Many authorities on human learning and memory believe that everything attended to and stored is available for recall; that is, given the right prompts and cues, all experiences stored in long-term memory are available for recall. Of course, with the passage of time and the continual processing of new information, those memories may be distorted. Time has a way of helping us forget the bad and remember the "good ole days."

Movies and books with plots about public crimes, such as bank robberies, sometimes have the witnesses hypnotized to aid in their recall of the events. This is an accurate portrayal of some criminal investigations because sometimes the police do hypnotize witnesses to better reconstruct the crimes. Relaxation helps in the process of recall, and hypnosis is a state of suggestive relaxation. When a person is hypnotized, he is relaxed and calm, and this psychological state helps the hypnotist lead the person in a step-by-step re-creation of the crime. Under hypnosis, a witness can better recall how many perpetrators there were, what they were wearing, how many gunshots were fired, and other information related to the crime scene. Relaxation is helpful because it reduces the ability of psychological defense mechanisms to block from awareness unpleasant or threatening events.

Accounts in literature and media have described situations in which adults who when hypnotized could remember crimes perpetrated against them or others when they were children. Hypnosis was able to bypass the psychological defense mechanism of repression. Those subconscious memories were attended to and stored but blocked from recall. You can see the effects of relaxation on recall just before you go to sleep. When you are relaxed and comfortable and just prior to dozing off, you are better able to remember the details of personal events that happened in the distant past.

Retrieval can be involuntary or effortful, and it involves the transfer of information from storage to consciousness (Ylvisaker & Feeney, 1998). Involuntary retrieval of information is sometimes called *free recall* (Gillis, 1996) or *incidental memory* (O'Shanick & O'Shanick, 1994). In patients with TBI, incidental recall is often more functional than effortful memory (O'Shanick & O'Shanick, 1994).

Everyone has experienced incidental recall when a song on the radio prompts a pleasant memory of days-gone-by. Often when these memories are prompted, not only do we have the thoughts of the event, but we also experience the emotions associated with them. It is as if the song transports us back to that time. Certain odors are also good at prompting these types of memory. In the Vietnam War film *Apocalypse Now*, the statement "I love the smell of napalm in the morning" depicts the power of odors to recall events and the feelings associated with them.

The observation that memories are often stored and recalled with the feelings associated with them was demonstrated during early brain-mapping studies. Some studies involved conscious subjects who had parts of their brains stimulated with small electric currents, the object of which was to identify certain sites of the brain with specific brain functions. Researchers found that when parts of the brain were stimulated, the subjects would report a particular event. For example, the subject might say, "I am at my grandmother's house, in the kitchen, and I smell freshly baked bread." The subject not only remembered being at grandmother's house but also had the feelings of the youngster. These subjects communicated that they remembered the events *and* they relived the emotional experience. Those studies and others like them have yielded important psychological information. It appears that our memories are not only stored in our minds, but they, and the feelings that occurred when they happened, are also available for recall. Those memories can have major effects on the way we think and act.

Memories, Libraries, and Tests

One way of understanding the memory problems experienced by many TBI patients is to liken them to books in a college library. The components of attention, storage, and recall are analogous to the way books are housed and used in a library. For the purposes of this example, consider each memory a book. Initially, for a book to be chosen for the library, an acquisitions staff person must become aware of its existence and select it. As you know, some college libraries are larger than others, and there are specialized ones on some campuses, such as medicine, law, or dentistry. Consequently, not all books are chosen for a particular library, and some libraries are more likely to seek volumes in a speciality area. Books chosen for a library are selected from thousands that are available. This process is similar to the attention component of memory. People cannot possibly remember everything that occurs to the senses, and because of their interests, some people are more likely to remember certain events than others.

Storage of library books is done with the aid of computers and call numbers. The book, which has been chosen for storage, is placed with other volumes that are similar to it in content. It is designated in a particular area of the library: wing, floor, row, and shelf. It is even carefully placed in a numerical order next to other books on the topic. Once the book is placed on the shelf, it is available to be checked out. Individual memories are also stored systematically in the memory bank of our brains.

To check out a book, all a student has to do is to locate in the computer the call number of the desired book. Unless the book has been checked out by someone else, the library patron can easily find and use it. Most libraries have signs that say "Please do not re-shelve books." The library personnel do not want students to remove a book, browse through it, and re-shelve it when done. They are afraid that it will be replaced in the wrong order or shelf. If that happens, even though the book is still in the library, it may be lost because the system for checking it out is disrupted. With tens of thousands of books, re-shelving a book in the wrong place can cause it to be lost. Loss of memory for a particular event can be viewed in the same way. Although a person has the memory of a particular event in her mind, it might be lost because there is a disruption in the system for recalling it. Some TBI patients do not attend well enough to new events, store them only temporarily or inappropriately, and/or have problems with retrieval.

Memory and Test Taking

Another way of understanding the memory problems seen in many TBI patients is to examine how students perform successfully on a test. Suppose you are taking a midterm test on the anatomy of the speech and hearing mechanism. Many of the questions on an anatomy test require you to remember the names of muscles, nerves, cartilages, and bones. Your ability to correctly answer the questions depends on attention, storage, and recall.

It is unlikely that you will answer the questions correctly if you have not read the text or attended the classes. Even if you went to the classes but your attention was elsewhere during the lectures, the information on the examination will not be familiar. Perhaps you were daydreaming, talking to your neighbor, or bothered by outside construction sounds when a particular muscle, for example, was discussed. Because of lack of attention, the information about a particular test question was never attended to.

Maybe the name of a particular muscle was never stored properly or well enough. Perhaps you did not take notes, review, and study them. The name of the muscle never made it to short- and long-term memory. There was never purposeful storage when you memorized the word, nor was there incidental storage that often occurs during group study sessions as other students talk about the lecture material. You never internalized the muscle and name by relating them to other information you have about the anatomy of the speech and hearing mechanism.

Finally, you may not remember the muscle on the midterm exam because you tend to freeze up during important examinations. Although anxiety can be helpful in motivating you to study, too much fear and worry can be counterproductive. Your anxiety levels go to unbearable levels, and you cannot think clearly. You do not read the question carefully or forget to use the process of elimination. Maybe you are understandably anxious because you did not study enough and the material was not stored with the clarity for easy retrieval.

In memory problems seen in TBI patients, it is important to discover where the process breaks down and to rectify the situation. Therapies for improving attention, precision of storage, and ease of recall can be designed to improve functional memory in many patients.

Recognition and Recall

There are two types of retrieval of information: recognition and recall. Continuing with the example of remembering answers to a test, *recognition* is knowing the correct answer when provided with several options. Recognition is employed when you take a multiple-choice test. Usually you have four or five answers from which to choose. After reading the options, you select the one that you recognize to be correct. Often this is done through a process of elimination in which unlikely answers are systematically eliminated as possibilities. *Recall* is employed when you take an essay or short-answer test. You are given an open-ended question, and you must supply the relevant information. As a rule, recognition of the correct answer is easier because you have cues, and complete understanding of the question is not required. In recall, you are not supplied with cues and must completely retrieve all relevant information about the concept. (See Box 10.3 for a memory-recall technique.)

Recognition is easier than recall for many TBI patients. Recognizing the correct date, time, relative, and city in which they reside, when provided with several options, is easier

BOX 10.3 • *Mnemonic Devices*

Students sometimes employ *mnemonic devices* to help them remember lists of information. They are often used in anatomy and physiology courses to help remember large numbers of muscles and nerves. A mnemonic device helps refine the process of storage and retrieval. A common mnemonic device for remembering cranial nerves is the statement: "On old Olympus towering top, a Finn and German vended a hop." The first letters of each word correspond to the initial letters in each cranial nerve: olfactory, optic, oculomotor, trochlear, trigeminal, abducent, facial, acoustic, glossopharyngeal, vagus, accessory, hypoglossal. Although this mnemonic device is helpful in storing and retrieving the names of the cranial nerves on a test, it sometimes requires that the sentence be used to remember a particular cranial nerve during a clinical staffing or other professional meeting. It would be better to associate the names of the cranial nerves with their function or in another relevant way.

Another mnemonic device using visual associations can also be employed to remember long lists of information. Perhaps as a child, you frequently traveled a particular path to a store or to visit a relative. You are very familiar with the path—each corner, shrub, tree, or bend in the road. Some people can remember large lists of information if they carefully place each item in their mind's eye next to a landmark on that familiar path. Then, when required to remember the information, all that is necessary is to stroll along the path in their mind's eye and retrieve each item.

recalling the information without cues. When trying to remember the names of body parts, for example, it is easier for a patient to know the answer if the examiner points to an arm and provides choices such as "Is this your hand, foot, arm, or shoe?" Patients are more likely to recognize and say the correct word than to recall it when simply asked, "What is the name of this body part?" Patients who have much better recognition than recall for words probably have Wernicke's area largely unaffected by the TBI. Wernicke's area is the receptive language center in the temporal lobe of the left hemisphere. Patients who cannot recognize the correct word probably have suffered damage to Wernicke's and adjacent areas of the brain.

Behavioral Disturbances

The behavioral problems seen in TBI patients can be traced to the site and size of the injury, the patient's pre-existing personality, and the environmental demands placed on him. The research describing behavioral problems shows certain patterns of behaviors occurring even in patients with mild brain damage. Unfortunately, the research is inconsistent in classifying, describing, and defining the specific patterns of behaviors.

Many TBI patients say and do inappropriate things. These actions can be startling and unsettling for their family and friends. It is not uncommon for patients to make obscene remarks, engage in sexually provocative and inappropriate behaviors, or act aggressively. Some patients play with themselves in public or inappropriately touch visitors. Many patients lose modesty, and some even walk into the halls naked. Other behavioral problems include talking too loudly, boasting, and laughing or crying at inappropriate times. Some patients talk on and on about irrelevant things and demand the attention of the listener. These strange behaviors are the source of embarrassment for family and friends. And patients, when told of them after they have recovered from the injuries, are also understandably embarrassed. It should be remembered, however, that health care professionals who work with TBI patients often see these behaviors, and patients and their families should not be unduly distressed by them. They are considered a natural and even necessary part of the recovery process.

Corrigan and Jakus (1994) list five categories of commonly seen behavior deficits in TBI patients. Patients display *aggressive behaviors*, which include biting, harming self, spitting, swearing, yelling, hitting, scratching, and kicking others. Neglect of *self-care skills* includes refusal to eat, wash, brush teeth, and comb hair. Patients also will not make their beds or keep the area clean. Behavioral problems involving *interpersonal skills* include poor conversational abilities, lack of assertiveness, procrastination, lethargy, and reduced motivation. Behavioral problems involving *coping skills* include refusing to take medications, difficulty solving problems, and poor responses to stressors. Deficits with *cognitive-related skills* include poor attention, concentration, memory, reading, writing, and learning skills. Suicide rates are higher in people with brain injuries, and Kuipers and Lancaster (2000) report the need for multiple strategies to respond to it. According to Corrigan and Jakus (1994), TBI patients also have poor social comprehension. Many patients displaying these behavioral problems are unaware that they are acting inappropriately.

Even patients with brain concussions display behavior problems for months following their injury. Impaired attention, reduced concentration and memory, irritability, and loss of temper occur in patients with postconcussive syndrome (McAllister, 1994). According to McAllister (1994), there is significant resolution of symptoms in about one-half of the patients by 1 month and roughly two-thirds of them at 3 months. Most patients are symptom free by 12 months. Patients with mild brain injuries which are *not* synonymous with postconcussive syndrome, also tend to experience lingering cognitive and behavioral problems for months following their injuries (McAllister, 1994). Long-term behavioral disturbances associated with TBI include disorganized, tangential, or wandering discourse; disinhibition; socially inappropriate language; hyperverbosity; and ineffective use of social and contextual cues (ASHA, 1988).

Flat Affect

A patient with TBI sometimes displays shallow emotions. The reduction in mood, emotion, feeling, and temperament is called **flat affect.** This change in emotions is particularly noticeable to family members who report that the patient is "not herself" and does not have the emotions that were typical before the TBI. A patient with flat affect has reduced and narrowed emotions and often acts removed from typical reactions to people, situations, and thoughts. She does not appear concerned about the predicament and may act indifferent to family and friends. Flat affect is the opposite of emotional lability (see Chapter 8); in emotional lability the patient has exaggerated emotions to people, situations, and thoughts.

When TBI patients have flat affect, it is usually more apparent during the early stages of recovery. Although the patient may show agitation early on, he will not have appropriate emotional responses that are clearly connected to people, situations, and thoughts. Family and friends often report flat affect occurring for months after the brain injury. It may even be a permanent part of the patient's personality changes. Individual and family counseling can be helpful in helping the patient and his family cope with flat affect.

Psychosis

Patients with TBI sometimes break with reality. According to Smeltzer, Nasrallah, and Miller (1994), post-traumatic psychosis is a generic label for psychotic illness in a person who has had a brain injury. They note that there is little, and often discrepant, research on psychosis among TBI patients. Based on current research, determining the percentage of post-traumatic brain-injured patients with psychosis is difficult. In studies reviewed by Smeltzer et al. (1994), the reported incident rates of psychosis in TBIs were so variable as to be meaningless. The data providing accurate percentages of patients who become psychotic or display psychotic symptoms is unreliable due to research methodological issues. Some studies show as many as 20% of patients with post-traumatic brain injuries may be classified as psychotic, and 50% or more may have signs and symptoms of problems with reality testing.

As noted above, the incidence and prevalence figures of psychotic disturbance in TBI patients are highly variable. Researchers who study these psychological reactions often have different criteria for classifying patients' behaviors. Sometimes what is considered a report of an hallucination or delusion can be in error due to the types of word-retrieval behavior seen in aphasia. One patient with a serious TBI reported to a psychologist, "They put me in a car and drove me to the fire station." He was persistent in reporting this event and could not be convinced that it did not happen. It was clearly an unlikely thing to happen to the patient because of the seriousness of his physical injuries. And there was no reason to take him to a fire station. The psychological report in the chart stated that he suffered from "psychotic episodes." Careful analysis of the situation led to a more accurate diagnosis.

In this particular nursing home, patients were sometimes given the reward of being able to sit at the nursing station, converse with the staff, and watch the goings on of the facility. As it happened, the place where the patients sat was adjacent to a fire hose, which was enclosed in a glass case. The patient, who was thought to have psychotic episodes, was simply reporting that he was given this reward for good behavior. Unfortunately, he did it using semantic association errors. An association error is when an aphasic patient uses a word that is associated in meaning with the desired one (see Chapter 8). So, when the patient said, "They put me in a car and drove me to the fire station," he used associated words such as "car" for "wheelchair," "drove" for "wheeled," and "fire station" for "fire hose." He was not reporting a psychotic event; he was not delusional; it was a real occurrence that was expressed in the language typical of aphasia. (*The Cell*, a film about schizophrenia and psychosis, provides excellent special effects showing delusions and hallucinations.)

Pediatric Traumatic Brain Injury

"Closed-head trauma in children is a major public health problem. It is a leading cause of death among youth and results in substantial neurobehavioral morbidity for survivors"

(Yeates, 2000, p. 92). TBI in children often presents with different symptoms than those typically seen in adults because children are still developing physically, mentally, and emotionally. At the time of the TBI, they may not have fully developed speech and language and other cognitive and emotional abilities. Consequently, the neuropsychological manifestation of the brain injury is different from what is seen in adults. Damage to an immature brain, one that is in the process of development, causes different symptoms and has different outcomes than what is seen when a fully developed adult brain is injured. In addition, children have different perspectives and needs. For example, they depend more on their families and care more about peer acceptance.

As with TBI in adults, the number-one cause in children is high-speed automobile accidents (Snow & Hooper, 1994). Other causes include falls and bicycle, motorcycle, and car–pedestrian accidents. In preschool children, accidents in the home and child abuse are frequent causes of TBI (Christoffel, 1990). Brain injury and death can be caused when an adult shakes a child to stop her from crying or as punishment. Like adults, male children tend to be more at risk for serious head injuries. Although the Glasgow Coma Scale can be used for measuring the effects of head injury in children, several tests have been adapted to assess children under the age of 3. They consider the unique cognitive, speech, and language abilities of young children (Snow & Hooper, 1994).

Factors that influence outcomes in children with TBI include the type and severity of injury sustained, medical complications, premorbid functioning of the child and/or family, and the effects of rehabilitation (Snow & Hooper, 1994). Open-versus-closed and generalized-versus-focalized head injuries damage the brain differently and can have differing outcomes. The more severe the injury, the less optimistic is the outcome potential. Like adults, the younger the person, the better is the **prognosis.** However, younger children may be at greater risk for learning difficulties because most of their learning is new (Snow & Hooper, 1994). Finally, the premorbid functioning of the child and his family must be considered when determining outcomes. Dysfunctional families and children with preexisting learning and emotional difficulties have more problems with rehabilitation.

As noted above, the age at which brain damage occurs is an important factor in deciding the prognosis for the child with TBI. Neurologically, this has to do with brain plasticity. In the young child, the brain is more plastic; that is, it is more flexible and capable of having other areas compensate for the damage that has occurred. In young children, the **cortex** is not as committed to a particular function as what is seen in adults, thus allowing for better compensation. This is particularly true with speech and language. Children with damage to Broca's and Wernicke's areas are more likely than adults to have adjacent areas of the brain, or the nondominant hemisphere, assume the primary role of speech and language functioning. However, in young children, evidence shows that brain plasticity and compensation is not equally likely for all cognitive functions. "The mounting evidence that young children may be more rather than less vulnerable than older people in certain critical areas of functioning is sobering and should motivate rehabilitation professionals to redouble their efforts for this group" (Ylvisaker, 1998, p. 7).

Unlike head trauma in adults, rehabilitation for the child must include objectives for transition back to school. Teaching and learning strategies for the child must be adjusted to accommodate the cognitive and emotional changes that have resulted from the head trauma. In addition, children are often placed in special education programs, and individualized education plans must reflect the myriad of cognitive deficits that can result from serious head trauma. Teachers, nurses, and school counselors must become active members of the special education program. Of course, the child's parents are pivotal members of the team and provide continuity of goals, objectives, and procedures at home.

Audiology and Traumatic Brain Injuries

Traumatic brain injuries can result in damage to the hearing mechanism. Both open- and closed-head traumas can impair hearing, depending on the site and type of injuries. According to Mackay et al. (1997), "Ideally, all patients admitted with a diagnosis of traumatic brain injury should undergo some type of risk assessment screening to establish the likelihood of damage to auditory structures" (p. 483). An audiological evaluation is necessary in determining the extent and severity of the head injuries. Audiological testing is an important part of a comprehensive neurological and otological assessment of certain patients with TBI. It is also essential that a patient's hearing be considered when assessing speech and language. Rehabilitation professionals must be able to rule out hearing loss and deafness before determining memory, orientation, cognitive, speech, and language impairments. For example, if patients wrongly answer questions dealing with orientation, they may be suffering from a hearing loss rather than disorientation. Similarly, when assessing auditory memory, it is essential that hearing loss and deafness be eliminated as a causal factor for deficient performance on those tests.

Head injuries can damage the external ear canal. There can be tearing, bleeding, and inflammation of the external ear canal, and sometimes the pinna itself can be damaged or torn off. In the middle ear, the ossicular chain can be disrupted, and the tympanic membrane can be ruptured. According to Northern and Downs (1991), bleeding in the middle ear or disruption of the ossicular chain can create a maximal 60-dB conductive-type hearing loss. When there is sufficient impact to the skull, the inner ear can also be compromised. Permanent sensorineural hearing loss can be caused by relatively moderate trauma to the skull (Northern & Downs, 1991). Acceleration and deceleration forces are one cause of laceration and hemorrhage injury to cranial nerve VIII in TBI (Mackay et al., 1997). The type and severity of central hearing losses depend on the areas of the brain that are damaged. Meningitis (inflammation of the **meninges**) may be a late complication of temporal bone fracture (Northern & Downs, 1991).

The testing conducted by an audiologist is usually done early in the rehabilitation program. The goal is to find where along the hearing mechanism the process of energy transformation is disrupted (see Chapter 6). Appropriate tests are conducted to determine whether the TBI has impeded the acoustic, mechanical, hydraulic, or electrochemical energy or transformation. The tests used to assess the hearing in patients with TBI include pure tones, tympanometry, acoustic reflex, otoacoustic emissions, and brainstem auditory evoked-potential assessment (Mackay et al., 1997). Because of the sophistication of some of these tests, they can be conducted on patients who are unconscious and unresponsive.

If a patient is found to have suffered a hearing impairment due to TBI, then the audiologist can suggest intervention strategies to compensate for the loss during hospitalization (Mackay et al., 1997). Rehabilitation team professionals can be told of the type of hearing loss and how to speak to the patient. Amplification devices can also be provided. These can include temporary amplification devices, which can be purchased at many commercial electronic establishments. Some hospitals also have access to donated, used hearing aids. They can be temporarily used during rehabilitation while waiting for proper hearing aid assessment and fitting. Family counseling by the audiologist may also be indicated. The audiologist is an important resource person for the patient, family, and rehabilitation professionals (Mackay et al., 1997).

Principles of Rehabilitation for Traumatic Brain Injuries

Some rehabilitation facilities provide an experimental treatment to patients called *coma stimulation therapy*. The patient is given multisensory stimulation including placing different odors and fragrances under the nose, providing several tastes on the tongue and lips, applying temperature and textures to the skin, massages, range-of-motion exercises, attempts to track lights or fingers, and presenting speech and nonverbal sounds to alternate ears (Gillis, 1996). Other activities include reading to the patient, providing her with information about family and current events, and engaging in familiar routines.

Although some authorities on TBI believe that coma stimulation therapy improves the patient's responsiveness and overall ability to benefit from rehabilitation, no definitive studies clearly support it. Although it is well intentioned, coma stimulation therapy is an experimental treatment that has not been proved to benefit patients. A major problem with the treatment is that it tends to give family and friends false hope. "Families are often desperate for hope and may grasp at any technique that sounds like an active process designed to speed recovery" (Gillis, 1996, p. 180).

The disabilities seen in TBI range from mild, barely perceptible changes in cognitive abilities to patients who never move beyond coma. Patients might present with mild communication disorders, which are only a minor nuisance, or be completely deprived of functional expressive and receptive abilities. Because of the range of severity and the many dimensions that can be affected, designing and implementing a treatment program is challenging. However, certain principles of treatment are applicable to the majority of patients with communication disorders resulting from TBI.

Ylvisaker and Szekeres (1994, pp. 552–553) have developed several critical principles of treatment for TBI patients. These principles focus on the patient's self-concept and incorporate all members of the rehabilitation team, including the family. The application of the principles varies with the stage of the patient's recovery.

1. Success, resulting from planned compensation and appropriately adjusted expectations, facilitates progress while building a positive self-concept.
2. The systematic graduation of activities, demands, and support . . . carefully adjusted to meet individual needs with withdrawal of support as individuals demonstrate increased capacity, facilitates improvement.
3. Generalization to real-world settings and activities must be a central component of intervention. The model could be either (a) focusing intensively on generalization after a skill has been acquired in a clinical context or (b) focusing on generalization from the outset, using functional activities and a variety of settings and everyday people.

Furthermore, individuals should be addressed as strategic problems solvers, actively involved in the process of generalization.

4. Sensitivity to executive system themes must be part of therapy sessions and the rehabilitative environment in general. This includes engaging individuals with CHI in self-appraisal, goal setting, decision making, planning and organizing, monitoring and evaluating, and practical problem solving in a variety of functional contexts.

5. Integration of treatment (including daily interaction and behavioral intervention) among all staff and family members facilitates the individual's orientation, learning, and generalization of learned skills. A key role for speech–language pathologists is to train everyday people (family, friends, and direct-care staff) in basic communicative competencies.

6. Whenever possible, personally meaningful activities and natural settings should be selected for cognitive and communicative intervention. Although individual sessions can be useful for diagnostic therapy, for training in personally sensitive areas, and for highly specific interventions, group therapy and community-based intervention are necessary components of social skills and social cognition therapy and for generalization training.

7. As much as possible, tasks should be designed that are consistent with the individual's pretraumatic personality, interests, and education/vocational background as well as goals for the future.

Ylvisaker and Szekeres (1994) emphasize the importance of systematic and gradual exposure to more demanding activities. The patient's premorbid personality and interests must be considered when working on generalization from clinical activities to real-world experiences. Treatment of neurogenic communication disorders must involve improving the patient's self-esteem (Tanner, 2003; Ylvisaker & Szekeres, 1994).

Two statements can be made about head and neck trauma rehabilitation. The first statement emphasizes the importance of getting an early start: "Rehabilitation begins at the accident site." An early start ensures that all that can be done will be done for the patient. Whether it is rapid transportation from the accident scene for lifesaving surgeries or audiological assessments in the intensive care unit, rehabilitation of patients with traumatic head and neck injuries needs to be aggressive and proactive. The second statement made about rehabilitation is "Communication is 90% of the job." Meaningful communication among the rehabilitation staff is essential for the design and implementation of a coordinated and effective treatment program. Regular communication with the family is also necessary; they must be brought into the rehabilitation program and made active members of the team. Finally, the quality and quantity of communication with the patient dictates whether a bridge or fence is created in achieving a meaningful and satisfying life following a traumatic head or neck injury. For example, Curran, Ponsford, and Crowe (2000) found that coping strategies focusing on problem solving and having a positive outlook were related to lower levels of anxiety in TBI patients and orthopedic patients.

Literature and Media Stereotypes

Christopher Reeve is a poignant example of the irony of head and neck injuries. In many ways Reeve demonstrated off screen the characteristics of his screen character, Superman. As a pilot he could soar with grace and ease. In the ocean he could experience the freedom of weightlessness while scuba diving. As a skier he happily accepted the challenges of steep slopes and white powder. He also delighted in the thrill of harnessing the power and strength of a thoroughbred horse. As can be the case for skilled athletes, pushing the athletic envelope led to his confinement to bed and wheelchair.

Jan Berry loved and sang about powerful cars, the thrill of a Stingray's acceleration, and the danger of four tires clinging to the pavement in a fast turn. But this need for speed also led to his own "deadman's curve." Gary Busey valued the sense of freedom found in riding powerful motorcycles. One of his arguments for not wearing motorcycle helmets was that they restricted the freedom of the rider's head movements. Had he been wearing a helmet at the time of the accident, it is probable that it would have saved him from his TBI.

Literature and the media are good at connecting high-risk activities with their consequences. Reeve's, Berry's, and Busey's accidents were covered in great detail. Books, movies, and television shows were made about them. They were also interviewed on television programs such as *The Larry King Show*. The interest in these people and other public figures who suffer serious head and neck disabilities does not go away after their injuries. For the most part, there is no attempt by the television or the film industries to hide or minimize the effects of their injuries. There are factual accounts of the ramifications of them, including the psychological, physical, social, and occupational effects. In addition, all examples used in this chapter have Web sites that address the nature and extent of the disabilities. They are either created and maintained by the public figures themselves or by people clearly friendly to them. The Internet has proved to be a powerful vehicle in providing personal and detailed information about people with these types of communication disorders.

Books and films can sometimes create unrealistic expectations about patients in a coma or who are stuporous. For example, there is no reason to question the accuracy of the effects of the drug L-dopa on the patients with encephalitis lethargia in the book and film *Awakenings*. However, anxious family members of comatose patients may have unrealistic ideas based on the book and film. They may jump to the conclusion that a magical drug can be given to their loved ones that can reverse serious brain damage and remove them from their stuporous or comatose state. Without counseling and accurate information provided by members of the rehabilitation team, these family members erroneously conclude that all coma and stuporous states are like the ones portrayed in *Awakenings*.

The power of literature and the media to inform and persuade is illustrated with James Brady. His tragic head injury and resulting communication disorders are used to show the damage, pain, and disability that can be caused by handguns. It gives a personal face to gun control legislation. Gun control advocates were persuasive in getting the "Brady Bill" enacted, and they continue to use him as a "poster child" for more laws governing the purchase and possession of firearms. They believe that more laws will remove guns from violent criminals. They point to Brady and in effect say, "This would have been prevented by more legislation; John Hinckley, Jr., would have obeyed them and, consequently, never have been able to do this harm. This tragedy would have been prevented." And when the victim himself, replete with his communication disorder, advocates for additional firearm legislation, there is a powerful persuasive effect.

Literature and the media show the promise of more freedom from severe head and neck injuries to millions of disabled persons with films like *The Bone Collector*. This movie did a wonderful job of showing how advances in technology can improve the quality of lives of people with serious spinal injuries and head trauma. Through technology, Lincoln Rhyme was again able to contribute to society and find meaning in his life. Technology has indeed opened doors for many communication-disordered people.

Old stereotypes of people with head and neck injuries are being attacked by literature and the media. In the not-so-distant past, people with communication disorders resulting from serious head and neck injuries were thought to be unproductive and unable to contribute to society. Often, they were considered burdens on family and society. Literature and the media, particularly the Internet, are positively influencing a change in those outdated and inaccurate stereotypes. Many of the people with serious head and neck injuries are powerful forces, as well, in helping destroy those negative and unrealistic beliefs. Their energy, persistence, and courage in confronting their disabilities are tributes to the human spirit.

Summary

People who have traumatic head and neck injuries were often vital and athletic and find themselves confined to a hospital bed or wheelchair as a result of their injuries. The typical head-injured person is a low-income, young man who had probably been admitted to a hospital previously with a head injury. Alcohol is often associated with these serious injuries. Patients with TBI often have reduced levels of consciousness, disorientation, and behavioral problems. A common symptom of TBI is a memory deficit. Patients have problems attending to information and/or storing and recalling it. Rehabilitation of the head-injured person requires cooperation and communication of all involved, including family and friends. Technology has improved the ability of head- and neck-injured persons to more fully participate in society. When the literature and media portray head or neck injuries, they often describe the courage and determination shown by these people in overcoming their impairments.

Study Questions

1. Why is it ironic that many people who suffer TBIs and neck injuries are young, vital, energetic, and athletic?

2. Discuss the "window of opportunity" with regard to TBIs.

3. Describe the typical head-injured person.

4. Compare and contrast *open-* and *closed-head injuries.*

5. Discuss *consciousness* as it relates to TBI.

6. Define and discuss *coma.*

7. List the lobes of the brain and discuss the possible symptoms of traumatic damage to them.

8. What is *executive functioning*?

9. List and discuss the four types of disorientation.

10. How is the "ability to profit from experience" related to the patient's memory?

11. Compare and contrast *recall* and *recognition*.

12. What are some reasons why TBI patients have behavioral problems?

13. Discuss how TBIs affect children and adults differently.

14. How do literature and the media typically portray people with head and neck injuries?

Suggested Reading

Curran, C. A., Ponsford, J. L., & Crowe, S. (2000). Coping strategies and emotional outcomes following traumatic brain injury: A comparison with orthopedic patients. *Journal of Head Trauma Rehabilitation, 15*(6): 1256–1274. This article examines coping strategies and emotional outcomes in TBI patients.

Ghajar, J. (2000). Traumatic brain injury. *Lancet, 356:* 923–929. This seminar reviews improved care and decreased mortality for patients with severe TBI.

11

Questions and Answers about the Profession

Chapter Preview

This chapter answers questions typically asked by students in an introduction to communication sciences and disorders course. Addressed are the professions of speech–language pathology and audiology, which are exciting, rewarding, and challenging. The scope of practice for speech–language pathologists and audiologists is summarized, including educational, clinical, and ethical requirements. There is a discussion of employment opportunities in the profession, various work environments, and typical salaries and opportunities. Students are urged to consider important factors should they become interested in entering the field of speech–language pathology and audiology, such as the job market, research opportunities in the field, and requirements for certification as a clinician. The Code of Ethics and a discussion of the responsibilities of a speech–language pathology assistant are also presented.

Understanding the Profession

QUESTION: What do speech–language pathologists do?

ANSWER: Speech–language pathology, an exciting and rewarding profession, carries much responsibility. Speech-language pathologists are *autonomous* professionals. The services they provide need not be prescribed by other professionals. Speech–language pathologists are independent practitioners and the primary providers of services to people with speech, voice, and language disorders. A summary follows of the major services and responsibilities of practicing speech–language pathologists, taken from the American Speech-Language-Hearing Association (ASHA) Web site (see Appendix A).

Speech–language pathologists provide screening, identification, assessment, diagnosis, treatment intervention, and follow-up services for people with disorders of speech, voice, and language and the cognitive and social aspects of communication. These services include consultation, counseling, making referrals, and preventive activities. Training and supporting family members of individuals with communication disorders is an important aspect of the profession. Clinicians develop and establish effective alternative and augmentative communication techniques and strategies including selecting, prescribing, and dispensing prosthetic/adaptive devices for speaking and swallowing. Prosthetic and adaptive devices include electrolarynges and speaking valves in the neck (see Chapter 3). Although audiologists are the primary providers of audiological services, speech–language pathologists conduct pure-tone air-conduction hearing screening and screening tympanometry as part of the diagnosis and treatment process (see Chapter 6). Also in the scope of practice are activities to reduce accents, collaboration with teachers of English as a second language, and improvement of patients' singing voices. Speech–language pathologists train and supervise support personnel. They also conduct, disseminate, and apply research in communication sciences and disorders. Speech–language pathologists serve many different kinds of people and are of course prohibited from discriminating in the provision of professional services based on race, age, gender, religion, national origin, and sexual orientation. The services provided to people with communication disorders are usually on a one-to-one basis or done in small groups, and therapies can continue for months and even years. Consequently, speech–language pathologists often develop close relationships with the people they serve. For many clinicians this is a rewarding aspect of the profession.

The process of diagnosing and treating a speech, voice, or language disorder is challenging. Speech–language pathologists use sophisticated instruments to diagnose and treat communication and swallowing disorders, including scopes that can be inserted into the mouth and throat and moving picture X rays of the speech and swallowing mechanism. Orofacial examinations are conducted to determine normal from abnormal oral structures and function, and psychometric tests assess whether speech and language are developing properly and the effects of treatment. The clinician's judgment is the ultimate tool used in the diagnostic and treatment process. Given the complexity of human communication, the process of diagnosing and treating these disorders is a complex, challenging, and rewarding endeavor.

Check out ASHA's Scope of Practice in Speech–Language Pathology Web site for a conceptual framework, definitions, and a detailed listing of the practice of speech–language pathology (see Appendix A).

QUESTION: What does an audiologist do?

ANSWER: Like speech–language pathology, audiology is an autonomous profession. According to ASHA's Scope of Practice in Audiology (see Appendix A), audiologists identify, assess, and manage disorders of the auditory, balance, and other neural systems. They select, fit, and dispense hearing aids and related devices. Audiologists work to prevent hearing loss through providing and fitting hearing protective devices, educating people to the effects of noise on hearing, and engaging in audiological rehabilitation. Audiological rehabilitation includes teaching speech reading, communication management, improving language development, auditory skill development, and counseling for people with hearing loss and their families. This may necessitate the screening of speech-language, use of sign language, and other factors affecting communication as part of an audiologic assessment. They engage in research on the prevention, identification, and treatment of hearing loss and balance system dysfunctions. Audiologists also train and supervise support personnel.

Audiologists consult with individuals, public and private agencies, industry, governmental bodies, and attorneys about the effects of noise and hearing loss. They are often members of interdisciplinary education and medical teams about communication management, educational implications of hearing loss, educational programming, classroom acoustics, and habilitation and rehabilitation issues. An increasingly important part of the practice of audiology is newborn screening. Audiologists use sophisticated testing instruments to determine the status of the hearing mechanism in babies who may be only hours old. Like speech–language pathologists, audiologists serve diverse populations and are prohibited from discriminating in the provision of professional services. Audiologists work in private practice, hospitals, physicians' offices, community speech and hearing centers, the military, rehabilitation facilities, and public and private schools. Many audiologists are members of the American Academy of Audiology (Box 11.1).

QUESTION: How do I know if the profession is right for me?

ANSWER: Students should consider all aspects of any discipline before declaring it as a major. Choosing a career is one of the most important life decisions you will make. Do not be hurried into declaring a major. Many college juniors and seniors do not know what they want to do for a living. One of the best things you can do, especially in your freshman and sophomore years, is take introductory courses in a variety of majors. As well, your university's counseling and testing office has aptitude tests that can predict careers for which you are best

BOX 11.1 • *The American Academy of Audiology*

Founded in January 1988, the American Academy of Audiology (AAA) is the world's largest independent, freestanding national organization for audiologists. The mission of AAA is to provide quality hearing care to the public, enhance the ability of members to achieve career objectives, provide professional development through education and research, and increase public awareness of hearing disorders and audiologic services. To be a member requires a minimum of a master's degree in audiology from an accredited university. The AAA publishes *The Journal of the American Academy of Audiology*, *Audiology Today*, and *Audiology Express*. It has approximately 7,000 members. You can get more information from its home page: http://www.audiology.org/about.

suited. Such tests can be valuable in helping decide whether a career in speech–language pathology and audiology are right for you.

You should consider many factors when deciding on a profession. Certain traits, aptitudes, and interests are important in the profession of speech–language pathology and audiology. First, you should ask yourself if you are people oriented. Most jobs in this profession involve frequent contact and interaction with people, although some specialty areas have less contact with people. For example, speech and hearing scientists and those involved in developing alternative communication devices typically spend more time doing research. Second, ask yourself if you like helping people. Are you a nurturing type of person? Like nurses, teachers, and physicians, do you want to use your knowledge and skills to help people? Third, are you untroubled working with the sick, hurt, or disabled? Does the thought of working in a hospital or nursing home distress you? Do you feel comfortable being around children and adults with multiple disabilities?

The most important questions to ask yourself relate to the nature of this discipline. Do you find the human ability to communicate, and its disorders, interesting, exciting, and worthy of your commitment? Do subjects such as neurology, anatomy and physiology, psychology, linguistics, phonetics, acoustics, and articulation spark your interest? Do you want to know how to evaluate and treat articulation, voice, language, hearing, and fluency disorders? Are you attracted to these concepts?

Consider many other factors also before committing to a career. Research the specific job market, salaries, and working conditions in the area of the country where you want to work. (Mean salaries for practitioners are provided later.) Talk to several practicing professionals and, if possible, spend time shadowing them at work. Also try to project what the future will bring for the profession. Will it fall as a casualty to technological advances and become obsolete or limited in opportunities?

Choosing a career can cause anxiety. It can be stressful trying to decide what to do with your life. It can also be an exciting time in which you carefully and thoughtfully commit to a profession that can bring great rewards and personal satisfaction. But remember that this decision, like many others in life, is not irreversible and permanent. During college many students reconsider careers as they learn more about the world of employment opportunities. Many people also change careers in later life.

QUESTION: Are there research opportunities in speech–language pathology and audiology?

ANSWER: Yes. Research is the foundation of speech–language pathology and audiology. Both professions rely on the scientific method to advance information about the causes, nature, diagnosis, and treatment of communication disorders. Scientists conduct research on every facet of normal communication, not just on communication disorders. Comprehensive knowledge of normal communication is required before we can understand and appreciate the variety of disorders that occur. Speech–language pathologists and audiologists rely on research conducted by speech and hearing scientists and researchers from other professions. Scientists in education, psychology, genetics, neurology, linguistics, anatomy, physiology, and acoustics also conduct research into communication and its disorders. Speech and hearing clinicians use this information to provide the best diagnostic and therapeutic services possible to individuals with communication disorders.

Research into normal communication is conducted on people of all ages. For example, research is done on newborns to find out at what ages they can recognize and understand the speech of their mothers and the acuteness of their sense of hearing. Toddlers and preschoolers are studied to learn stages of speech and language development. Research is conducted to learn when phonological processes and speech sounds are learned. Scientists study fluency in people of all ages. Currently, much research is being conducted to see what parts of the brain and nervous system are important to various aspects of speech, voice, hearing, and language functioning in normal individuals. Researchers are investigating the anatomy and physiology of normal speech. In the elderly, studies are conducted to see what normally happens to language, memory, thinking, hearing, and voice quality as a normal part of the aging process. Cultural, gender, and socioeconomic factors are investigated to see what roles they play in normal communication development and usage. Research into normal communication is highly sophisticated and involves the newest tests, instruments, and procedures available to scientists. Communication is one of the highest functions performed by humans, and research into it is exciting. This type of scientific inquiry is often *pure research* because it is done to quench the thirst for knowledge about the nature of communication. *Applied research* is done to answer specific questions about the causes, diagnosis, and treatment of communication disorders.

Applied research involves looking at the diseases and disorders that cause speech and hearing pathologies. Scientists study syndromes, disorders, and diseases that can affect speech, voice, language, and hearing to determine the effects they have on the ability to communicate, procedures for evaluation, and methods of treatment. These studies are conducted on fetal alcohol syndrome, Parkinson's disease, muscular dystrophy, multiple sclerosis, polio, acquired immunodeficiency syndrome (AIDS), head trauma, and stroke, to name a few. Currently, exciting research is being done on laryngectomy transplants and cochlear implants. Studies are conducted to discover therapies and treatments for communication disorders and whether patients can benefit from them.

The majority of research in communication sciences and disorders is conducted at universities by professors, and many graduate programs require research projects of their students. Consequently, students often participate in cutting edge research, and many conduct experiments as part of their graduate requirements. Many of these studies are published in scientific journals or presented at professional conferences. After graduation, research continues to be conducted by practicing speech–language pathologists and audiologists.

Understanding and doing research is a integral part of the practice of speech–language pathology and audiology.

QUESTION: What is the job market like for graduates in speech–language pathology and audiology?

ANSWER: The job market, the availability of employment, fluctuates over time. It is a direct result of supply and demand, depending on how many people seek the available jobs. This is true for virtually all professions. For example, in some years, the demand is great for engineers, and at other times, students with degrees in business administration are aggressively sought. The demand for graduates in speech–language pathology and audiology also changes over time.

Over the past 50 years, the job market has been very favorable; this trend continues today. Most speech–language pathologists and audiologists who want to work can find employment. Historically, there have been several jobs for each person seeking one. Certainly, there have been times where finding employment was difficult. Periods of layoffs and reductions in force have occurred due to financial constraints in the public schools. At times, jobs in a medical environment have been tight due to Medicare and other cutbacks or caps on services. Nevertheless, these were exceptions to the rule, and such things happen in all professions. The supply–demand factors affecting employment have typically favored the job seeker. Sometimes, employers offer generous signing bonuses and other perks to job hunters. *Perks* are job benefits that go beyond the typical ones usually offered by an employer. They can include use of a company car, expense accounts, college tuition payments for continuing education, access to executive facilities, private parking spaces, personal days off, child care, and other benefits. As far as the availability of jobs is concerned, the profession of speech–language pathology and audiology has regularly been an excellent career choice.

QUESTION: Where do people work once they get their degrees?

ANSWER: An appealing aspect of this profession is the variety of employment settings. Graduates get employment in two primary fields: medical and educational settings. The need for professionals to work in these environments fluctuates. Some years, more jobs are available in hospitals, nursing homes, home health agencies, and the like, and in other years, more jobs are available in public and private schools.

Employment in medical environments includes hospitals, nursing homes, home health agencies, and physicians' offices. These typically are day jobs on 12-month contracts. They often have generous benefit packages including paid vacations, sick leave, life and disability insurance coverage, and medical care. Some positions are primarily with pediatric patients, but most involve older people (geriatrics). Specialized employment possibilities include evaluating and treating a particular type of communication disorder. For example, speech–language pathologists and audiologists can work only with pediatric head-trauma patients or only with children with birth defects or orofacial anomalies. Some clinicians work primarily with adults with voice disorders or head traumas. Most individuals in a medical environment, however, see a wide range of patients and disorders. (See Appendix B for the short story, "Preponderance of Evidence," and an example of what it is like to work in a hospital.) When working in a medical environment, speech–language pathologists and audiologists have frequent professional interaction with physicians, nurses, psychologists, social workers, dietitians, physical and occupational therapists, and other medical personnel.

In the educational environment, most job opportunities are in the public schools. Typically, these are 9- or 10-month contracts. These positions also often include generous benefit packages with health care, life and disability insurance, and time off for holidays, snow days, and sick leave. One benefit of employment in an educational setting is that many employees have a large part of the summer off, but consequently the salary may be accordingly lower. In educational environments, clinicians also see a wide range of disorders. Caseloads of public school clinicians depend on where they work. Most clinicians work with children in preschool through the elementary grades. Some work with middle and high school students with communication disorders. Clinicians in the public schools see children with articulation, phonology disorders, language delay, stuttering, cleft lip and palate, mental deficiency, and learning disabilities. Some clinicians focus on a specific disorder such as autism, Down syndrome, or learning disabilities. (See Appendix B for the short story, "A Day at JFK," and an example of what it is like to work in a public school.) When working in an educational environment, speech language–pathologists and audiologists have frequent professional interaction with principals; school nurses; special education and classroom teachers; dental, educational, and psychological specialists; counselors; teachers' aides; and other school personnel.

Certified speech–language pathologists and audiologists also work in other sites and types of employment. Graduates find employment in mental retardation facilities, schools for the deaf and hard-of-hearing, public health clinics, Bureau of Indian Affairs boarding schools, United Way agencies, research organizations, and private and group practices. Job opportunities also exist in colleges and universities. Most graduate programs in communication sciences and disorders have on-site clinics in which students provide services to individuals with communication disorders under careful supervision of clinical supervisors. Clinic work gives students valuable experience in working with patients who have a variety of disorders. Clinical supervision in a college or university is a potential employment opportunity for experienced clinicians. Jobs are available overseas in military hospitals and schools, and other countries seek graduates with degrees in communication sciences and disorders.

QUESTION: How do I know if my professional interest is in medical or educational settings?

ANSWER: There is a simple way to consider this question: Do you prefer working with children or adults? Most jobs in education involve working with children with communication disorders. Conversely, most of the patients seen in medical settings are older adults who have had strokes or other age-related diseases and disorders. Of course, exceptions occur in both employment settings. Some clinicians in a medical center work exclusively with pediatrics patients, and school clinicians also see adults with mental deficiency and other disorders. However, as a rule, educational settings involve working with children, and medical environments involve evaluating and treating adults and geriatrics.

QUESTION: Does this profession have status and prestige?

ANSWER: Will this profession be one that will bring you recognition and respect? Measuring the intangible aspects of any profession is difficult. Several years ago, *Money* magazine listed the public's opinion of various professions. They gave 50 professions letter grades from A+ to C–, based on how the general public viewed their status and prestige. The highest grade, A+, was given to high-profile professions such as physicians and lawyers. The lowest grade, C–, was given to occupations such as hairstylists and bakers. Speech pathologists/audiologists received a grade of A–, placing them in the same category as accountants and auditors, computer programmers, dental hygienists, people in marketing and advertising, registered nurses, and public relations specialists.

Educational Preparation, Certification, and Licensure

QUESTION: What are the courses like in communication sciences and disorders?

ANSWER: Challenging. With few exceptions, the courses are exciting, demanding, and rewarding. Students learn about the marvelous human ability to communicate—exploring the entire process from putting thoughts into words to understanding spoken statements (see Chapter 1). The courses cover cognition, language, phonetics, motor speech functioning, acoustics, and hearing. Courses address specific disorders such as stuttering, phonological disorders, swallowing problems, and hearing loss. Other courses deal with medical syndromes, specific diseases, or birth defects. Evaluation and therapeutic methods are also taught.

Because these disciplines are based on the scientific method, courses in how to conduct and understand research are offered. Many graduate programs offer the option of a master's thesis. For students taking the research option, courses in research design and statistics are required, and students design and complete a research project related to speech and hearing, a valuable aspect of professional preparation. The master's research project is especially important for students who want to pursue a Doctor of Philosophy (Ph.D.).

QUESTION: What are the educational and clinical requirements to become a speech–language pathologist or audiologist?

ANSWER: Certificates of Clinical Competence (CCC) in speech–language pathology (CCC-SLP) or audiology (CCC-A) are issued by the American Speech-Language-Hearing Association. When a person is granted the certificate, he has met the basic educational, clinical, and professional requirements to practice the profession of speech–language pathology or audiology. The CCC is recognized by most states as meeting the minimum requirements to receive a license to practice. Additionally, most countries recognize the CCC as meeting or exceeding their educational, clinical, and professional requirements to practice.

To obtain the CCC in either speech–language pathology or audiology requires a master's degree or its equivalent from an accredited program (Box 11.2). The equivalent of a master's degree is met by some individuals who have advanced degrees in other professions. As long as they have the course and clinical work required by ASHA, a master's degree specifically in communication sciences and disorders, or similar degree title, is not required. Like all majors, students majoring in communication sciences and disorders must take a specified number of courses in particular areas. Students complete course work that addresses normal communication. These courses include anatomy and physiology of the speech and hearing mechanism, phonetics, language development, and so on. Each candidate for the CCC also must take courses addressing major communication disorders such as stuttering, aphasia, motor speech disorders, and language delay. Effective January 1, 2005, a minimum of 75 semester credit hours must be completed in a course of study addressing the knowledge and skills associated with communication disorders, and 36 of those hours must be earned at the graduate level. A strong clinical training requirement is required, which is usually completed at the master's level.

Under supervision, students work directly with children and adults with a variety of disorders. They evaluate and treat people who have aphasia, apraxia

BOX 11.2 • *The Council of Academic Accreditation*

The Council of Academic Accreditation (CAA) accredits institutions of higher learning that offer graduate degree programs in speech–language pathology and/or audiology. CAA accreditation ensures that the academic and clinical practicum offered by an accredited program meets nationally established standards. Accreditation is given initially for a 5-year period and then for a maximum period of 8 years for reaccreditation. Accredited programs have engaged in extensive self-study, submitted a complex application, undergone an on-site visit by a team of specially trained peers, and submitted annual reports during the period of their accreditation. Check out a listing of the CAA programs for your state: http://professional.asha.org/academic/council.cfm.. The area in which a program has been accredited is indicated by SLP (speech–language pathology), A (audiology), or SLP/A (both). Their status in the review process is also listed.

of speech, dysarthria, language delay, hearing loss, deafness, and so on. These clinical experiences, called the *practicum* (see the next question), occur in several different work environments such as clinics, schools, hospitals, and nursing homes. After the rigorous educational and clinical requirements at the master's level, students undergo the Clinical Fellowship.

The Clinical Fellowship (CF) occurs after the candidate for the CCC has received the master's degree or its equivalent. During the CF, she is employed in clinical practice. During the first 36 weeks of full-time clinical practice, there is also supervision by a certified speech–language pathologist or audiologist. (For those working less than full-time, the CF lasts longer.) The supervisor need not be affiliated with a college or university. This supervision is not as intensive as that provided during the master's degree, but it does involve site visits, monitoring of patients, and regular communication with the applicant. The CF provides mentoring for the candidate by a practicing professional.

Candidates for the CCC in speech–language pathology or audiology must also pass national examinations, which are comprehensive assessments of the candidate's knowledge of communication sciences and disorders. A national testing company administers the tests, and although students can take the tests at any time, most do so after the completion of their course requirements. The candidate can take the test three times. Once all requirements are met and the candidate agrees to abide by ASHA's Code of Ethics, he is granted the CCC. ASHA's Code of Ethics is a very important set of rules governing ethical aspects of the profession. The Code of Ethics gives specific rules to speech–language pathologists and audiologists, detailing what is considered ethical and unethical conduct. The document is designed to protect the rights of consumers of speech and hearing services and to ensure that they receive the highest quality of professional services. Typically, the average undergraduate takes 4 years to obtain a bachelor's degree. Some colleges and universities have accelerated undergraduate programs in which the student can graduate with a bachelor's degree in 3 years. For people who have an adequate undergraduate preparation in communication sciences and disorders, a master's degree can usually be completed in 2 or 3 years.

QUESTION: What is the practicum?

ANSWER: With the practicum, students learn to apply in clinical situations what they have learned in their academic program. Most practicum training occurs during the master's program, although some colleges give undergraduates clinical experiences. During the practicum experience, students are supervised while they provide clinical services. Currently, 375 hours of direct patient/client contact and 25 hours of observation are required. Supervision of the applicant is never less than 25% for any clinical activity. Practicum experiences are very costly to colleges because there is much individual student–professor contact, and it is an important but time-consuming aspect of professional training for speech–language pathologists and audiologists.

QUESTION: Are there other requirements to work as a speech–language pathologist or audiologist?

ANSWER: States also have licensing laws for speech–language pathology or audiology. Most of these states accept the CCC to meet their licensing guidelines, although some states have additional requirements to become licensed. These additional requirements can include continuing education, background checks, and other minimum education and practicum standards.

QUESTION: Is there an organization for students in communication sciences and disorders?

ANSWER: Yes. It is called the National Student Speech-Language-Hearing Association (NSSLHA). There are chapters of NSSLHA at most colleges and universities. Students run NSSLHA, although there is usually a faculty advisor. Students are strongly encouraged to join NSSLHA once they have declared communication sciences and disorders as a major. Both undergraduates and graduate students can benefit from membership in NSSLHA. Membership provides an opportunity to meet with other students majoring in the discipline and helps create a sense of community. NSSLHA publishes a journal and newsletter providing information important to students about the communication disorders and the profession of speech–language pathology and audiology. NSSLHA is active in promoting the interests of students in such areas as educational and clinical requirements and university, local, state, and national political issues.

QUESTION: Are there job opportunities for students with bachelor's degrees in communication sciences and disorders?

ANSWER: Yes. Although a master's degree is required to practice speech–language pathology and audiology, an undergraduate degree prepares a student for many career options that do not directly involve clinical practice. Like any general studies degree, a bachelor's in communication sciences and disorders is a broad degree considered valuable by employers who want to train their own college-educated employees. An undergraduate degree in communication sciences and disorders provides the educational background to enter the job market in a variety of occupations such as pharmaceutical sales, publishing, and educational product development. It qualifies the graduate for many administrative positions in governmental programs such as Head Start, Bureau of Indian Affairs schools, and health agencies. An undergraduate degree in communication sciences and disorders meets many of the requirements that business and industry want for positions that simply require a bachelor of science or arts degree. There is also the opportunity to work as a speech–language pathology assistant (discussed later).

QUESTION: What are the admission requirements for graduate school?

ANSWER: Getting into graduate school is competitive. Individual colleges and universities have different requirements to be admitted to their graduate schools. Most colleges and universities require a minimum cumulative grade point average (GPA), usually a 3.0. This is the average grade of all courses that an undergraduate has taken. Some departments have higher GPA requirements that are set by their graduate school. Departments sometimes require that only the courses taken in the major, or the major GPA, meet or exceed minimum requirements. Many colleges and universities also require the Graduate Record Examination (GRE), which is an admission test for graduate school. (Sidebar 11.1) Because the profession of speech–language pathology and audiology requires a master's degree, students need to get good grades, especially in the professional courses.

Some colleges and universities admit students to their programs with undergraduate degrees in disciplines other than communication sciences and disorders. Usually, these students must then take the professional undergraduate courses before they can be formally admitted to the graduate program. This process is sometimes called *leveling*. Once the leveling or prerequisite courses are taken, the student begins the graduate course sequence similar to graduate students who have undergraduate degrees in the discipline.

The attrition rate in graduate programs is low. The *attrition rate* is how many of the applicants do not successfully complete the degree either because they drop out or fail their course work or practicum studies. Because of the high standards and stringent admission requirements, most students enter graduate school well prepared and with a history of successful academic careers. A very high percentage of those admitted to a graduate program eventually graduate.

QUESTION: What is a Doctor of Philosophy (Ph.D.) in communication sciences and disorders?

ANSWER: The Doctor of Philosophy is a research and scientific degree. Currently, the highest degree necessary to practice in the profession of speech–language pathology and audiology is the master's degree. The master's is the terminal degree. A *terminal degree* is the highest education needed in a particular occupation or profession. Many schools offer a Ph.D. in speech and hearing sciences and/or speech–language pathology and audiology. (Some universities also offer an educational doctorate, or Ed.D.)

Although both Ph.D. degrees are similar, there are fundamental differences. A Ph.D. in speech and hearing sciences focuses more on normal aspects of speech, voice, language, and hearing. A Ph.D. in speech–language pathology or audiology also addresses normal aspects of communication, but the focus is on

SIDEBAR 11.1 • *The Graduate Record Examination*

The Graduate Record Examination (GRE) is like the college entrance test that students take to be admitted as an undergraduate. It is designed to predict how well one will do in graduate school. There are three sections to it; some departments require the whole test, whereas others require only one or two sections. Departments either have a set minimum score on the GRE or rank all applicants to their program.

diagnosis and treatment of speech, voice, and language pathologies. Students at the Ph.D. level specialize in a particular area such as acoustics, voice science, stuttering, phonological disorders, or orofacial anomalies. Both degrees require a dissertation. A dissertation is like a master's thesis, but the research is more elaborate, complex, and detailed.

QUESTION: Is there an advantage to having a degree in another profession in addition to speech–language pathology and audiology?

ANSWER: It depends on the degree. For example, a certified speech–language pathologist who has a teaching degree has more job opportunities. Smaller school districts often seek people with multiple degrees who can both teach special education courses and serve as speech–language pathologists. Similarly, smaller hospitals and rehabilitation centers often will seek employees who have both speech–language pathology and occupational or physical therapy degrees.

QUESTION: What are the requirements to work as a speech–language pathology assistant?

ANSWER: ASHA has recently established the criteria for becoming a speech–language pathology assistant. Effective January 1, 2003, applicants must have an associate degree with specific course work in the field of communication disorders. In addition, each applicant must complete 100 hours of supervised fieldwork experiences.

QUESTION: What are the responsibilities of a speech–language pathology assistant?

ANSWER: ASHA is very clear about the responsibilities of a speech–language pathology assistant. Generally, a speech–language pathology assistant can help with hearing screenings; follow treatment plans established by a certified speech–language pathologist; document patient/client performance; assist in assessment, clerical duties, and collecting data; and help with the maintenance of equipment. Speech–language pathology assistants cannot do testing, screening, or diagnosing patients with feeding/swallowing disorders or participate in professional conferences without the presence of a supervisor. Other activities beyond the job responsibilities for a speech–language pathology assistant include writing treatment plans, signing formal documentation, selecting patients for services or discharge, and counseling patients about their status or services. Speech–language pathology assistants must not represent themselves as speech–language pathologists.

Professional Practice

QUESTION: Does ASHA require continuing education after it grants the CCC?

ANSWER: ASHA requires its members to continue their professional education by obtaining continuing education units (CEUs) (Box 11.3). In addition, many states, with their licensure laws, require that the licensee obtain a specific number of CEUs. According to ASHA, as of 2001, 40 states require continuing education for renewal of licensure in audiology, and 38 require continuing education for renewal of licensure in speech–language pathology (see Appendix A).

QUESTION: What are the salaries for graduates?

ANSWER: The salary range is difficult to evaluate because so many variables are involved. The state speech and hearing association or university employment office can provide average salaries in one's state. Generally, salaries for new graduates in communication sciences and disorders are competitive with those of other disciplines. Most graduates in communication sciences and disorders receive starting salaries in the upper half of the range of salaries received by their graduating classes. According to ASHA, in 1997, the starting salary for a speech–language pathologist was $30,000 for an academic year and $38,000 for a calendar year. Typically, those who work in a medical environment get higher salaries than those in the school systems. One reason for this disparity is that medical employment is usually on a 12-month contract, whereas public school employment is on a 9- or a 10-month academic year. According to ASHA, in 1997 the median annual salary for a certified speech–language pathologist employed on 9- or 10-month contract was $39,950. The median annual salary for those working on a calendar-year basis was $44,000. Audiologists reported a median academic-year salary of $40,000, whereas those on a calendar-year basis was $43,000. Currently, there are no data on speech–language pathology assistant salaries. However, the salary for speech–language pathology assistants is likely to be consistent with occupational and physical therapy assistants. Typically, they make about 60–75% of the professional level salaries. When one considers salaries, knowing the cost-of-living statistics for a particular locale is also important. A high salary in a city with high housing, food, and transportation expenses may not go as far as a seemingly low salary in some small towns and rural areas. When seeking employment and negotiating

BOX 11.3 • *Continuing Education and the Continuing Education Unit*

The continuing education unit (CEU) was established in 1968 by a U.S. Department of Education task force. It is a nationally recognized standard unit of measurement for participation in a continuing education activity that is not offered for academic credit. ASHA CEUs must meet certain educational content requirements, including that they are related to the scientific basis of speech–language pathology and audiology, speech/language/hearing sciences, and/or the contemporary practice of speech–language pathology and audiology. The content level must go beyond that which is required for initial certification by ASHA. Check out the CEU Web site for more information (Appendix A).

for salary, a graduate must consider the cost of living in the area. Check out Appendix A for a Web site that addresses professional salaries.

QUESTION: What opportunities are there for speech–language pathologists and audiologists in private practice?

ANSWER: The potential to develop a successful private practice is an attractive aspect of majoring in communication sciences and disorders. Some speech–language pathologists and audiologists maintain full-time private practices. Others have part-time practices in which they are employed by hospitals or schools full-time but see patients privately after work or on weekends.

It takes several years to develop a full-time private practice, and there are financial risks to consider. Startup costs include rent, security deposits, testing and equipment purchases, diagnostic and therapy supplies, and salaries for office personnel. Some private practices have contracts with small schools, hospitals, or nursing homes. Under the terms of the contract, the speech–language pathologist or audiologist provides speech and hearing services, and the organization or facility reimburses them on a patient or student basis or on a per-day, per-week, or annual basis. Some private practices grow into large business organizations with many contracts, patients, students, and clients. They have many employees and consultants. Others stay small, either by design or circumstance. Even small private practices have many benefits that go beyond financial ones such as being one's own boss, setting schedules, and deciding which patients to see.

Students often ask how much money a typical private practice generates. This is an important but difficult question to answer. First, there is really no "typical" private practice. Private practices are as diverse and unique as are the professionals who establish them. Some prefer to work part-time and treat only one disorder such as stuttering. Some clinicians maintain a home office. Other private practices are in larger buildings with several offices, therapy suites, and a reception area. Second, the business savvy of the entrepreneur partly determines the income potential of a private practice. Some private practices are extremely successful and generate large incomes, whereas others fail. Factors affecting the success of a private practice include governmental policies, supply and demand, and the general economy. According to the latest figures published by ASHA, in 1997, the median calendar-year salary was $46,250 for a full-time private practitioner in audiology and $48,000 for speech–language pathology (see Appendix A).

Of course, not everyone wants a private practice, nor is everyone suited for one. Private practice involves much uncertainty. Unlike employment with a set salary, private practice has no guarantee of an income. Private practice is competitive and requires hard work and long hours. Some private practitioners remark that their businesses are either "feast or famine." Sometimes there are generous financial rewards, and at other times, covering day-to-day expenses is difficult. Record keeping is an important aspect to a practice. The private practitioner can deduct or receive tax credits for most expenses related to her practice. Expenses for a home office, automobile, clinical and office supplies, travel, dues, insurance, and other aspects related to a private practice are usually deductible. Self-employment individual retirement accounts (SEP-IRAs) are available to the private practitioner to set aside money for retirement. Full- or part-time, private practice is a viable option for speech–language pathologists and audiologists.

QUESTION: How do certified speech–language pathologists and audiologists keep current about professional issues?

ANSWER: After finishing the required formal education, speech–language pathologists and audiologists can keep current in several ways. Many ASHA members continue to take college courses throughout their careers. They take extension, night, or Internet courses to improve their diagnostic and therapeutic skills. Workshops are also valuable sources of continuing education. Many specialty workshops address current topics in autism, aphasia, attention deficit disorders, newborn hearing-screening procedures, phonology, diagnostic principles, and so on. One of the most valuable sources of continuing education is the annual ASHA convention.

ASHA conventions are well attended by its members. They are held in November, usually in major U.S. cities. Because of the size of the convention, an entire city's convention center and several adjacent hotels are utilized. Short courses are given on particular topics, along with seminars, minicourses, and poster sessions. Hundreds of scientific papers are presented. Committees meet, plan, and direct the course of the profession. There are also job interviews. An interesting aspect of the annual convention is the exhibits. Hundreds of companies that publish books, manufacture technical devices, and develop diagnostic tests and therapeutic programs have displays and exhibits. Annual conventions also involve parties, dinners, keynote speakers, balls, gatherings for college alumni, and tours of the city. Most state speech and hearing associations also have conventions, which are smaller but also offer scientific papers, exhibits, and other opportunities for continuing education. Conventions are lively, exciting events for speech–language pathologists and audiologists and a valuable source of continuing education.

Other sources of continuing education are journals and books. Scientific journals present theory and current research about a particular professional topic. ASHA publishes several journals such as *Language, Speech and Hearing Services in the Schools (LSHSS)* and journals of clinical practice. State associations, publishing companies, and professional interest groups also publish journals; through reading journals, professionals keep current about recent scientific advances in their particular area of interest. Professional books are also a source of continuing education. Several publishing companies have clubs that promote new books in a particular area.

QUESTION: Is there an advantage for a speech–language pathologist or audiologist to be bilingual or multilingual?

ANSWER: Because the caseloads of speech–language pathologists and audiologists are increasingly multicultural, a clinician who speaks and understands more than one language has an advantage. This is particularly true in speech–language pathology in the area of language testing and therapies. Being able to test and provide therapy in a patient's native language is an important, if not necessary, skill.

QUESTION: What will the future bring to the professions of speech–language pathology and audiology?

ANSWER: Speech–language pathology and audiology are professions that rely in part on technology for research, diagnostic, and therapeutic services. Consequently, the computer revolution has had and will continue to have a significant effect on them. (See Appendix B for the short story, "Welcome to the Cyber Speech and Hearing Clinic," addressing likely technological advances.) In addition to the effects of technology, the demographics of the United States will continue to play an important role in the supply-demand for clinicians. It is likely that as the United States continues to grow and age, more speech–language pathologists and audiologists will be required, especially in medical environments (see Chapter 1).

Suggested Readings

Tanner, D. (1997). *Handbook for the speech–language pathology assistant.* Oceanside, CA: Academic Communication Associates. This handbook provides a review of communication disorders and valuable information for the speech–language pathology assistant.

Tanner, D. (2001, December 2). Welcome to the brave new world of the cyber speech and hearing clinic. *ASHA Leader.* This article discusses what technology may bring to the clinical provision of speech and hearing services in the future.

Glossary

The following books and dictionaries were consulted in selecting and defining some of the terms in this glossary.

Anderson, K. (Ed.). (1998). *Mosby's medical, nursing, and allied health dictionary* (4th ed.). St. Louis: Mosby.

Bear, M., Connors, B., & Paradiso, M. (1996). *Neuroscience: Exploring the brain.* Baltimore: Williams & Wilkins.

Culbertson, W., & Tanner, D. (1997). *Speech and hearing anatomy and physiology workbook.* Boston: Allyn & Bacon.

Dirckx, J. (Ed.). (1997). *Stedman's concise medical dictionary for the health professions* (3rd ed.). Baltimore: Williams & Wilkins.

Kent, R. (1997). *The speech sciences.* San Diego: Singular.

Nicolosi, L., Harryman, E., & Kresheck, K. (1996). *Terminology of communication disorders* (4th ed.). Baltimore: Williams & Wilkins.

Shames, G., Wiig, E., & Secord, W. (1998). *Human communication disorders: An introduction* (5th ed.). Boston: Allyn & Bacon.

Tanner, D. (1999). *The family guide to surviving stroke and communication disorders.* Boston: Allyn & Bacon.

Tanner, D. (2003). *The psychology of neurogenic communication disorders: A primer for health care professionals.* Boston: Allyn & Bacon.

Zemlin, W. (1998). *Speech and hearing science* (4th ed.). Boston: Allyn & Bacon

In addition to other terms defined in the text, this glossary defines terms that you may need to know.

a- A prefix indicating the complete inability to perform a function.

abduction The movement away from the body's midsagittal plane. In voice, the movement away from the midline of the two vocal folds; opening of the glottis.

abductor In voice, the muscle that performs abduction; the posterior cricoarytenoid muscle.

abstract attitude The ability to symbolize, understand, and categorize verbal and nonverbal information; generalized ability to understand relationships.

abulia The chronic inability to make decisions or to preform voluntary activities; chronic procrastination.

acalculia In aphasia, the inability to perform and understand simple mathematics due to brain damage.

accent Phonetic traits of a person's native language carried over into a second language; in phonetics, the application of stress to a syllable.

acoustic agnosia   The inability to perceive differences in speech sounds; the inability to perceive salient auditory features.

acoustic impedance audiometry   A hearing test measurement of opposition or resistance of sound energy through the middle ear.

acoustic nerve   The cochlear branch of cranial nerve VIII; the vestibulocochlear nerve.

acoustic neuroma   A tumor of the auditory nerve.

acoustic reflex   The automatic contraction of the stapedius and tensor tympani muscles in response to a loud tone; also called the stapedial reflex.

acoustic reflex threshold   The lowest intensity or loudness of a tone producing the acoustic reflex.

acoustics   A branch of physics that deals with sound.

acquired aphasia   The loss of language occurring after birth because of disease or injury.

acquired hearing loss   Hearing loss that is not congenital; hearing loss occurring after birth because of disease or injury.

addition   In speech articulation, an unnecessary sound placed in a word.

adduction   The movement of a body part toward the midsagittal plane. In voice, the drawing toward the midline of the two vocal folds; closing of the glottis.

adductor   In phonation, a muscle that performs adduction.

adventitious deafness   Deafness occurring after birth because of disease or injury; acquired deafness.

affricate   A speech sound that consists of a plosive and a brief fricative.

agnosia   A perceptual disorder in which a person has trouble recognizing and appreciating information coming from the senses; usually specific to one modality of communication.

agrammatism   In aphasia, the loss of the ability to understand and use the grammar of a language due to neurological damage; the omission or misuse of the grammatical units of language.

agraphia   In aphasia, the inability to write secondary to central language deficits and *not* due to limb paralysis; the inability to express oneself in writing.

air–bone gap   In audiology, the difference, measured in decibels, that an air-conduction threshold exceeds the bone-conduction threshold at any frequency.

air-conduction testing   A measurement of the auditory system by presenting tones of different frequencies and loudness levels.

alaryngeal speech   Any type of speech produced without a larynx.

alexia   In aphasia, the inability to read *not* due to visual acuity deficits or blindness.

alveolar   The tissue just behind the upper incisors.

amnesia   The loss of memory; the partial or complete inability to recognize or recall past events.

amplification   In audiology, the process of increasing auditory input to enhance perception.

aneurysm   The ballooning, or swelling, in a weakened area in the wall of an artery.

anomia   In aphasia, the loss of the ability to recall words; not limited to nouns.

anosognosia   The inability to perceive, recognize, and accept body parts; the denial of disability.

anoxia   Lack of oxygen to the brain.

anterograde amnesia   The loss of the ability to store and recall new memories.

aperiodic   Without periodicity; irregular.

aphasia   The multimodality inability to encode, decode, and/or manipulate symbols for the purposes of verbal thought and/or communication; the loss of language due to damage of the speech and language centers of the brain.

aphemia   The inability to speak due to loss of language; aphasia.

aphonia   The loss of the ability to vibrate the vocal cords to produce voice. The complete lack of phonation; without voice.

apoplexy   A cerebral vascular accident; a stroke.

apraxia   The loss of the ability to plan and sequence voluntary body movements due to a stroke or other neurological disorder.

apraxia of speech (AOS)   The loss of ability to conceptualize, plan, and sequence motor speech due to a neurological disorder.

aprosody   The loss of the rhythm, cadence, and melody of speech.

artery   A vessel that carries blood from the heart to other parts of the body.

articulation   Shaping compressed air from the lungs into individual speech sounds; the act of moving the vocal tract structures so that speech sounds are produced.

articulator   An organ of the speech mechanism that valves the compressed air coming from the lungs.

aspiration   In phonetics, the addition of the whispered glottal sound source to the normal sound of a phoneme. In dysphagia, ingestion of food or liquid into the respiratory system.

assimilated hypernasality   Too much nasality on sounds following or preceding nasal phonemes.

assimilation   The phonological process of combining characteristics of adjacent phonemes.

association   The internalization of information and the process of making it personally relevant; relating of experiences, perceptions, and thoughts.

ataxia   The loss of the ability to engage in smooth motor activities. The loss of muscle tone, balance, and coordination of muscle groups primarily due to damage to the cerebellum and/or the tracts leading to and from it.

ataxic dysarthria   A subtype of dysarthria associated with damage to the cerebellum and the tracts leading to and from it. Speech is ill coordinated and produced with improper timing and stress.

athetosis   A type of neuromuscular disorder characterized by tremor and discoordination often occurring in cerebral palsy.

atrophy   When a body structure withers, shrinks in size, and becomes weak due to disuse or disease.

audible inspiration   Perceptible sound produced during the act of drawing air into the lungs.

audiogram   A graph for recording air- and bone-conduction hearing thresholds.

audiology   The branch of science concerned with the study, diagnosis, and treatment of hearing disorders.

audiometrist   An audiology technician working under the supervision of an audiologist or otologist.

auditory acclimatization   The gradual process of becoming accustomed to the increased loudness of a sound.

auditory agnosia   The inability to perceive differences in speech and environmental signals; the inability to perceive salient auditory features.

auditory closure   The integration of auditory stimuli into a perceptual whole.

auditory cortex   An auditory area in the superior temporal lobe of the cerebral cortex, also called Heschl's gyrus.

auditory discrimination   The ability to perceive differences in sounds.

auditory perception   The process of detecting salient features from the hearing mechanism; the mental awareness of a sound and organization of sensory data received from the ears.

auditory training   Therapy provided to a patient with a hearing loss to maximize the use of residual hearing.

aural habilitation   Therapies and procedures to improve communication abilities in individuals born hearing impaired.

aural rehabilitation   Therapies to improve a hearing-impaired person's ability to communicate; includes speech and language therapy, speechreading, manual communication, and amplification.

automatic speech   Utterances made with little or no thought including songs, verses, and profanity.

bel   A unit of sound intensity measurement where 10 decibels equal one bel; a logarithmic unit named after Alexander Graham Bell.

benign   A nonmalignant neoplasm or tumor; noncancerous.

Bernoulli principle   A principle of physics that describes the decrease in air pressure associated with increased airflow velocity. The Bernoulli principle helps close the glottis during phonation by lowering air pressure on the medial vocal fold surfaces and drawing them toward the midline.

bifid uvula   A uvula divided into two sections; a cleft of the uvula.

bilabial   Pertaining to two lips. Sounds produced with both lips, such as /b/ and /p/.

bilateral   Referring to two sides of a structure; the opposite of unilateral.

bilateral adductor paralysis   Inability of both vocal cords to close; both vocal folds fixed in an open position.

binaural   Pertaining to both ears.

bisyllable   A word with two syllables.

blend   Two or more consonant sounds without a vowel separating them; also called a consonant cluster.

block   In stuttering, an abnormal obstruction of speech valving.

Blom-Singer prosthesis   In a laryngectomy, a surgical procedure in which a plastic tube is placed into the pharynx to serve as a voice source.

body image   Awareness of one's own body and bodily behaviors; a composite vision of oneself.

bone-conduction testing   An assessment of sound transmission to the inner ear by use of a vibrating oscillator in contact with the mastoid process of the temporal bone, thus bypassing the air-conduction mechanism.

Boyle's law   A principle of physics describing the inverse relationship of the volume of a fixed amount of gas to its pressure. In respiration, expanding the thoracic cavity decreases the air pressure and draws air into the lungs; relaxing the thorax increases internal air pressure, expelling air.

brainstem   The upper part of the spinal cord located where the neck meets the skull.

breathy   The voice quality created by excessive leakage of air when the vocal cords vibrate.

Broca's aphasia   The loss of speech and language expression due to an acquired lesion of the dominant cerebral hemisphere.

Broca's area   The part of the brain largely responsible for expressive communication; located in the frontal lobe in the dominant cerebral hemisphere and named after the French neurologist Paul Broca. Cortical area associated with expressive language and motor speech production.

bulbar palsy   Weakness and impaired movement of the larynx, pharynx, tongue, and/or lips, secondary to disease or injury of the brainstem motor nuclei.

carry-over   In stuttering, the habitual use of the tools of fluent speech in everyday situations.

CAT   *See* computerized axial tomography.

catastrophic reaction   In aphasia, a psychobiological breakdown resulting from excessive stimulation, frustration, and anxiety. A sudden overwhelming feeling of anxiety and the reaction to it, including irritability, withdrawal, fainting, or other nonadaptive behavior; an anxiety attack.

central hearing loss   The loss of hearing resulting from damage to the central nervous system.

central nervous system (CNS)   The brain and spinal cord.

central sulcus   The fissure that divides the frontal and parietal lobes, also called the fissure of Rolando.

cerebellum   The part of the brain responsible for muscle tone, balance, and coordination.

cerebral cortex   The thin layer of gray matter surrounding the cerebral hemispheres.

cerebral dominance   The tendency for one cerebral hemisphere to be dominant over the other for a particular function.

cerebral hemispheres   The two sides of the cerebrum.

cerebral vascular accident (CVA)   A sudden interruption of blood flow to the brain; a stroke.

cerumen   The waxlike secretion in the auditory canal.

CHI   *See* closed-head injury.

circumlocution   Using a substitute word for the one that cannot be remembered or spoken. The substitution of a word to avoid a feared one; rearranging or rephrasing the original thought.

clavicular breathing   A type of shallow breathing accomplished primarily with the upper thoracic muscles.

cleft lip   A congenital craniofacial malformation of the upper lip involving failure of fusion during gestation; may be unilateral or bilateral.

cleft palate   A congenital craniofacial malformation involving a failure of maxillary fusion during gestation, resulting in a complete or incomplete fissure in the hard palate, velum, and/or uvula; may be unilateral or bilateral.

clinical phonetics   The use of phonetics in the diagnosis and treatment of communication disorders.

clonic blocks   In stuttering, repetitive blocks at the same valving site.

closed-head injury (CHI)   Cerebral trauma of the nonpenetrating variety in which one or more cognitive functions are impaired or destroyed.

cluttering   A thought-organization fluency disorder characterized by short attention span, an excessive rate of speech, omissions and substitutions of sounds and words, and a lack of awareness of the problem.

CNS   *See* central nervous system.

coarticulation   Overlapping articulatory influences during connected speech.

cochlea   The sensory mechanism of hearing in the inner ear; the end organ of hearing.

cochlear implant   An electronic device surgically implanted into the ear to enhance cochlear function.

cochlear nerve   The auditory branch of cranial nerve VIII.

cognates   In phonetics, consonants produced in the same manner and place and differing only by voicing.

cognition   Higher mental functions that include reasoning and information processing; mental processes of thinking, judgment, and abstraction.

cognitive prerequisite   The thought processes that underlie language.

communication disorder   The abnormality, impairment, or inability to exchange information between speaker and listener.

communicative stress   Anxiety and fear associated with speaking to authority figures, large groups, or under conditions of temporal urgency.

complete cleft   Cleft extending from the lip through the velum; may be unilateral or bilateral.

compliance   In audiology, the ease of energy transfer through the outer or middle ear.

compression   In acoustics, the stage in which particles are compressed from their resting position in a sound wave.

compulsivity   Unwanted, recurring urges to perform an act.

computerized axial tomography (CAT)   Scanning of a body structure and gathering anatomical information obtained from computed tomography.

confabulation   Giving answers to questions with little or no regard for their truthfulness or accuracy; making up false stories.

confirmed stuttering   The diagnosis of stuttering made by a certified speech–language pathologist; also called true stuttering.

congenital deafness   The loss of hearing occurring before or during birth.

connotation   The affective or evaluative meaning of a word derived by the speaker or listener.

consonant   The speech sound produced with or without voicing by movements of the articulatory structures that modify the airstream. They are characterized by vocal tract constriction and by articulatory gestures toward or away from the syllabic nucleus.

consummation of communication   The satisfactory completion of a speech act.

contact ulcer   In voice, ulceration of the vocal folds; abrasions or holes on the vocal cords.

content word   Words that carry the most meaning in an utterance, such as nouns and verbs.

continuant   Speech sounds (such as /s/ and /v/) produced by continuous, uninterrupted airstream modulation during articulation.

conversion aphonia   The loss of voice resulting from psychic trauma; psychogenic aphonia.

conversion deafness   Deafness resulting from psychic trauma; psychogenic deafness.

conversion reaction   The somatization of an emotional conflict and resulting disorder.

coping style   The habitual method of adjusting to anxiety, stress, and unwanted changes.

coprolalia   The unprovoked use of obscene or profane language; excessive swearing.

core behavior   In stuttering, repetitions, prolongations, and blockages of speech.

cortex   The layer of gray matter covering the surface of the cerebral hemispheres; the thin outer layer of the brain is also known as the gray matter.

covert reaction   In stuttering, the feeling, reaction, and attitude occurring during a moment of stuttering.

cranial nerves   Twelve pairs of neuron bundles emerging from the cerebral hemispheres, thalamus, and brainstem.

croup   An inflammatory laryngeal condition with hoarseness, barking cough, audible inhalation, and inhalatory stridor.

CVA   *See* cerebral vascular accident.

DAF   *See* delayed auditory feedback.

damping   The decrease of acoustic energy over time and distance or because of impedance or opposing energy.

deaf   Without the sense of hearing; hearing that is nonfunctional.

deaf mute   The slang term for one who can neither speak nor hear.

decibel   One-tenth of a bel; a logarithmic unit for measuring loudness.

decode   The process of breaking down and analyzing a signal, such as speech and language, into its meaningful component parts.

degenerative disease   A condition that results in deterioration of the ability to function normally over time.

déjà vu   The belief or illusion that an event has occurred before.

delayed auditory feedback (DAF)   The time delay in perceiving one's own speech; associated with increased dysfluency in normal speakers.

dementia   A generalized cognitive deterioration including disorientation, impaired judgment, and memory defects; generalized intellectual deficits.

denasality   A voice quality characterized by lack of nasal resonance on normally nasal phonemes; reduced nasality.

denial   The refusal and unwillingness to perceive and recognize threatening, unpleasant, and intolerable realities.

denotation   The objective referent for a word. The unemotional, nonaffective, and nonevaluative meaning of a word.

dental phoneme   A speech sound made by approximating the lip or tongue with the upper incisors.

desensitization   In stuttering therapy, the gradual and systematic presentation of anxiety-evoking stimuli when the client is otherwise relaxed and comfortable.

developmental stuttering   During the developmental period, speech containing more frequent and severe dysfluencies than what would be considered normal; also called incipient stuttering.

deviated uvula   Leaning or deflection of the cone-shaped muscle hanging from the velum.

diagnosogenic theory of stuttering   The theory that stuttering occurs because of misdiagnosis of normal dysfluncies in a child's speech; labeling a child a stutterer causes him to stutter [Wendell Johnson].

dialect   A phonological, semantic, and/or syntactic variation of spoken language associated with geographical and social factors.

dichotic listening   The presentation of different signals to both ears at the same time.

diphthong   A phoneme produced by moving the structures of articulation from one vowel articulatory gesture to another.

diplophonia   The simultaneous vibration of the vocal cords and the ventricular folds producing two distinct tones.

direct laryngoscopy   A diagnostic procedure in which a laryngoscope is guided downward to view the vocal folds.

discomfort level   In audiology, a loudness level perceived to be uncomfortable.

disguise reaction   Attempting to minimize the stuttering moment by hiding or concealing the stuttering behaviors.

disorientation   Inaccurate perceptions and judgments about time, place, person, and/or situation (predicament).

distinctive features   A set of phonetic attributes that distinguish one phoneme from another.

distortion   In speech articulation, the indistinct production of a sound.

Doppler effect   In acoustics, a change in pitch caused by movement toward or away from the source of a sound.

dys-   A prefix indicating impaired, faulty, deficient, and/or diseased.

dysarthrias   A group of neuromuscular speech disorders; impaired speech due to neurological and muscular deficits.

dyscalculia   In aphasia, the impaired ability to comprehend and perform simple arithmetic.

dysfluency   A breakdown in the rhythm and flow of speech caused by repetitions, prolongations, blocks, and/or pauses.

dysgraphia   In aphasia, problems with writing *not* due to hand or arm paralysis.

dyskinesia   Abnormal voluntary movements.

dyslexia   Problems with reading *not* due to visual acuity deficits.

dysnomia   In aphasia, word-finding problems; *not* limited to nouns.

dysphagia   Problems with the ability to chew, suck, and/or swallow.

dysphonia   Any impairment or defect in voice production.

dyspraxia   The impaired ability to plan and sequence voluntary movements due to a neurological disease or disorder.

dysprosody   An impairment in the melody, cadence, and rhythm of speech.

dystonia   An abnormal, involuntary rhythmic twisting of body structure.

ear   External, middle, and inner aspects of the organ and structures of hearing.

echolalia   Automatically repeating or parroting something heard.

-ectomy   A suffix indicating surgical removal.

edema   Swelling due to too much fluid in cells, tissues, or cavities.

ego   One of the three aspects of the personality that is involved in evaluating, directing, and controlling thoughts and actions in response to reality.

ego restriction   Narrowing of self-involvement.

ego weakness   The reduced strength of the aspect of the personality involved in evaluating, directing, and controlling thoughts and actions in response to reality.

egocentric Self-centered.

electrolarynx An electrical device used to produce voice in a patient with a laryngectomy; an artificial larynx.

embolism A mass obstructing a blood vessel that develops in one part of the vascular system and ends up in another. *Emboli* means more than one plug, as in a "shower of emboli."

empathy Feeling the emotions of another person; recognition and understanding of the emotional state of another person.

encephalitis An inflammation of the brain.

encode The process of putting an idea or thought into a signal system, such as speech and language.

engram A physical representation of a memory.

enunciate To articulate speech sounds precisely.

equal-loudness contour The sound pressure necessary to produce equal loudness across frequencies.

ERA *See* evoked response audiometry.

escape behavior An attempt by the stutterer to remove himself or herself from a stuttering moment.

esophageal speech A type of alaryngeal speech in which compressing air in the esophagus and releasing it through a construction produces a pseudovoice; also called belch talking.

esophagus The tube leading from the throat to the stomach.

etiology The cause of something.

euphoria A heightened sense of well-being.

eustachian tube The air passageway from the nasopharynx to the middle ear, allowing equalizing of pressure.

evoked response audiometry (ERA) A special type of electroencephalic audiometry measuring electrical responses of the cerebral cortex.

executive function The cognitive skills involved in planning, organization, self-monitoring, and strategy formulation for complex behaviors; metacognition.

experimental phonetics A branch of phonetics utilizing laboratory instruments and the scientific method.

experimental stuttering Stuttering produced under laboratory conditions.

expiration During breathing, the process of expelling air from the lungs.

expressive aphasia A type of neurologically based language disturbance involving the expressive components of language: speaking, writing, and gesturing.

expressive language Use of socially shared encoded symbols to communicate spoken, gestured, or written concepts, ideas, and emotions; expression of the speaker's psychological state.

external auditory meatus The passageway extending from the auricle (pinna) to the tympanic membrane.

external ear The most distal parts of the ear, including the pinna and the external auditory meatus.

extrapyramidal system Cell nuclei and nerve fibers involved in automatic, unconscious aspects of motor coordination, posture, and movement; other than those of the pyramidal system.

extrinsic laryngeal muscles   Those laryngeal muscles with their origin outside the larynx.

extrinsic tongue muscles   Those tongue muscles with their origin outside the tongue.

facilitation   Enabling desired behaviors, reactions, and adjustments.

false negative   A test result indicating the absence of a pathology when in fact a pathology exists.

false positive   A test result indicating a pathology when in fact a pathology does not exist.

falsetto   The highest voice register; produced by vibration of the medial parts of the vocal folds.

fear   The expectation of unpleasantness.

fiberscope   A flexible fiberoptic tube with the tip providing its own light source and magnifying capacity.

filler   An interruption of the flow of speech by sounds such as "uh," "um," and "er."

filter   In acoustics, a device that amplifies certain frequencies and attenuates others.

flaccid   A weak or limp muscle that is relaxed and without tone.

flaccid dysarthria   A neuromuscular speech disorder associated with lower motor neuron damage.

flat affect   Narrowed mood, emotions, and temperament; reduced subjective experience of emotion.

fluent speech   Smooth and effortlessly produced speech without hesitations, interjections, or repetitions; the act of speaking easily and effortlessly.

foreign accent   Speech characteristics of nonnative speakers of a language.

formant   On a spectrogram, a frequency band in which there is a relatively high degree of acoustic energy or resonance for vowels and voiced consonants.

frequency   In acoustics, the number of compressions and rarefactions of a sound wave during a period, usually one second. In voice, the number of vocal fold vibrations occurring in a period, usually one second.

fricative   A speech sound made by forcing air through a constricted area, resulting in turbulence and a continuous, aperiodic sound.

function word   A word with an obvious grammatical function, such as a preposition, an article, a pronoun, and a conjunction.

functional communication   The ability to express and understand basic wants, needs, ideas, and emotions.

fundamental frequency   In voice, the average frequency of vibration of the vocal folds. In acoustics, the lowest frequency of a complex periodic sound wave.

gag reflex   The automatic tendencies to gag, choke, retch, or heave when stimulated.

gain   In audiology, the output minus the input of a hearing aid.

general phonetics   The study of speech sounds.

gentle onset   In stuttering, a light, easy onset of speech.

gesture   A formal or an informal movement of the body to describe or reinforce verbal communication.

glide   In speech articulation, a sound requiring movement of the articulators from one position to another.

glossal   Pertaining to the tongue.

glossectomy   Surgical removal of all or part of the tongue.

glottal   Pertaining to the glottis.

glottal fry   A gravelly sound produced by the vocal cords, usually low pitched; pulsating or creaking voice quality.

glottal opening   The space between the vocal cords.

glottal stop   A sound made by stopping and releasing the airstream at the level of the vocal folds.

grammar   The rules of the form and usage of a language.

grammatical morphemes   Units of meaning; suffixes and function words.

grapheme   Printed or written symbols.

gray matter   The collection of neuronal cell bodies in the central nervous system; gray-colored tissue of the brain and spinal cord, primarily made up of cell bodies.

grief response   Predictable stages in the process of accepting unwanted change.

gustatory   Related to the sense of taste.

gustatory agnosia   A disorder relating to the perception of taste.

guttural   Produced in the throat; pertaining to the throat or voice.

gyrus   A convolution, ridge, or elevation of the cerebral cortex.

habilitation   A therapeutic intervention to develop a deficient function, such as communication.

habitual pitch   A pitch used most often during spontaneous speech; also called modal pitch.

hard contacts   Speech produced with excessive pressure or force.

hard glottal attack   Forceful initiation of phonation.

hard-of-hearing   Reduced hearing sensitivity.

hard palate   The bony roof of the mouth.

harmonic   In acoustics, whole-number multiples of the fundamental frequency of a complex sound wave.

harshness   A voice quality caused by excessive force and hypertension of the vocal cords.

hearing aid   A device that amplifies sound and directs it to the ear.

hematoma   A blood clot.

hemiparesis   Weakness of the muscles on one side of the body.

hemiplegia   Paralysis of the muscles on one side of the body.

hemorrhage   The rupture and escape of blood from a vein or artery.

Hertz (Hz)   Cycles per second.

hesitations   Unusually long pauses during speech.

hippocampus   A structure in the brain that plays a role in learning and memory.

hoarseness   Raspy voice quality; a combination of harsh and breathy voice qualities.

homonymous hemianopsia   A disorder in which the visual field is limited to one-half of the total visual world; blindness or visual impairment in the same one-half fields of both eyes.

hydrocephalus   An excessive accumulation of cerebrospinal fluid within the cranial cavity; also known as "water on the brain."

hyper-   Prefix meaning "too much."

hyperacusis   Abnormally sensitive hearing; sounds perceived as excessively loud.

hyperkinetic dysarthria   Speech pathology associated with damage to the extrapryamidal system and characterized by unwanted speech movements occurring slowly or rapidly.

hypernasality   Excessive perceived nasality; too much nasal resonance.

hypo-   Prefix meaning "too little."

hypokinesia   Slow or diminished movements.

hypokinetic dysarthria   Speech pathology associated with damage to the extrapyramidal system involving slow rate of speech, monopitch, voice tremor, monoloudness, and indistinct phoneme production.

hyponasality   Too little perceived nasality on the nasal consonants; densality.

hysterical aphonia   The loss of voice because of psychogenic factors.

hysterical deafness   Deafness occurring because of psychogenic factors.

hysterical dysphonia   Impaired voice because of psychogenic factors.

hysterical stuttering   Late onset stuttering that usually results from extreme anxiety and other psychogenic factors.

ideation   The creation of ideas into formal concepts.

ideational apraxia   The disruption of the ability to conceptualize and program a motor impulse.

idioglossia   A private, distinctive language invented by an individual or individuals, especially twins.

idiolect   An individual speaker's variation in phonology, semantic, or syntactic aspects of language.

idiopathic disorder   A disease arising from no apparent organic cause.

image   A mental representation of some aspect of reality.

immittance   In audiology, measurements made of tympanic membrane compliance or impedance.

impedance   Resistance to a flow of energy.

impedance bridge   An instrument to measure tympanic resistance to acoustic energy.

incidence   The frequency of occurrence.

in-class substitution   In articulation, the substitution of a speech sound within the same category, e.g., fricative for fricative, glide for glide.

incus   One of three bones comprising the ossicular chain; the anvil.

indirect laryngoscopy   The technique of viewing the interior of the larynx indirectly with a mirror and a light source.

infarct   The sudden death of tissue because of a lack of blood supply.

inflammation   A swelling of part of the body due to injury.

infraglottic   Those parts of the larynx below the vocal folds.

inhalatory stridor   A glottic sound produced during inhalation.

inner ear   That part of the ear where mechanical energy is transformed into hydraulic and electrochemical energy.

inspiration   During breathing, the process of taking air into the lungs.

insufficient palatal vault   An inadequate arch of the hard palate for housing the resting tongue.

intelligence   The abilities to reason, abstract, problem solve, acquire, and retain knowledge.

intelligibility   The ability to be understood by a listener, usually measured in percent; the degree a person can be understood by others.

intensity   In acoustics, the force by which a sound is produced. In audiology, the power of a sound wave, usually measured in decibels.

interdental   A consonant produced with the tongue approximating the upper teeth.

internal monologue   Talking with oneself; self-talk or inner speech.

interrupter device   In stuttering, a sudden surge of tension, jerk, or other muscular movement used by the stutterer to terminate the stuttering moment.

intrinsic laryngeal muscles   Muscles having both their origin and insertion within the larynx.

intrinsic tongue muscles   Muscles having both their origin and insertion within the tongue.

intrusive sound   An extraneous sound produced between other speech sounds.

intubation   Insertion of a tube into the body.

ipsilateral   Pertaining to the same side; on the same side of the midline.

ischemic   An inadequate flow of blood to a part of the body.

jargon   Fluent but unintelligible speech; fluent speech that makes no sense.

jargon aphasia   A type of aphasia in which the patient utters fluent speech but it makes little or no sense.

jitter   In voice, rhythmic variations in the frequency of a sound.

JND   *See* just noticeable difference.

just noticeable difference (JND)   The minimal difference in characteristics between two stimuli detectable by an observer.

kinesthesia   The perception of one's body movement. In speech, the perception of movement and direction of the speech musculature.

Korsakoff's syndrome   Confusion, disorientation, apathy, and confabulation resulting from chronic alcoholism.

labial   Having to do with the lips. In phonetics, a sound produced by one or both lips.

labialization   Using the lips in the production of a sound.

labiodental   A consonant produced by approximating the lower lip with the upper incisors.

language   The multimodality ability to encode, decode, and manipulate symbols for the purposes of verbal thought and/or communication. Rule-governed, socially shared code for representing concepts with symbols.

laryngeal   Pertaining to the larynx.

laryngeal block   During stuttering, the involuntary closure of the vocal cords.

laryngeal prominence   Anterior projection of the thyroid cartilage, especially noticeable in some adult males; the "Adam's apple."

laryngectomy   The surgical removal of the larynx.

laryngology   A medical specialty addressing the diseases and disorders of the larynx.

laryngopharynx   The division of the pharynx lying below the oropharynx.

laryngoscopy   Observation of the interior of the larynx by any optic device equipped with a light source.

larynx   The organ of voice between the pharynx and trachea.

lateral   In phonetics, a consonant produced by air pressure around one or both sides of the tongue.

lax   In phonetics, sounds produced with reduced muscular tension; the opposite of tense.

light contact   In stuttering therapy, easy, relaxed approximations of the articulators.

limb apraxia   The inability to purposefully perform a movement with an extremity; body apraxia.

limbic system   A group of interconnected structures involving emotion, memory, and learning.

lingua-dental   Using the teeth and tongue in the production of a speech sound.

lingua-alveolar   Relating to the tongue and the alveolar ridge.

lingua-palatal   Relating to the tongue and the hard palate.

lingua-velar   Relating to the tongue and the velum.

lingual   Having to do with the tongue. In phonetics, speech sounds made with the tongue.

lingual frenulum   The cord of tissue running from floor of the mouth to the middle of the undersurface of the tongue.

linguistic competence   Knowledge of the rules of language, its grammar, semantics, phonology, and syntax.

linguistic form and structure   The combination of sounds into words and grammatical inflections, and the creation, organization, and understanding of sentences.

linguistic performance   The actual usage of language. How a person uses linguistic competence.

linguistic phonetics   A branch of applied phonetics that analyzes the sound system of a language; phonology.

linguistic relativity   The notion that language affects and facilitates thought.

linguistic stress   The emphasis on certain syllables and words.

linguistics   The study of language.

lip rounding   In phonetics, production of a sound with the lips in a rounded position.

liquid   A generic term for /l/ and /r/ sounds.

listening   Reception, perception and association of acoustic events.

localization   In neurology, the idea that all brain functions can be discovered and mapped. The identification of areas of the brain responsible for specific aspects of physical, mental or emotional functioning.

loci of overt stuttering   The particular sounds or words on which stuttering behaviors occur.

loft register   Falsetto.

logorrhea   Continuous fluent incoherent production of words; pathological, uncontrolled talkativeness.

Lombard effect   The tendency to raise the level of speech loudness to compensate for background noise.

loudness   The psychological perception of amplitude or intensity of an acoustic signal.

lung capacity   The potential amount of air contained in the lungs; also called respiratory capacity or forced inspiratory volume.

lung volume   The space occupied by the air in the lungs at a given time; respiratory volume.

macroglossia   An abnormally large tongue relative to the oral cavity.

magnetic resonance imaging (MRI)   A scan of any part of the body in which the patient is exposed to a magnetic field and a computer creates images of the structure.

malignant   A tumor resistant to treatment; cancerous.

malleus   One of three bones comprising the ossicular chain; the hammer.

malocclusion   Deviation from normal occlusion.

mandible   The lower jaw.

manner of articulation   The characteristics of speech-sound production by changes in airstream modulation and amount of vocal tract constriction.

manual communication   The use of the fingers and hands to communicate; sign language.

masking   Noise that interferes with the detection of another acoustic signal.

mastoid process   A bony protuberance of the temporal bone behind and below the external ear.

maxilla   The upper jaw.

Meniere's disease   Inner ear syndrome that includes hearing loss, tinnitus, and vertigo.

meninges   The three membranes surrounding the surface of the central nervous system; the dura mater, arachnoid mater, and pia mater.

metacognition   Knowledge about all cognitive processes, their products, and anything related to them; thinking about thinking.

metastasize   The spread of a disease from one location to another.

microbar   Unit of pressure; one-millionth of a bar.

microcephaly   An abnormally small head.

microglossia   An abnormally small tongue relative to the oral cavity.

middle ear   The tympanic cavity where acoustic energy is transformed into mechanical energy.

midline   The center point or line.

minimal contrasts   A bisyllable containing two vowels and slightly different acoustic features.

minimal pair   Two words differing only by a single phoneme.

modality   Any avenue or mode of communication.

modulation   In voice, alteration of the voice quality and loudness during connected speech.

monaural   Pertaining to one ear.

monosyllable   Having one syllable.

morpheme   The smallest unit of meaning in language; the minimal unit of speech that is meaningful.

morphemics   A branch of linguistics that studies the morphemes of a language.

motor cortex   The areas of the brain directly involved in control of voluntary movement.

motor neuron   A nerve that passes from the central nervous system to a muscle and causes movement.

motor speech disorders   Pertaining to disorders of motor tracts and muscles; apraxia of speech and the dysarthrias.

motor strip   A term used to represent motor control areas in the precentral gyrus.

motor unit   A muscle fiber and the lower motor neuron that causes it to contract; a muscle and the nerve closest to it.

MRI   *See* magnetic resonance imaging.

multiple dysarthria   Two or more dysarthrias occurring concurrently or the changing of dysarthria type over time; mixed dysarthria.

mutational falsetto   In males, the failure to change from the higher-pitch voice of a child to the lower-pitch voice of the adult male.

mute   The inability to phonate and articulate.

mutism   Completely without speech; inability to phonate and articulate.

myopathic   An abnormal disease or condition of a muscle.

myringotomy   A surgical procedure to open the tympanic membrane and allow reduction of pressure in the middle ear.

nasal   Pertaining to the nose; rhinal.

nasal coupling   A lowering of the velum to allow airflow through the nasal passageway.

nasal emission   Air escape from the nose during speech, usually resulting from velopharyngeal incompetence or insufficiency; air flowing out of nose.

nasal resonance   A coupling of the nasal to the oral cavities and the subsequent modification of the glottal tone.

nasality   The production of phonemes with the acoustic properties of nasal resonance.

neologism   A made-up or invented word; a conventional word used in an unconventional manner.

nerve deafness   Deafness resulting from disease of the cochlea or auditory nerve.

neuron   In the nervous system, cells that transmit electrochemical impulses.

neuroscience   The interdisciplinary science that studies the brain, emotions, and behaviors.

neurotransmitter   A chemical involved in synapses.

nodule   A small node; benign tumor.

noise   Any signal that competes with the perception of a stimulus; unwanted sound.

nonfluency   The disruption of fluent speech; speech produced with complications.

nonverbal communication   Communication without using spoken words.

normal dysfluency   Naturally occurring repetitions, prolongations, and hesitations during speech.

nystagmus   Abnormal oscillations of the eyes.

obsessive–compulsive disorder (OCD)   The persistent adherence to thoughts and beliefs and the need to perform certain rituals to excess.

OCD   *See* obsessive–compulsive disorder.

olfactory   Related to the sense of smell.

olfactory agnosia   A disorder relating to the perception of odors.

omission   In articulation, the lack of a sound in a word where one would be expected.

open-head injury   Head trauma caused by a missile or projectile penetrating the skull.

open syllable   A syllable ending with a vowel.

optic chiasm   An area in the brain where the right and left optic nerves converge.

optimal pitch   The pitch that is most efficient for a given person to use; the pitch level best suited to an individual that produces the voice with the least effort.

oral apraxia   The loss of the ability to conceptualize, plan, and sequence voluntary oral nonspeech movements due to a neurological disorder.

organ of Corti   Part of the cochlea containing sensory receptors.

organic   In medicine, the physical basis for a disorder.

organic depression   Feelings of despair, sadness, isolation, hopelessness, and helplessness caused by brain chemical imbalance or deficiency.

orientation   Awareness of time, place, person, and situation (predicament).

oscillation   Rhythmic repetitive movements.

oscillator   A device for producing vibrations.

OSHA   Occupational Safety and Health Administration, a federal government agency.

ossicles   Bones of the middle ear.

otitis   An inflammation of the ear.

otoacoustic emission testing   Measuring sounds generated within the cochlea.

otolaryngology   A medical specialty concerned with diagnosis and treatment of diseases and disorders of the ear and larynx.

otology   A branch of medicine concerned with the diagnosis and treatment of diseases and disorders of the ear.

otorhinolaryngology   A medical specialty concerned with diagnosis and treatment of diseases and disorders of the ear, nose, and throat.

otosclerosis   Hardening of the middle ear, impeding the movement of the ossicular chain.

otoscope   A device for visual examination of the external ear canal and tympanic membrane.

overlearning   In speech–language pathology, the practice of a speech motor skill beyond what is necessary for production, retention, or recall.

overt features   Fully developed obvious features of stuttering; those readily apparent.

palatal lift   A prosthetic device that elevates and extends the soft palate to help achieve closure.

palpate   To stimulate or evaluate a body structure by touch and pressure.

palsy   The paresis or paralysis of a muscle.

paralysis   A condition in which a muscle loses its ability to contract or move due to muscular deficits or neurological lesions.

paraphasia   An aphasic-naming disorder characterized by choosing the incorrect word that either rhymes or has a semantic relationship to the correct one; literal and verbal paraphasias.

paresis   Partial paralysis.

Pavlovian conditioning   A form of learning, especially emotional learning, in which a previously learned neutral stimulus becomes a conditioned stimulus when presented repeatedly with an unconditioned stimulus. In stuttering, the way negative emotions are associated with dysfluent speech.

perception   An awareness and appreciation of the salient aspects of a stimulus. Selection, organization, and interpretation of sensory stimulation.

perceptual-motor   The interaction between perception and motor activities.

peripheral   Away from the center.

peripheral nervous system (PNS)   The part of the nervous system made up of the cranial and spinal nerves and the autonomic nervous system. Parts of the nervous system other than the brain and spinal cord.

perseveration   The automatic continuation of a speaking or writing response seen in some patients with neurogenic communication disorders. Sensorimotor responses that persist for a longer duration than what the intensity and significance of the stimuli would warrant.

pharyngeal flap   A surgical procedure used to help velopharyngeal closure.

phonation   Any voiced sound that occurs at the level of the vocal cords; also called voicing.

phonatory apraxia   The loss of the ability to conceptualize, plan, and sequence voluntary laryngeal movements due to a neurological disorder or disease.

phoneme   A speech sound.

phonemic analysis   The act of analyzing speech sounds in a given language.

phonemics   The study of a language's sound system.

phonetic analysis   The study and analysis of speech sounds relative to their acoustic and perceptual features.

phonetic practice   Improvement of motor control and intelligibility by using a sound repeatedly.

phonetic variation   Phoneme differences.

phonetically balanced words   Lists of monosyllabic words that approximate the incidence of phonemes in the English language. Phonetically balanced words are used in speech discrimination testing.

phonetics   The science concerned with the perception, classification, description, acoustics, and production of speech sounds of a language.

phonics   A method of teaching reading by addressing the phonetic pronunciation of letters.

phonological approach   Therapy for speech disorders that considers speech sound development as the discovery and fusion of syllable formation principles.

phonology   The study of the sounds of a language and the way they are combined into words; the study of the sound system of a language.

phonotactics   Rules for sequencing speech sounds in words.

physiological phonetics   The study of the anatomy and physiology involved in speech.

pitch   The psychological perception of frequency of vibration.

pitch range   In voice, the distance between the lowest and highest glottal frequency; usually expressed in Hertz (Hz) or musical notes.

place of articulation   The location of greatest vocal tract constriction caused by the approximation of the speech articulators.

plosive   A consonant produced with complete cessation of the airflow and often occurring with an audible burst of air on release.

PNS   *See* peripheral nervous system.

polyp   In voice, a fluid-filled blister on the vocal cord; a mass of tissue projecting outwardly.

polysyllable   Having multiple syllables.

posterior   Toward the back or behind.

postlinguistic deafness   Deafness occurring after the development of speech and language.

pragmatic stuttering therapy Stuttering therapy in which the context, purpose, and environment are emphasized during fluency training.

pragmatics Rules governing how language is used. Linguistic acts involving the purpose, environment, and context in which they are performed.

prelinguistic deafness Deafness occurring before the complete development of speech and language.

presbycusis Age-related hearing loss.

prevalence The extent that a disorder occurs in a population or a group.

prognosis An educated guess or prediction about how well a patient will recover.

progressive relaxation Systematic reduction in tonus of muscle groups to attain specific and general levels of muscular relaxation.

projection Attributing one's own intolerable wishes, thoughts, motivations, and feelings to another person.

prolongation In stuttering, the abnormal increased duration of the production of a sound.

propositionality The meaningfulness and amount of content in an utterance.

proprioception Sensory data providing conscious and unconscious awareness of bodily positions in space.

prosody Acoustic patterns of speech such as stress, intonation, rhythm, melody, pitch, and voice quality; includes fluency, cadence, inflection, and emphasis aspects of speech.

prosthesis A fabricated artificial substitute for a missing part of the body.

pseudobulbar palsy Neuromuscular deficit resulting from upper motor neuron damage or a disease process.

pseudoglottis An artificially created pair of vocal cords; neoglottis.

pseudostuttering In stuttering therapy, deliberately faking stuttering to reduce the fear and anxiety associated with it.

psychoacoustics The study of psychological responses to sound.

psychogenic Of emotional or affective origin.

psychology The study of human consciousness; methods of measuring, explaining, and changing behavior in humans and other animals.

puberphonia The voice of an adolescent.

pure tone A sound wave having only one frequency.

quadriplegia Paralysis or weakness of all four extremities.

quality In voice, the perceptual correlate of complexity. In acoustics, the psychological impression of the spectral characteristics of a sound.

quality of life The combination of factors that contribute to satisfaction with life.

rarefaction In acoustics, the separation of air particles in a sound wave from their neutral or resting positions.

rate of speech The speed of speaking, usually measured in words per minute.

receptive aphasia A type of neurologically based language disturbance in which the person has problems reading and understanding the speech and gestures of others.

receptive language   The decoding of phonemes, words, gestures, and graphemes into recognizable language patterns.

recruitment   A disproportionate increase in the loudness of a particular sound.

referent   The aspect of reality referred to by the symbol.

reflex   An involuntary reaction in response to a stimulus.

register   The pitch range and resonance properties of the voice.

rehabilitation   The therapeutic restoration of a deficient function, such as communication, to normal or near-normal levels.

reinforcement   The positive or negative consequences of a behavior.

repetition   In stuttering, the abnormal and unwanted repetition of sounds, syllables, words, and/or phrases.

residual hearing   The amount of hearing remaining in an individual with a hearing loss.

resistance block   A device used in dysarthria therapy to provide tongue, palatal, or jaw resistance.

resonance   In speech, the sympathetic vibration of vocal tract tissue and air columns in response to a vibrating source.

resonance frequency   A system's natural frequency.

respiration   The act of breathing: inspiration and expiration; the driving force for speech.

respiratory capacity   Potential contents of the lungs and airways leading to and from them.

respiratory tracts   An air passageway to and from the lungs.

respiratory volume   The space occupied by the air in the lungs and the passages leading to and from them.

retrocochlear   Neural structures of the auditory system beyond the cochlea.

retrocochlear deafness   Deafness resulting from a lesion beyond the cochlea.

retrograde amnesia   Amnesia for events before an illness or traumatic brain injury.

rhythm of speech   Melody of speech.

rigidity   The quality of not bending; inflexibility. Muscular resistance to passive motion.

rolfing   Deep massaging of stiffened muscle groups.

saliva   A secretion from the salivary and mucous glands of the mouth.

scanning speech   Slow or measured verbal output.

schedules of reinforcement   The duration and frequency in which reinforcements are administered.

schwa sound   The sound "uh," as in "understand."

screening test   A gross measurement of a function to determine the need for additional testing.

secondary gain   The resistance to eliminate a disorder because of neurotic gains associated with being disabled.

secondary stuttering   Stuttering associated with awareness of the disorder and subsequent escape and avoidance behaviors.

seizure   A spontaneous excessive discharge of cortical neurons.

self-concept   An awareness of oneself, particularly in relation to others; images and definitions of self.

self-esteem   The positive belief and feelings about one's self-concept.

semantics   The meaning of words; the relationship between a symbol and what it represents.

senility   The cognitive and intellectual deterioration associated with pathological aging.

sensitivity   The ability to sense and respond to a stimulus.

sensorimotor   A combination of motor activity and sensations or feedback accompanying them.

sensorimotor approach   Therapy for speech disorders that considers speech sound development to be the result of several maturation factors especially auditory perception and fine motor skills.

sensorineural hearing loss   Impaired hearing resulting from cochlear or retrocochlear lesions.

shimmer   In voice, the cycle-to-cycle variations in amplitude of a glottal sound.

short-term memory   The temporary storage of information limited in capacity and requiring continual rehearsal.

sibilant   A high-pitched speech sound produced by pushing air through a constricted area, such as /s/ and /z/. A consonant produced with acoustic energy in the mid- to high-frequency ranges.

signal   In perception, the important part of sensory information; that which is attended to as opposed to noise.

simple harmonic motion   Periodic oscillations of a body, resulting in a sine wave.

simple tone   Pure tone.

simple wave   A sinusoidal wave.

social-communicative development   The development of the functional processes that underlie language. Learning the way language communicates needs, desires, feelings, and ideas.

soft palate   The soft part at the back of the roof of the mouth; the velum.

sonant   A phoneme produced with accompanying vocal fold vibration; a voiced phoneme.

sound discrimination   The auditory ability to perceive the difference between two sounds, especially similar ones.

sound field   The area into which sound is introduced through a loudspeaker.

sound-level meter   A device for measuring the loudness of sound.

sound pressure level   The decibel level relative to 0.0002 dyne/cm^2.

sound spectrogram   Graphic representation of sound by time, frequency, and energy; readout of a sound spectrograph.

spasm   An involuntary contraction of a muscle or a muscle group.

spastic   A form of paralysis in which a muscle is contracted all the time, due to a neurological injury or disease; hypertonicity.

spastic dysarthria   A neuromuscular speech disorder associated with bilateral upper motor lesions.

speaking rate   The number of works spoken per minute.

spectrography   In acoustics, an electronic instrument or computer program that analyzes the speech signal by passing it through a series of filters and graphically representing its frequency, duration, and intensity.

spectrum   A graphic representation of sound, showing the frequencies and amplitudes of the individual components of a wave.

speech act   The verbal expression of an intent; an act of propositional verbal communication.

speech audiometry   A hearing test measurement of speech awareness.

speech frequencies   Frequencies at which the majority of speech energy occurs.

speech–language pathologist   Professional involved in the diagnosis and treatment of communication disorders.

speech reading   Using visual cues to comprehend speech; lip reading.

spirometer   A device used to record and measure air capacity of the lungs. Measurement of pulmonary volumes and capacities.

split-brain study   A study of brain functioning following disconnection of all or part of the corpus callosum.

spontaneous recovery   In aphasia, the period of time post-onset in which the brain naturally resolves part or all language disturbances.

stammering   A term used to describe stuttering in many countries outside the United States.

stapes   One of three bones comprising the ossicular chain; the stirrup.

stimulability   The ability to produce a targeted speech sound by attending to visual, auditory proprioceptive, and kinesthetic feedback.

stoma   A small opening into a body passage or cavity. In laryngectomy, the opening into the trachea.

stop   In articulation, speech sounds made by momentarily and completely ceasing the air stream and subsequent acoustic energy in the speech tract.

stop consonant   A speech sound produced by momentarily stopping the air flow, such as /p/, /t/, and /k/.

stress   In speech, the variations of intensity and force of a syllable when compared with adjacent ones. The total amount of acoustic energy in the production of one syllable when compared to another.

strident   A sound produced by directing the airstream against a hard articulator and creating high-frequency acoustic energy.

stroboscope   In voice, an instrument that provides intermittent light used to slow and illuminate the vibrating vocal folds.

stroke   The sudden interruption of blood flow to the brain; a cerebral vascular accident.

stuttering   A word improperly patterned in time and the speaker's reaction thereto [Van Riper].

subcortical   The area of the brain below the cerebral cortex.

subglottal air pressure   Pressure below the glottis.

subglottic   Below the vocal folds.

submucous cleft   A cleft in the hard palate but covered with tissue and appearing normal.

substitution   In speech articulation, replacing the correct sound with another one.

supraglottic   Above the vocal folds.

suprasegmental   Intonational, stress, and durational features of a language that extend across one or more segments; prosody.

surd   A sound of a language produced without accompanying vocal fold vibration; voiceless.

syllable   The basic physiologic and acoustic unit of speech.

syndrome A combination or cluster of symptoms that usually occur together.

syntax Linguistic rules for arranging morphemes into connected utterances. The grammatical structure of language, especially word order.

systematic desensitization In stuttering, a method of reducing negative emotions associated with certain speaking stimuli through relaxation training, counseling, hypnosis, role-playing, and meditation.

tachylalia An excessive rate of speech.

tactile Relating to the sense of touch.

tactile agnosia Disorder relating to the perception of touch.

tangential speech Utterances lacking continuity and consistency in a train of thought.

tap A speech sound resulting from brief contact between articulators, usually the tip of the tongue and the alveolar ridge.

TBI *See* traumatic brain injury.

teacher of the hearing impaired Professional involved in the education of deaf and hard-of-hearing people.

telegraphic speech Communication using a minimum of function words and using many content words; similar to a telegram.

tempo The rate or speed of speaking.

thorax The chest.

threshold shift In audiology, the change in hearing sensitivity caused by exposure to noise.

thrombosis A plug that stops the flow of blood. Unlike an embolus, it does not form elsewhere and migrate.

TIA *See* transient ischemic attack.

tic A sudden twitch; an involuntary contraction of a muscle or muscle group.

timbre The perceptual correlate of a sound spectrum.

timing device In stuttering and apraxia of speech, activating behavior or responses designed to compel utterances at a specific moment in time.

tinnitus The sensation of ringing, buzzing, or humming in the ear without an external source.

tonic A contraction of a muscle that is not sufficient to produce movement.

total communication approach A comprehensive habilitative process for patients with severe hearing loss and deafness.

trachea The windpipe.

tracheotomy A surgical procedure in which an opening is made into the trachea and a tube inserted to help respiration.

transient ischemic attack (TIA) Like a stroke but does not result in permanent damage to the brain and lasts less than 24 hours.

traumatic brain injury (TBI) An injury to the brain caused by an outside impact or a penetrating object.

tremor A vibration of a muscle or structure of the body; rhythmic shaking or trembling of a muscle group.

trill A speech sound produced by vibrating an articulator by the airstream.

tympanic membrane   A thin membrane, found between the external and medial sections of the ear, that transmits acoustic energy to the ossicles.

tympanogram   A chart of the results of acoustic impedance audiometry depicting eardrum and middle-ear compliance.

ultrasonic   The frequency of vibrations not perceived as sound; above approximately 20,000 cycles/second.

unilateral   Pertaining to one side of the body.

unilateral abductor paralysis   Inability to separate the vocal folds due to neuromuscular damage to one of them.

unilateral adductor paralysis   Inability of one vocal cord to close; one vocal fold is fixed in an open position.

unilateral neglect   Problems attending to one side of the body.

unvoiced   A sound produced with no vibration of the vocal cords, such as "sh" and /h/.

uvula   The small, midline muscular process hanging from the posterior border of the velum; the muscle that hangs down at the back of the soft palate.

vein   A blood vessel carrying blood to the heart.

velopharyngeal closure   The closing off of the nasal cavity by the actions of the velum and pharynx.

velopharyngeal incompetence   The inability to separate the nasal cavity from the oral cavity by the velum and pharynx.

velopharyngeal insufficiency   Insufficient tissue or movement to effect closure of the velopharyngeal sphincter.

velum   The soft palate.

ventricle   An interconnected, fluid-filled cavity in the brain.

verbal   The spoken word.

vertigo   Dizziness; sensation of spinning or falling caused by abnormalities of the vestibular system.

vibrato   The rise and fall in pitch and loudness of the voice.

vibratory cycle   One cycle of periodic acoustic or of vocal fold vibration.

visual agnosia   The inability to appreciate the significance of written words or objects.

visual neglect   Lack of attention to a particular space or visual field.

vocal   Pertaining to the voice.

vocal cord (chord)   The paired folds in the larynx containing the vocal ligament that produces sound when vibrated.

vocal resonance   The modification of the laryngeal sound source by sympathetic vibration of the column of air in the speech tract.

voice   Any sound produced by the vibration of the vocal folds.

voice onset time (VOT)   The time between the release of an obstruent consonant and the start of voicing.

voiceless   A sound produced without vibration of the vocal folds.

VOT   *See* voice onset time.

vowel   A voiced speech sound resulting from relatively unrestricted passage of the airstream though the vocal tract.

waveform   In acoustics, the graphic representation of molecular displacement.

wavelength   The distance a wave travels during each cycle of vibration.

Wernicke's aphasia   The loss of speech and language reception due to an acquired lesion of the dominant cerebral hemisphere; sensory aphasia.

Wernicke's area   The cortical receptive language center in the temporoparietal area of the dominant cerebral hemisphere, named after the German neurologist Karl Wernicke. The part of the left side of the brain largely responsible for receptive communication (understanding).

white matter   The part of the brain that is white in appearance because it contains more nerve fibers; a collection of axons below the cerebral cortex.

white noise   A broadband aperiodic sound with similar energy levels across the audible range of hearing.

yawn-sigh   In voice therapy, a method of obtaining soft glottal attacks to reduce vocal abuse.

zero-hearing level   Minimum sound pressure level necessary to make any frequency audible.

Appendix A

Professional Issues and Informational Web Sites

ADA home page: http://www.usdoj.gov/crt/ada/adahom1.htm

Incidence and Prevalence of Speech, Voice, and Language Disorders in the United States, 2002 Edition:
   http://www.professional.asha.org/resources/factsheets/speech_voice_language.cfm

Code of Ethics of the American Speech-Language-Hearing Association:
   http://www.professional.asha.org/resources/ethics_index.cfm

Continuing Education and the Continuing Education Unit (CEU):
   http://www.professional.asha.org/continuing_ed/

Frequently Asked Questions about Speech-Language Pathology Assistants:
   http://www.professional.asha.org/information/faq_careers.cfm

Requirements for Certification by the American Speech-Language-Hearing Association:
   http://www.professional.asha.org/certification/membership.cfm

Salaries: http://www.professional.asha.org/careers/careers.cfm

Scope of Practice in Audiology of the American Speech-Language-Hearing Association:
   http://www.asha.org/careers/audiology.cfm

Scope of Practice in Speech-Language Pathology of the American Speech-Language-Hearing Association:
   http://www.asha.org/careers/slp.cfm

States' Continuing Education Requirements:
   http://professional.asha.org/continuing_ed/resources/states/index.cfm

Appendix B

Short Stories

A Day at JFK

Ah, school days, school daze. Twelve years of desks, lunchrooms, chalkboards, friends, crayons, recesses, rejections, loves, loves lost, bullies, nerds, holidays . . . each day a drama for teachers and students alike. There are hundreds of cast members, each with their own script, and as they say in theater, there are no small parts.

What follows is a story about some of the teachers, parents, and students whose lives intersect at John F. Kennedy Elementary School. Take a few minutes and read about the best of times and the worst of times for Alex, a child who stutters; a young boy and girl with delayed language; little lisping Blake; and Kevin, a child born with a cleft lip and palate. See what it is like to be young and different when it comes to communication. Meet children with articulation problems and Wendy, a speech–language pathologist, whose job it is to help all of them. See how communication disorders affect these children, their parents, and classroom teachers. Before you read the rest of this book and learn of stages, norms, diagnoses, and treatments, read this story and the drama that happens every day at JFK and thousands of schools just like it.

Alex

You can hear a pin drop. Try as he would, Alex cannot look up from his brand-new white running shoes. They are the kind with red lights that flash on the heels every time he steps down. His mother had not been happy about their cost and had said something about having to get a second mortgage to pay for them. Alex has no idea what a mortgage is, but he suspects that it might be where parents get money for kids' shoes. (Maybe a third mortgage will pay for the 21-speed mountain bicycle he had seen in the window of the Broken Spokes Bicycle Shop.) As Alex stares at his shoes, he wishes that they could somehow magically transport him from the front of this classroom to his tree house high atop the backyard oak tree. The silence is deafening. Finally, he hears some kids at the back of the class talk and laugh, and he knows it is about him when he hears the whispered words: "Porky Pig." His stomach tightens into a knot.

Mrs. Lawson also feels the tension and wonders how to handle the situation. She knows Alex is going through a stage in which he stumbles and struggles with his speech. Over the years, she has seen many of her pupils repeat and hesitate as they spoke in front of her first-grade classroom. But Alex is having more trouble than most, and she has never had a child just stop in the middle of a sentence and stare at the floor. "Thank you, Alex," Mrs. Lawson says more to the classroom than to him. "Children, it's only 10 minutes until lunch break. Return crayons to your cubby and get in line for lunch." In an instant, the quiet of the classroom is transformed into the familiar sounds of first graders talking, milling, and laughing as they prepare for lunch. Some children reach for plastic lunch boxes, with their names boldly printed in black marker, while others grasp stained brown bags. Meal tickets are pulled from the tiny pockets of the children whose parents prefer that they eat a hot lunch.

As Alex walks to his cubby, his shoes flashing red lights with every step, Mrs. Lawson asks him to come to her desk. She can see the embarrassment on his little face and wishes that she had never asked him to present his "show and tell" to the rest of the class. But what was she supposed to do? All the other children had stood in front of the class and proudly told of pets, toy cars and trucks, leaves, and unusual mechanical objects. Alex had brought the "bug in a jar" to class and to have never given him the opportunity to share the adventure of capturing it would have drawn even more attention to his speech problem. She tells Alex how well he'd done and pretends to be fascinated by the black-and-yellow bug.

Lunchtime at John F. Kennedy Elementary School starts at 11:15 and ends at 1:00 when the "commons" area is finally vacated. Row after row of chattering children walk through the cafeteria as food servers plop, stack, and pour federally subsidized meals to them. Kindergartners can barely reach the top of the serving counters, and many sixth graders have already outgrown the tables. There is no shortage of energy as hordes of children fall upon the common. Lunchtime at John F. Kennedy school is a treat for all the senses. Today, the smell of loose meat, tomato sauce, milk, and bread saturates the area, as do the sights and sounds of youngsters learning and exploring everything new.

Steven stakes out a place at the lunch table for him and his friend, Alex. His jacket, lunch box, and "49ers" cap are placed on it to clearly deter other children from sitting there. Alex is always late getting to the table, and as usual it is Steven's job to claim it. Steven and Alex's friend, Stacy, looks in his direction as she and her usual group of friends walk to the end of the long lunchroom. Although they are neighbors and often play together on weekends, Stacy has little to do with them during the week. She prefers her girlfriends, and that is just fine with Steven and Alex. To the boys, groups of girls are as foreign and strange as aliens from another planet. Stacy is fun to play with alone, but when she is with her friends, it is just too complicated. Besides, Steven and Alex have a serious problem to deal with this high noon. There is a stranger in town, and he apparently wants to befriend them. His name is Kevin. This is the third day in a row he has sat next to them at lunch. It was time to see what this stranger is all about.

Kevin

Brent and Maggie Byrne had moved from California last June. Both had quit high-paying jobs and pulled their children out of excellent schools to leave the Golden State. Like thousands before them, they had just gotten tired of the California stress. Certainly, California is a wonderful state, an economic powerhouse. The state is blessed with warm temperatures, theme parks, the Pacific Ocean, and huge, sprawling centers of culture. There was never a weekend in which the Brynes had wanted for something to do. But California had been getting to be too much. There are riots, mud slides, earthquakes, floods, crime, and worst of all, mile after mile of gridlocked freeways. It was just one thing after another, and they finally had just had enough. After searching maps and travel brochures, and taking several "scouting" trips, they had finally settled on this small town and the simple life it promised. One of the first lessons they had learned was that the simple life was often accompanied by culture shock. It was amazing how many services they had taken for granted that were simply not available in small towns. One of the biggest concerns was the special needs of their 7-year-old son, Kevin. He had been born with a cleft lip and palate.

It was 7 years ago that Maggie breathed a sigh of relief as she literally counted fingers and toes. It wasn't until she looked carefully into Kevin's face that she saw the gaping hole; it extended from his lips to the back of his throat. It was certainly a shock, but she had already known that nothing would ever detract from the love she felt for this little helpless baby. She glanced at Brent and no words were spoken . . . no words needed to be spoken. As if with mental telepathy, they both communicated their resolve to love this child not only in spite of but in many ways because of his facial anomaly. And Kevin had proved to be a little trooper. Although he suffered surgery after surgery to bring his lip and hard and soft palates together, he had done little crying and even less complaining, especially considering what he went through. The surgeries and the weeks of healing had been painful for Kevin physically and for Maggie emotionally excruciating. The earaches Kevin had every time he got a head cold had almost been as painful as the surgeries, but the tubes put in his ears by the otologist had helped. Maggie had quickly learned that frequent earaches are also a part of cleft lip and palate.

The cleft palate team at the Children's Hospital had been the most professional group of people Maggie and Brent had ever known. Surgeons, dental specialists, audiologists, pediatricians, speech–language pathologists, social workers, and psychologists met regularly with the family to review and plot the course of Kevin's habilitation. It seemed that every aspect of Kevin's life had been considered and every problem related to the birth defect had been anticipated. The plastic surgeons were the ones that brought the most visible changes. It was wonderful how "normal" Kevin's face and mouth had become. With the help of dental braces, his teeth were also moving normally into place. Now he looked like many of the children at this small school, with shiny metal braces and rubber bands bulging from their mouths.

Although the surgeries to repair Kevin's appearance had been in the category of a miracle, the ones to repair the soft palate and the way it moved to the back of the throat on certain sounds had not been as successful. Kevin still spoke with too much nasality, and you could often hear a "sssss" coming from his nose. It was left to the speech–language pathologists to help Kevin's speech sound normal. The gains in this aspect of his cleft lip and palate habilitation were slow, but they were happening nonetheless, at least while they lived in California. It was still an unknown what this small town would bring. Maggie and Brent had been surprised to find that there was no cleft palate team and that there had never been one. It appeared that Kevin was the only child in this rural community with this type of problem. As their new pediatrician had noted, "We never had a need to create a team." She had convinced them that although they had a different way of doing things, Kevin would continue to get very good care.

Steven and Alex look over at Kevin. Without a second thought, Steven asks, "May I have one?" He points to Kevin's "Eatables." As Steven mooches the food, Alex thinks, "The new kid's got style." He looks over at the latest rage in first-grade lunches. It is a box with all the fixings. All a kid has to do is to put the stuff together and, bingo, there is a sandwich, pizza, or Mexican meal. Alex had brought Eatables to school a couple of times earlier in the year, but his mother had said they were too expensive and had once again commented about going to the mortgage store for money. In a generous gesture to Steven's question, Kevin pushes the box in his direction and tells him to help himself. Steven, never one to turn down another kid's meal, finishes it in seconds. After a few first-grade pleasantries are shared, the three of them run down the stairs to the playground for a quick ritual of "prowl the yard." The friendships that are made that day would last for years. After the threesome break to attend the afternoon classes, Steven remarks that the new kid is nice but seems to have a funny accent. Maybe he is from the Deep South. Alex figures that he had also been in a bike accident, what with that scar on his lip. That is all they ever said about Kevin's cleft lip and palate.

Michelle

Michelle is a sweet child. She opens her heart to everyone, but she especially loves that cat. The sight of her carrying that big, black-and-white neutered tomcat from room to room brings a smile to everyone who sees it. Michelle had always been smaller than the rest of her friends, and how she manages to carry him from room to room without assistance is amazing. And the fact that Michelle has cerebral palsy makes the feat even more remarkable. Michelle and that cat look quite the sight . . . this tiny girl carrying a huge cat, sometimes with his feet and tail dragging. You just can't hold back a smile when you see the look on that cat's face. It is one of benign feline tolerance. He obviously doesn't want to be girl-handled, but somehow he accepts the violation as his "job" in the family. He runs from everyone else, but not from Michelle. She loves that cat . . . a warm doll with fur and a heartbeat.

Michelle's cerebral palsy is mild, and according to the doctors, it is the type that would primarily affect her walking and talking, or motor skills, and then only a little bit. Jim and Cathy had gone through the expected emotional roller-coaster ride when the news was given to them. But over the past 8 years, they had learned to accept her disability and the day-to-day inconveniences it brought. She can get around without a wheelchair or walker, feed herself, go to the bathroom, and brush her long, reddish brown hair without much help. Oh, it takes a little longer and seems to be more awkward, but she gets the jobs done. Her speech patterns are typical of this type of cerebral palsy; sounds and words are slooooly draaaawn out as she forces spastic muscles into speech positions. To strangers, her slow, drawn-out speech sounds abnormal, but to Jim, it is music to his ears. After three strapping boys, this delicate, loving child is the apple of his eye. Jim and Michelle have that special father–daughter relationship, and the cerebral palsy only makes it more special.

The realization that Michelle was also delayed in her mental abilities didn't happen suddenly; it took years for Cathy's nagging suspicions to be confirmed. Michelle just didn't do the little things that Cathy had seen the other children do, or they were done much later.

From holding her head up when she was an infant to the extra 8 months it took for her to say "Mama," Michelle appeared slower than her brothers. At first she just assumed it was the cerebral palsy, a result of the spastic muscles' refusal to move as easily as normal ones. But there was more to it than just the physical. Michelle's language development seemed different from that of the other children. The first indication Cathy could not ignore happened when she was picking up Michelle from day care. When Cathy was watching Michelle and the other children chatter about the class hamster, "Bud," the delay became apparent. The other children were putting three and four words together and even making adult sentences, but Michelle would point to the brown and white rodent and say, "Bud run." The biggest indication that all was not well with Michelle's thinking was her lack of understanding. She just couldn't follow complicated directions. Although the other children her age had begun to follow step-by-step instructions, Michelle still seemed to get hung up on the first one. None of the day-care teachers had said anything about Michelle's mental development, but a conference with her kindergarten teacher revealed that Michelle might be "mentally challenged." When Cathy had been young, it was called "retarded," but now the words were "challenged" or "special." But Cathy knew what the words meant. Her youngest child and only daughter was going to have a more difficult life. For Michelle, the road to an education at JFK would be uphill.

Mikey and Nicole

Wendy, the speech–language pathologist, had originally majored in education at a small northwestern college. It wasn't until her junior year that she realized that she loved children but not classrooms full of them. Teaching a classroom full of children was different from teaching a child or a small group of them. She liked the individual contact. She wanted to make a difference. To Wendy, the one-to-one interaction was what teaching was all about. It didn't take her long to realize that teaching a classroom full of 25 or more students did not lend itself to this close pupil–teacher relationship. She had stumbled upon the major of speech pathology and audiology when there was a guest lecture in one of her education courses. Although Wendy was never impulsive, she had formally changed her major by the end of that week, and she had never regretted it. It took her an extra year to get the undergraduate degree in communication sciences and disorders, and she discovered that getting accepted into a master's program was very competitive. She was finally accepted into a small college in the Midwest, and 2 years later, she had the coveted degree. She had done well on the national test and had completed her clinical fellowship last year. The supervisor of her clinical fellowship was one of her professors who had been happy to travel to her small school for the site visits. He had said that getting out of the academic environment once in a while was pleasant, and he looked forward to visits to the real world. At last, she was a fully certified speech–language pathologist, a card-carrying member of the American Speech-Language-Hearing Association, or ASHA, as everyone called it.

Wendy looks forward to the morning sessions and is unhappy that a meeting would cut into them today. She particularly likes the time spent with Michael. Little Mikey has a language delay. The testing that Wendy had done found that, although he is as bright as can be in most areas, his vocabulary is significantly reduced. He just does not understand as many words as other children his age, nor can he use language to express himself as well as other kindergartners. Even the psychological testing done by the school psychologist showed his only problem to be with expressive and receptive language. After meeting with his parents, Wendy traced the problem to environmental deprivation. Actually, in many ways Mikey is far from environmentally deprived; he has a rich home life, full of stimulation. It just lacks enough interaction and communication with adults and other children. Mikey lives on a farm, a 2-hour bus ride to school, and he has a pony, a pet goat, a large red barn, and acres of rolling countryside to explore. Mikey is an only child, isolated from other children, and is not developing communication abilities well enough. It is certainly a mild language delay, but a language delay nonetheless. Wendy knows Mikey will spend only a few months in the speech program.

   Nicole is a different story. Also a second grader, Nicki has a serious articulation problem. Wendy knows that they are going to have a long-term relationship. At first, Wendy couldn't understand anything the child was saying. It never ceases to amaze her how well parents can understand their children, even the ones with major intelligibility problems. The first time Wendy met the family, Nicki had a long discourse punctuated with smiles, frowns, and expansive hand gestures. Unfortunately, all Wendy could understand was a couple of words in the long string of unrecognizable sounds. After Nicki had completed the monologue, her mother turned to Wendy and matter-of-factly summarized: "Nicki said her little sister broke her ankle in a sledding accident." How Nicki's mother was able to decipher meaning from that unintelligible string of sounds still stuck in Wendy's mind. Over the months, Nicki had begun to learn the rules by which sounds were placed into words. Her speech is now beginning to be intelligible, even to strangers.

The IEP Meeting

"He's so ADD." Wendy turns to see a sixth-grade girl give the diagnosis to other girls who eagerly agree with her. As Wendy hurriedly continues on her way to the IEP conference room, she thinks of Mr. Palcich's sixth-grade class and wonders if he is now teaching a theory of disabilities module to the 10-year-olds. Then it hits her that the words *attention deficit disorder* have now become like the word *neurosis*. ADD has now entered the general vocabulary to refer to someone disliked or who creates problems. Actually, there are two types of ADD: There are children with attention deficits who are hyperactive and those who are not. Clinically, the classification criteria are hard to meet, and specific scores on tests and clear behaviors must indicate that a child has ADD. Nowadays, it seems that every child with a lot of energy is diagnosed by his or her parents, teachers, or sixth-grade girls as ADD. Wendy suspects that both Tom Sawyer and Huck Finn would have had similar diagnoses.

   Individualized education plan (IEP) meetings are usually scheduled for late afternoon. Occasionally, there are necessary exceptions, and this morning's meeting is one of them. IEPs are important aspects of special education, and the faculty makes every effort to attend them. They are designated times when the professionals get together with a child's parents and discuss issues, plot a child's course of special instruction, and review progress. The meetings are usually held in the conference room—that is unless the director of Resource Programs, Ms. Hacking, forgets to schedule it, as she frequently does. Wendy painfully remembers last month's IEP meeting held in a vacant classroom and how uncomfortable she was . . . adults were never intended to sit in those small classroom chairs. That meeting seemed to drag on forever. And there was the memorable exchange between Mr. Palcich and Ms. Hacking.

Bob Palcich is a sixth-grade teacher and has been one forever. Apparently, he thinks that the computer-generated sign "Files Must Be Signed Out" prominently displayed over the rows of filing cabinets does not apply to him. Not only had he not signed for a child's file, but he had also taken it home for review, another no-no right up there with treason. Whenever there were spats, Wendy, along with most of the team, just sat quietly and watched the drama. To Wendy, these dramas are rich entertainment, unless she is forced to be a participant. Mr. Palcich and Ms. Hacking had a lively discussion about procedures, confidentiality, responsibilities, tenure, "mindless bureaucratic rules," and seniority. Wendy had given both entertainers credit for a fine show and considered the conflict a tie. By the end of the meeting, both had cooled down, with egos intact. Wendy knows that Mr. Palcich will continue to take home the unsigned files for review, and Ms. Hacking will continue to object. There will be another act.

Wendy sits at the end of the conference table, opposite Ms. Hacking. Ms. Hacking is the consummate professional, and takes her job very seriously. Rumor has it that, before being promoted to administration, she was one of the best resource teachers ever. However, in true Peter Principle form, she had been taken out of the classroom and is now an administrator with the jobs of scheduling, budgeting, signing student files, coordinating IEP meetings, and the inevitable one-act plays with Mr. Palcich and others. Although she performs her duties well, it seems that she has to work very hard at them. According to the academic grapevine, teaching children with special needs had come very naturally to Ms. Hacking, much more naturally than administration. Wendy thinks it sad that good teachers are sometimes promoted away from that which they do best: teaching.

Mr. Palcich walks into the conference room. His mussed hair and shirttail hanging from his belt suggest that already he has had a challenging morning. He smiles at Wendy and sits next to her. From his old brown leather briefcase, he pulls a handful of papers to be graded. He obviously is going to use the time before the start of the meeting to his advantage.

Bob Nettell is the school psychologist. Actually, he is the only one for the entire school district. He spends a lot of time on the road, traveling from school to school. The word for a traveling educational professional is "itinerant," and in rural communities, many people find themselves on the road a lot. Even Wendy has had to travel to a small elementary school 30 miles away. On Tuesdays and Thursdays, she leaves early in the afternoon in the school district's small, white, gas-efficient car. At first, she had resisted the "traveling speech show," but recently, Wendy has looked forward to the 40-minute trip. It gives her precious time alone, an opportunity to listen to the only rock station in earshot, at maximum decibel levels, and to enjoy the sights of the crisp fall foliage. Dr. Nettell spends most of his days in a similar car, and she wonders if he listens to the same radio station blasting tunes from The Rolling Stones to Britney Spears. When he isn't traveling from school to school, he is stooped over papers, intensely scoring IQ, aptitude, and achievement tests. He is also getting that "spare tire" that goes with a sedentary job. Wendy had taken courses in college with aspiring school psychologists. She is convinced that they view the entire world, and all the people in it, in terms of standard scores, stanines, means, age equivalents, and percentiles. They have a very statistical way of looking at things.

Marsha Marlow and Edna Hoopes walk into the conference room together. Edna is the resource teacher and Marsha the idealistic, enthusiastic student teacher . . . a role she plays well. They appear to have developed a close professional relationship. Although Marsha is also from the small college where Wendy had received her master's degree, they had not known each other. Most of Wendy's courses were in the College of Health Professions, and Marsha is in the College of Education. Marsha is learning a lot from Edna, and many of the children in the resource room are benefiting from the additional personal contact. Marsha had also brought new information and ideas to this little school, especially on current ways of treating reading problems and how to handle kids with ADDs, perhaps even that unruly sixth-grade boy.

The schedule shows that the first child up for review is neither in Mr. Palcich's class nor in Wendy's speech program. Ms. Hacking has to make accommodations for this child's busy parents, both of whom are here for the meeting. To make room for the participants, both Wendy and Mr. Palcich sit in the not-so-comfortable couch next to the wall. The parents are understandably anxious and listen intently to the reports from the professionals at the table. The child is a bright boy with above-average intelligence. In fact, according to Dr. Nettell, he scored 2-standard deviations above the average on a recently administered IQ test. Both parents breathe a sigh of relief when they are told that this means he resembles gifted children more than average ones on most of the IQ subtests. He appears to do very well in school except for writing. He just can't seem to put his ideas on paper. He has dismal spelling and struggles with all but the easiest writing tasks. His parents are happy that he met the guidelines for inclusion in the resource program. He will leave his homeroom for an hour each day to get the special services he desperately needs.

The second child on the list is Alex. Wendy, leaving Mr. Palcich on the lumpy couch, takes her place at the table and prepares her notes. Mrs. Lawson and Alex's mother, Jan, enter the room together and sit next to the resource teachers. Wendy is happy that the schedule is being followed and that Alex's IEP is to happen on time.

Alex's Mom

Jan had been concerned about Alex's speech for the past year. She hated to admit it, but she needed professional help in dealing with his stuttering. She had always been very independent about child rearing, and learning to speak correctly was no exception. In fact, when Alex had trouble mastering his /r/ sound, she had simply given him examples of how to say it and corrected him occasionally. Except for the stuttering, he now talked like other children his age. However, during the final few weeks of summer vacation, he had been stuttering much worse. She had tried to help by telling him to slow down and think before he talked, but this seemed to make matters worse. Lately, he had been sounding more and more like her brother-in-law, who has stuttered all his life. She actually welcomed the sealed note from the school speech pathologist requesting a meeting. She had readily given permission for the stuttering evaluation and had completed the long medical and educational questionnaire. She had also filled out a stuttering questionnaire asking detailed questions about how many sounds he typically repeated, how long the stuttering silences were, and whether or not he struggled to get the words out. She had answered them as carefully as possible.

During the short drive to the school's special education annex, Jan had to admit that she was nervous about the meeting. She had never been to an IEP meeting. She knew she would be meeting with Alex's teacher, a school psychologist, the resource teacher, and Wendy, the school speech pathologist. Over the telephone, Wendy had given her some information about what was to be discussed and how IEPs worked, but this was to be a new experience for her. She felt more than a little intimidated. As she pulled into the parking lot, she realized that her feelings were similar to the ones she had when she was a little girl in school. It was like being called to the principal's office.

Jan is greeted by Mrs. Lawson. They had met briefly when she brought Alex to his first day of school. Jan had been happy to learn that Alex was going to be in her classroom. Mrs. Lawson had the reputation of being a superb first-grade teacher, and Jan knew how important first experiences and getting off to a good start are. They sit next to each other at the conference table as introductions are made.

Jan scrutinizes the people at the table, as she is certain they are scrutinizing her. They all seem pleasant enough as they are joking and talking with one another. As introductions are made, Jan is brought into the world of IEPs. She is also introduced to Dr. Nettell and a special education teacher. There is also a student teacher present. They share handshakes and smiles.

Ms. Hacking, the one doing the introductions and apparently the leader of the group, begins by reviewing Alex's file. They quickly get down to business. For the next 20 minutes, histories are reviewed, tests explained, opinions offered, goals established and refined, and problems anticipated. Like a morning fog, Jan's fears lift as it becomes clear that these people are genuinely concerned about her one and only child. He is not just another pupil, one of many. And every attempt is made to bring Jan into the discussions. Her ideas, observations, opinions, and feelings are sought by everyone at the table. But a lot of information is given, too. It is like a breath of fresh air to hear from Wendy and what she knows about stuttering. The goal is to detour Alex from the road to becoming a stutterer, one taken years ago by his uncle. The IEP team's professionalism also relieves the anxiety she has been feeling. Jan understands that the long- and short-term objectives she signed that morning are no guarantee of success, but she feels good about the steps that are being taken. With what she has learned, it all seems like common sense. As she leaves the parking lot that day, she feels relieved that Alex is in good hands.

"On the Road Again"

Sometimes the speech teacher, who travels twice a week to his school, calls Blake out of class, and they take that long walk to the speech room; other times, she simply sits next to him and helps with his desk work. Blake prefers the help with his desk work. He had found that the speech teacher also knows a lot about third-grade math. Oh, she spends a lot of time on numbers beginning with "his" sound, but she is also very helpful in getting the answers, too. "Six," "seven," "seventeen," "seventy," and "subtraction" are words that she requires him to think about and occasionally repeat, and he is learning to make the "steam" sound like she wanted. All he has to do is remember to keep his tongue behind his teeth. On the days when they work on "his" sound in the speech room, there are cards after cards with pictures containing the /s/ sound. Sometimes "his" sound is at the first of the word, and other times it is in the middle or at the end. When he says "his" sound correctly, he usually gets praise from her in the form of a broad smile and a very sincere "Good job, Blake," "Good talking," or "Very good." He enjoys making her so happy by saying the names of the pictures correctly. He is certain that he makes her day by talking with his tongue in the right place. If that is all it takes to make her happy, he will continue to do it. She is easy to please.

On the way back from the small elementary school and with the radio blasting, Wendy thinks about Blake. She always sees him at the end of the day because it is such a treat for her to work with him and she savors the moment. He sits so intently, hanging on every word she speaks, and does everything a third grader is capable of doing to produce the "sssss" that so many children lisp. His improved speech is gratifying for Wendy, and she particularly enjoys the walk with him back to the noisy classroom. They talk of things so important to third graders and so often forgotten by adults. From baseball to tall Trudy who taunts and teases him, Wendy relishes her brief window into the life of this little third grader with a lisp.

As Wendy pulls her car into the parking lot of John F. Kennedy Elementary School, she prepares mentally for the next day. Hopefully, tomorrow, there will be no interruptions of the morning sessions and the time she spends with Michelle and Nicki. Michelle will learn new concepts and how to manage spastic speech muscles. Nicki will learn the more advanced rules by which sounds are combined into words. She will work with Mikey on his nonfarm vocabulary list and with Kevin on talking with his mouth opened wider, a way of reducing too much nasality. And there will be the first session with Alex and her new mission to remove self-consciousness and struggle from this first-grader's speech. These children, and all of the others carefully placed on her caseload, will benefit from her knowledge, concern, and skills. As Wendy turns the lights off in her office and walks down the long hallway, through the common, smelling the lingering, familiar smell of tomato sauce, she remembers that guest lecture about communication disorders and the career decision she had made so long ago. She knows that she is making a difference in the young lives with whom she has been entrusted. As Wendy walks to her car, she bids "Good evening" to Mr. Palcich, realizing that he probably has yet another child's file hidden deep in that old, beat-up, brown briefcase. Tomorrow will be another day at JFK.

Preponderance of Evidence

Chapter 1

"Madam Forewoman, has the jury reached a verdict?" A well-dressed woman in her early 30s stood in the jury box and faced the judge. Obviously nervous, but with a sense of resolve in her voice, she replied, "We have Your Honor. The jury finds for the plaintiff." As sighs of relief saturated the oak and mahogany courtroom, the judge acknowledged the verdict by writing something on a small notepad. Then, for 10 gratifying minutes, the forewoman continued to list the charges and verdicts against the defendants. The courtroom again resonated with sighs when the forewoman decreed that punitive damages should also be awarded. The final award would be in the millions.

Michael Blake and Margaret Hunter turned to each other at the plaintiff's table and hugged in relief. After the jury was dismissed and the courtroom emptied, Mike and Maggie were greeted by Mason Sommerness, the senior partner and namesake of the firm. Mason lavished them with praise for a job well done and offered assurances of vacations, bonuses, and perks. "The mother of all cases," he had called it.

The case had lasted 3 years and had just about financially gutted the small law firm. Expert-witness fees, travel costs, depositions, autopsy reviews, and expense after expense had nearly depleted the firm's resources. Last month a bridge loan from a friendly bank had kept salaries forthcoming for the office staff. Fortunately, there would be no appeal, and within 6 weeks, Albert Anderson's estate and the law firm of Sommerness, Blake and Magnum would receive their just rewards. For Mike and Maggie, month after month of 12-hour days would be rewarded. Of course, for both the firm and the family, the settlement was bittersweet. No amount of money could return the spark of life that was Albert Anderson. No settlement would ever return him to his loving children and adoring grandchildren. Nothing would ever erase the memory of his unnecessary, premature, and tragic death. The huge medical industry defended his death as yet another "acceptable" casualty. After all, he was in his 70s. After all, he was sick. After all, he had undergone heart surgery. After all, people die. But to the people who mattered, the judge and jury, Albert Anderson's demise was the result of an arrogant, uncaring, negligent nursing home and a series of sloppy medical decisions. The nursing home—and its larger, deep-pocketed parent company, Southwest Healthcare Systems—would pay dearly for his death, and just maybe because of it, future lives would be saved. Albert Anderson's death would not have been in vain. As Mike had told the jury in the summation, "After all, people deserve better."

Three years ago, Nina Miller, a woman in her late 40s, entered Mike Blake's office and said her father had just died. She talked about his heart surgery, depression, and loss of weight. She told of the months she desperately tried to help him. She spoke of the love she had for her "daddy." She told of the nursing home that had promised to help him gain weight and recapture his rugged, athletic frame. The grief-ridden daughter also produced a picture of Albert Anderson proudly sitting atop a horse, with snow and pine-covered mountains in the distance, apparently taken 2 years before his death. She also showed Mike the nursing home brochure that boasted of its ability to help people like him. Then, Nina told him a woeful tale of misdiagnoses, broken lines of communication, improper care, indifferent doctors and nurses, and a nursing home that didn't give a damn. As she sobbed quietly, she told of an emergency room doctor, who upon seeing her emaciated father, threatened to call the police, to bring charges against her! When she told the ER doctor that she was bringing him from a local nursing home, Palo Verde Eldercare, he had uttered "criminal." Two days later, Anderson died a death of starvation, fever, and suffocation. He had drowned in his own fluids, and his heart had given out.

At first, Mike had agreed just to look into the case. He knew this would be a big commitment and that the financial risks to the firm would be substantial. At 53 years of age, Mike was comfortable. After years of struggling, his practice had blossomed into a small but secure firm specializing in accident and disability law. He still worked long hours but enjoyed what he did. A new home had just been purchased, and a grandchild was on the way. So, he decided, he would begin with a simple look-see. He would test the legal waters carefully before committing his firm's future.

His first stop was the emergency room and a quick discussion with the ER physician. The doctor had indeed remembered Anderson and had confirmed the report by the daughter. A review of the medical records showed his weight to be 97 pounds; his height was 5 feet, 11 inches. The county pathologist also remembered Anderson's body and the "infiltrates" found in his weak lungs. Death was listed as congestive heart failure. The pathologist had also remarked that something was medically awry. Something was not right in the death of Albert Anderson.

By the end of the month, Mike and his legal secretary and investigator, Maggie, had completed their initial investigation. There were several tense meetings with the staff and other partners of the firm. On a Friday afternoon, at precisely 4:15, they met with Nina and agreed to take the case. On behalf of Albert Anderson's estate, the small law firm of Sommerness, Blake and Magnum would sue two physicians, the administration and medical staff of Palo Verde Eldercare, and its parent company, Southwest Healthcare Systems. David would take on Goliath.

Chapter 2

Kendra Coons, Corrine Erickson, Seth Stubblefield, and two assistants were the entire Speech–Language Pathology Service for the 230-bed hospital and the two adjacent nursing homes, one of which had just been purchased by the parent company, Southwest Healthcare Systems. As recently as 2 years ago, their department was double that size, but corporate, insurance, and Medicare changes had resulted in personnel cutbacks. To say they were overworked and understaffed gave new meaning to the word *understatement*. But, as Kendra said at the close of each weekly staff meeting, "Ours is not to question why. . . ."

Corrine and Seth, with the help of the two speech pathology assistants, did the majority of evaluations and therapy for the inpatients and outpatients at the hospital. Kendra, as chief of the service, had some clinical duties, but about 50% of her time was taken by important and not-so-important administrative responsibilities. With the acquisition of the adjacent nursing home, Palo Verde Eldercare, or PVE as the staff was now calling it, she had assumed some clinical transition duties. Prior to the acquisition, PVE had relied on private contract suppliers of speech–language pathology services. Understandably, the private practice group was unhappy at losing the nursing home contract but was cooperative and helpful during the recent transition period. Actually, Kendra was impressed at their professionalism and the way they put the patients' needs above all other concerns during this difficult and awkward period. Kendra hoped she, and her overworked staff, could continue to provide the high-quality services for the 66 residents of the nursing home.

Kendra was approaching retirement age. Although the idea of unlimited days of golfing, traveling, and gardening was appealing, she knew she was not one who could idle away time. Time was too precious. Her professional life had been too full, too rich, and too rewarding. Kendra knew, for her at least, the so-called golden leisure years would be a fool's gold paradise, dull and boring without the professional stimulation to which she had grown accustomed. Her profession was too much a part of her life to simply walk away and not look back. It wasn't a matter of money, either. The greatest bull market in history, a diversified 401K plan, and her disciplined monthly IRA investments had paid off. Kendra was a wealthy woman. Oh well, she still had 3 years to ponder options and possibilities, and in the back of her mind, she added part-time private practice to them. Ah, to be her own boss.

Corrine and Seth made a great team. The two saw eye to eye on just about everything related to the practice of speech–language pathology in a medical setting. This was even more remarkable given their different educations. Corrine had taken the standard route to the profession. Early in her undergraduate career, she had declared it as a major and had been accepted into graduate school on the first try. With an undergraduate GPA of 3.93 and an excellent GRE score, Corrine could have had her pick of graduate schools. However, a bearded young man, a biology major and passionate love interest at the time, had made it an easy decision to obtain both degrees from the same university. Maslow's hierarchy held true for 22-year-old Corrine. Love needs outranked all but safety and breathing on the road to self-actualization. Besides, it was an old and obsolete dictum that the graduate degree should be obtained elsewhere from the undergraduate one. With faculty turnovers, the revolution in information technology, and the fact that the American Speech-Language-Hearing Association reviews and accredits graduate programs, one can get a fine education without jumping from one university to another. And, most important, Corrine had her *whole* future to consider, and the engagement ring had been a major part of the equation. Sadly, whether it was the result of the stresses of graduate school or a difference of opinion about the important things in life—children, religion, and where to set down roots—their future died a quick but painful death. To Corrine, the final year of graduate school was saturated with the grief of their lost future together. And in many ways, a future is the hardest to lose. The passage of time, her first professional job, and a move to the Southwest had healed much of the pain, as had a tall, soft-spoken computer analyst who worked in the hospital's business office. Time had helped Corrine realize that there are many wonderful roads beside the one not taken.

Seth's path to the profession had been nonstandard, to say the least. It seemed he just couldn't find a major that suited him. At the end of his junior year, he had finally majored in "general studies" as a desperate attempt to get a degree in something, anything. His advisor had told him that it was a fine, liberal-studies type of education that many employers sought. Today, employers simply want to train their own employees. The seasoned advisor had also confided that many juniors and seniors have yet to commit to a lifelong career. And perhaps, even the idea of committing to one discipline for an entire lifetime was as dated as the required blue suits and corporate allegiance to IBM and other paternalistic megacorporations in days gone by. After all, learning had become a lifelong pursuit, opening up many new employment possibilities. And when Seth's father had suffered the massive stroke and lost his speech, his lifelong learning path had taken yet another detour. In the 8 months before his father's death, Seth had a crash course on the nightmare that was aphasia. The massive stroke had taken his father's language, but it had also sparked an interest in this mysterious disorder. After taking "leveling" courses, Seth was admitted to a graduate program in communication disorders. Three years later, he found himself working with hundreds of patients with aphasia, all trying to navigate through a wordless world. Seth had finally found his calling.

Chapter 3

Helen Cutler is a delightful woman and Seth looked forward to the 50 minutes, a clinical hour, spent with her. A clinical hour is 50 minutes of direct patient contact and 10 minutes to chart the SOAPs. Subjective, objective, assessment, and progress was the structure the progress notes were to take when written in the chart, and everyone knew the job wasn't done until the paperwork was completed. However, over the years, clinicians had stopped the formality of carefully identifying the patient's status and progress in SOAP form, and now three or four lines on the yellow "Speech Pathology" notes sufficed. SOAPS had evolved to a simple short paragraph, to no one in particular, showing what goals and objectives are being sought and how well the patient is responding. And Helen is improving like gangbusters.

Helen always dresses for therapy, much like she dresses for dinner. The 86-year-old had suffered a stroke, which had caused the right side of her face to sag. Her tongue movements were slow and sluggish, and, at first, she sounded as though she was talking with a mouthful of peanut butter. However, Helen was more concerned with the drooling. Her self-esteem could handle the slurred, distorted speech, but the saliva that dripped from her mouth was most disconcerting to her. It was just too unladylike, and Helen is the consummate lady. Her hair is always sculpted impeccably, and her face is adorned with just the right amount of makeup. There is just the slightest wisp of perfume, as she gracefully takes her seat at the therapy table. Fortunately, therapy and nature's healing ways had stopped the drooling and cleared her mouth of the peanut butter speech. Helen was to be discharged soon, and both she and Seth were pleased with themselves.

The therapy for Helen had been a standard fare of muscle-strengthening exercises and sound-precision drills. Both Helen and Seth had found interesting ways to do the drills and exercises, to keep them from being boring childlike tasks. Today, Helen is articulately recounting time spent in her early 20s, which according to her, was a wonderful, wild time in Chicago. Helen had just calmly noted that she had proudly considered herself a "flapper" when Seth felt the vibration of his pager. The numbers 111 indicated that he had a visitor. The session with Helen was over, but Seth still wanted to find out what in the world was a "flapper." Helen had conversed with the precision and clarity demanded of this particular exercise and had met the goals for the session, but Seth was still curious about this woman's wild past. As he helped Helen gather her belongings and leave the office, he made a mental note to find out just what a "flapper" was in Chicago's roaring days of yore.

The woman introduced herself as an investigator with the law firm of Sommerness, Blake and Magnum and said she had a few questions of him. With those words, Seth's mental alarm went off. Up went his guard. She might as well have said she represented the Devil and was his senior Angel of Death. Seth wondered if he was being sued, and gratefully recalled that the hospital paid his, and the other clinicians, medical malpractice. It was one of the perks negotiated before the layoffs. Two million dollars protected him, his sparse savings account, and future earnings, from the legal eagles, or vultures, depending on which side of the law you are on. Legal birds of prey and scavengers always seemed to circle a hospital. The attractive, well-dressed woman, Margaret Hunter, was professional, polite, and to the point. Did he remember a patient by the name of Albert Anderson? Was there ever a staffing regarding this patient? Did he remember a referral for a swallowing evaluation? Did he conduct one? Was a video swallow study conducted on the patient? Did he keep medical records in the department, in addition to the ones in the patient's chart? Seth drew a blank. He told Ms. Hunter that he would need time to consult his records. As he walked to his next patient, he thought, "Who the heck was Albert Anderson?"

"Is there anything worse than a brain tumor?" Corrine thought as she began the initial evaluation on the 37-year-old woman sitting in the chair. Her head had been shaven, but new growth was just beginning to cover her scalp, which Corrine thought was remarkably smooth and even attractive in an unusual sort of way. Would it be out of place to remark that even without hair, the patient was still a pretty woman? It seemed the baldness accentuated her dark brown eyes and full lips. She decided not to remark about the patient's appearance. Over the years, she had learned that often the best thing said was nothing. As Corrine laid the test stimuli on the table in front of the patient, her mind focused on her own headache. "Great," she thought, "Now, I've got a brain tumor eating away at my gray matter?" Of course, Corrine knew this was a psychological downside to the job. When you are around sickness and disease 8 hours a day, 5 days a week, year after year, you don't have headaches, you have brain tumors. You don't mishandle eating utensils, you have early-onset symptoms of multiple sclerosis. The saliva on the pillow after an afternoon nap is an early indication of Lou Gehrig's disease. A little dizziness after standing up too fast is an impending stroke. Forgot your keys? Well, welcome to the world of Alzheimer's disease, where you meet new people every day.

Corrine went slowly with the patient. The evaluation would not be completed today, nor did it need to be. The patient tried her best to focus, but she was slow and often completely unresponsive. Even after completing the tests of her receptive language abilities, Corrine wasn't certain how much the patient understood what had been spoken. This was not the first patient she had evaluated with a brain tumor, and Corrine knew she would likely improve, often rapidly, after the surgery. Sadly, she also knew that brain surgery often only bought time for the patient, a few more months or perhaps a couple of years. Of course, there was always room for optimism, what with the new generation of drugs showing so much promise in cutting blood supply to tumors and even attacking their evil genetic core. Corrine's role in the cancer battle was all about the patient's quality of life. Others would try to destroy the army of out-of-control brain cells. Her job was to help the patient regain as much communication as possible. Her job was to help this woman navigate through the frightening changes in her speech and language abilities. Her job was to help restore speech and language and all the connections with loved ones that only communication can maintain. Her job was to make those additional years provided by the physicians and nurses as meaningful and rich as possible. No small task.

After completing the partial evaluation, she stopped at the cafeteria for a sandwich. It was 11:45, Corrine was hungry, and her stomach had announced it to all who rode with her in the elevator. After paying for the pastrami on rye and the diet drink, and automatically getting the generous employee discount, she took her usual table in the corner of the dining room, partially hidden by a huge support pillar. She liked to eat alone and cherished the time to read the latest mystery novel about a Navajo police detective named "Chee." But halfway through her solitary lunch, a woman approached her, apologized for the interruption, and began to ask her questions about a patient, Albert Anderson, of whom she had absolutely no recollection.

Chapter 4

At first glance, Palo Verde Eldercare (PVE) looked like any other average-sized nursing home. Maggie Hunter had been inside only two other nursing homes in her life, and this one didn't seem much different from them. Not much different except for the odor, that is. It was a mixture of food, sweat, sickness, and old age. The place smelled dirty. The halls were lined with old people. Some patients were shuffling slowly from one place to another, while others just sat in wheelchairs staring at her and into space. As she approached the first-floor nursing station, she noticed 8 or 10 people sitting in a communal television space, not really watching the old television set mounted high above their heads. The sound emanating from the television was too loud for normal ears but probably too soft for them to hear. A perky talk-show host was interviewing someone who felt deeply victimized by this, that, or the other fashionable thing. Tears were flowing from the guest, and an extreme closeup caught all her talk-show pain. The studio audience clearly commiserated with the poor, hapless victim, but for the PVE residents watching the show, her plight—broadcast to millions of people and sponsored by a new, improved toothpaste—seemed trite. Maggie wondered if Albert Anderson had sat in that same room, watching talk shows, wasting away, and silently passing time, until his days ended.

The director of nursing was defensive. Most people are defensive when talking to a lawyer or an investigator, especially when they are on the other end of the lawsuit. But this nurse was more defensive than most. She remembered Anderson and knew of his death. She also knew of the suit and had met twice with the administrator of the facility. She had also met with the lawyers who would defend them, their action, and inaction. She provided little information about his medical condition, standard of nursing care for him, diagnostic procedures, and therapies. In effect, she told Maggie that the only information she would receive about the case, at least from her, would be during a deposition or trial, under oath, and with her lawyers present. That was fine. After all, that is the way the system worked.

On the way out of the PVE, a nurse's aide approached Maggie and asked to have a few words with her. Lori—a woman in her early 40s, a bit overweight but strong and muscular—wanted to talk about Anderson. After looking around for spies, they slipped into a vacant room. Maggie took notes while Lori spoke of Anderson's care, or lack of it, indifference and incompetence in his treatments, and the thinly veiled frustration and anger many of the staff felt at him for not improving. She confessed she had grown to like Anderson. She also told of the "soup incident."

Chapter 5

After Albert Anderson's heart surgery, he began to lose weight and was depressed. These are not uncommon reactions after major bypass surgery. But Albert continued to waste away. After his surgery, his anxious daughter, Nina, had brought him home and tried to nurse him back to health. She regularly consulted with his doctor and did everything she thought was right. She fed him slowly and carefully 8 to 10 times a day. She created a warm, bright bedroom and was vigilant about his medications. She loved, nurtured, prodded, and tried to coax him back to health. She happily returned the love he had so unconditionally given to her. But it was to no avail. He just barely held his own weight. Then, one day she saw an advertisement in a newspaper. A nursing home, not far from her house, professed the staff, skill, compassion, and expertise in helping patients just like her father. Three days later he was admitted to Palo Verde Eldercare. Nina finally sought help from medical specialists. She breathed a breath of relief. Unfortunately, that breath of relief quickly turned to a gasp of exasperation.

At first, Albert Anderson's medical care appeared competent. He was placed in a private room, and medical professionals from all walks of life evaluated, interviewed, and planned for his care. The paperwork was completed in great detail, especially those dealing with the out-of-pocket expenses that she, with the help of a second mortgage on her home, would have to endure. However, within a week or so, Nina started to notice signs that all was not as it appeared. Meal trays were just left with her father, sometimes out of his reach, and picked up later with nary a bite taken. He continued to lose weight. His depression deepened, and his antidepressants were given at irregular times, if at all. Frequently, an entire day would pass without Anderson ever leaving his bed, except for the occasional trip to the bathroom, which required help from the scant number of busy, overworked nurse's aides. And more than once, to Nina's disgust, he had spent hours laying in his own waste; the call light had repeatedly been turned off at the nurses' station. And then there was the incident with the soup.

It was no secret that Albert Anderson was allergic to milk products. Nina had told everyone about his serious allergy, from the attending physician to the nurse's aide who brought him his tray. It was listed in every section of his chart. She had even printed a sign and placed it on the wall of his room. Milk products had always caused her father to have a violent reaction, often requiring an immediate, panicky drive to an emergency room. So, when Nina had unexpectedly visited him at lunchtime and found the bowl of New England clam chowder, loaded with whole milk and carelessly placed on his tray, she became furious. She immediately took the bowl of soup to the nurses' station. As she walked toward the three nurses and ward clerk, she got the usual unmistakable looks from them: "Here comes that pest with yet another complaint." When she showed the bowl of soup to one of the nurses and got the usual brush off, Nina simply threw the contents of the bowl on the counter. Five weeks later, a judge threw out the complaint from the two nurses who alleged of being scalded by the lukewarm soup. The judge had boldly stated that the action of Nina Miller, although inappropriate, was understandable and possibly justified.

Nina, a hands-on-kinda gal, was not reticent about continuing to complain to the powers-that-be about his lack of care. Oh, the nurse's aides listened to her and promised to do better. The nurses also said they would be more careful. The doctors assured her that all was well. Even the hospital administrator had reminded her that they, and not she, were the professionals and knew best. But nothing changed, and Albert Anderson slowly began to die.

Several times Nina had called The Doctor. Each time, it was a hurried, impatient, one-sided conversation. The Doctor was a busy man, and she understood that. He was also one of the finest heart surgeons in the Southwest, a fact she would never deny. After all, it was his skilled hands that had repaired her father's heart. But he just seemed too busy to talk to her about pressing postsurgery concerns. Several times, she had asked The Doctor if something might be wrong with Albert's ability to swallow. And several times he said that he would look into it. She got the same indifference from him as she did from the staff at PVE. As she told The Doctor, sometimes, when her father would eat, he'd panic and push the food away. But there were no signs of choking. He'd rarely coughed or gagged. After a meal, if you listened carefully, you could hear a gurgle deep in his chest. And he always seemed to have a low-grade fever.

So, to the medical specialists, if Albert Anderson didn't cough, choke, or gag, he obviously didn't have a swallowing problem. His refusal to eat, the occasional panic attacks during mealtimes, and weight loss were common problems associated with postsurgery depression. Sometimes, Nina got the distinct impression that had she gone to college like everyone else in the medical world, she would have known this simple truth. After a while, she stopped wondering, aloud that is, whether her father had a swallowing problem.

Chapter 6

Had the results not been so tragic, the botched orders could have been called a comedy of errors. On a chilly day in November, The Doctor had his nurse call in the orders, and the busy charge nurse at PVE dutifully noted them on the chart. No one will ever know for certain whether The Doctor's nurse misunderstood his words or whether the charge nurse at PVE made the mistake, but an upper GI was ordered rather than a video swallowing study. No one will ever know for certain whether The Doctor referred Anderson to the speech pathology service for an informal speech and language evaluation or whether he wanted a comprehensive dysphagia assessment. All that was written in the chart was "speech referral." No one will ever know for certain why Anderson didn't get a complete, comprehensive swallowing assessment. However, one thing was known for certain by the plaintiff's expert witnesses who testified 3 years later. Anderson was silently aspirating deadly food particles into his lungs for weeks, perhaps months, before his death. And according to one expert witness, a physician with a medical degree from a fairly decent school, Harvard University, those particles led to the congestive heart failure that killed Albert Anderson.

That Albert Anderson didn't choke, gag, or cough during mealtimes did not rule out a swallowing problem. Silent aspiration occurs when a patient appears to swallow normally, but food particles or liquids are breathed into the lungs. Usually, in silent aspiration, the patient swallows, but some food particles or liquids remain in the throat, either at the base of the tongue or around the vocal cords. Then, when the patient breathes after the swallow, they are sucked into the lungs. This problem is compounded if the patient doesn't have a productive cough. Often, weak and feeble patients can't build up the air pressure to blow the aspirated food particles from their lungs or the passages leading to them. It is called silent aspiration precisely because the patient doesn't cough, choke, or gag. It is a serious medical condition, which often leads to pneumonia, and it can be deadly.

There are several steps to a comprehensive swallowing evaluation. Usually, it is preceded by a bedside assessment. Here, the speech–language pathologist assesses the patient's oral–motor abilities and sensation. But there is only so much information that can be obtained at a patient's bedside. If the clinician suspects that the patient may be silently aspirating, he or she recommends the barium swallow study and actually goes to the Radiology Department to participate in the procedure. After donning lead aprons to protect from the radiation, the clinician watches the patient, actually his or her blurry skeleton, swallow a white liquid and other foods soaked in the stuff. During the procedure, the clinician can see whether the patient aspirates during any aspect of the swallow. Although there are false-positive and false-negative results to any medical tests, the majority of the expert witnesses opined that Albert Anderson would have survived his dysphagia had this procedure been followed.

Chapter 7

The depositions were taken in the Gold Conference Room of the hospital. Corrine, Seth, and Kendra were scheduled, in that order, to take a solemn oath to God that everything said was the truth and the whole truth. They agreed to provide all they knew about Albert Anderson. The depositions for each clinician lasted about an hour, but they were very long hours. The defendant's attorneys were present and conferred, objected, and moved to "strike" regularly during Mike's examination. Mike was always pleasant but very businesslike, as he sought to get to the truth. A court reporter took down every word, even every "ah," "um," and stutter, in frightening detail. By noon, Corrine, Seth, and Kendra were deposed and deposed well. Other depositions were taken that day, and even more were scheduled at different places and at different times. Nurses, nutritionists, social workers, doctors, administrators, and family members all experienced the ordeal of the deposition.

During the trial, neither Corrine, Seth, nor Kendra were required to testify, although their depositions were referred to several times. Lori, the nurse's aide, was examined and cross-examined for 6 grueling hours. Mike skillfully re-created the series of events that had led to Albert Anderson's death. Breakdown after breakdown in communication occurred between The Doctor and the other medical professionals. Mike proved, beyond a reasonable doubt, that the standard of care for Anderson was certainly inconsistent and inadequate. He created an accurate picture of Palo Verde Eldercare as a shoddily run, negligent nursing home. Although most of the staff tried to provide quality care, the nursing home's motivation for profit often torpedoed their efforts. Mike also showed how a patient, like Anderson, who fails to improve as expected can sometimes create a culture of resentment and negativity among the medical staff. This is especially true when there are stress and conflict with a family member. He told of the soup incident. Mike clearly portrayed The Doctor as a skillful surgeon who had dedicated his life to help the hurt and sick. But Mike also showed that The Doctor was not careful enough, nor did he keep up on important postsurgical medical treatments and therapies. And Mike provided a preponderance of evidence to the jury of seven women and five men, with two alternates, that the speech pathology staff never did get the referral on Anderson. They were never able to do the testing and therapies that "probably" would have saved his life. In the legal world, the distinction between "possible" and "probable" is an important one.

The orange, desert sun was setting over the top of the modest homes. You could hear children laughing and playing. Finally, it was beginning to cool down, and the thermometer read only 99 degrees. Of course, it is a dry heat, as if that's a comfort to desert dwellers. Nina Miller had just finished pouring herself another glass of sun tea, which had been brewing all day on the porch, when she saw a red, Pontiac Grand Am pull into her driveway. Maggie Hunter, dressed in a comfortable sundress, politely refused the large glass of iced tea and told of pressing after-work shopping that needed to be done. Then, Maggie pulled a very formal-looking check from her purse and gave it to Nina. The check, written to his estate, and the first of three to be delivered by Maggie, had five zeros behind a single digit. Both women began to cry. Later, as the red car drove off and the tears dried on her face, Nina sadly returned to the kitchen of her modest home. As she looked in the direction of the vacant bedroom where she had tried so desperately to nurse her loving daddy back to health, she knew just how empty this victory really was. She would gladly tear up this check, or any check, even one with fifty zeros behind double digits, to hear the laughter and see the smile and to be hugged, just one more time, by her daddy.

Welcome to the Cyber Speech and Hearing Clinic

It is the not-too-distant future. The computer revolution that started in the late twentieth century still raged and showed no sign of retreating. No other device had changed human-kind more than the silicon chip. It had affected virtually every aspect of human life. Some of the changes demanded by the computer chip were painful, but many were wonderful as well. Medicine, science, education, religion, entertainment, business, industry, and family struc-tures had all been transformed by this tiny electronic device. And the professions of speech–language pathology and audiology were no exception.

Nick and Jennifer sat quietly at the dinner table with little Andrea, their firstborn pride and joy. Lately, dinnertime with the small family had become too quiet, too lacking in com-munication. After weeks of concern, Jennifer had decided that something was wrong; all was not right with Andrea's speech and language development. At first, it was just a nagging sus-picion that Andrea didn't talk as well as her playmates. Lately, the signs had become more than Jennifer could ignore. While other children were making adult sentences and eagerly playing verbal games with one another, Andrea was distant and aloof. In communication abilities, Andrea just seemed delayed when compared to other children of her age.

Quiet saturated the dinning room as Jennifer reported her concerns to Nick. He lis-tened intently as she spoke in excruciating detail of baby talk lasting too long, inabilities to follow verbal directions, and constant difficulties keeping up with other children at recess. Jennifer told Nick of her fear that Andrea might be delayed, or God forbid, retarded in her development. She anxiously awaited Nick's feedback while Andrea sat in her booster chair, silently making colorful sculptures with her food.

"You're right. Her speech development seems slow," Nick admitted both to himself and his wife. "I've seen her play with other children, and she just doesn't seem to talk as well as they do. Maybe we should have her evaluated."

Jennifer found relief in his statement. At least Andrea's slow speech development wasn't just in her mind, a figment of her imagination. After all, Andrea was her first and only child, and she didn't have a lot of experience in these matters. "Then it's decided," resolved Jenni-fer, "We'll get her evaluated as soon as possible." Nick nodded and silently wondered how much the deductible and co-payments would cost; but his real fear was for his daughter and her future.

The next morning, Jennifer went downstairs to the most frequently used part of their house, the Cybercenter. It was a small but comfortable room, with brightly colored walls, large draping plants, and a thick, gray carpet. The computer was amazingly small, given its capabilities. The big semicircular monitor was the newest digital brand. It went from floor to ceiling and almost provided a 360-degree viewing area. Jennifer sat at the keyboard and voice-response station while Andrea played quietly with her favorite robotic toy.

Jennifer's words, "On computer," were automatically voice-printed and immediately brought the big screen to life. From a directory of programs, games, and Web sites, she used the mouse to select the Cyber Speech and Hearing Clinic icon. One click later, a pleasant male voice announced, "Welcome to the Cyber Speech and Hearing Clinic. How may we help you?"

Jennifer replied, "I'm concerned about my daughter's speech development. She is three years old and doesn't seem to talk like other children her age." The computer voice acknowledged her concern and stated that a form must be completed before the evaluation could be conducted. A few seconds later, a colorful form appeared on the big screen, and the computer voice stated, "Please complete this form. You may use voice or keyboard responses."

Jennifer began answering the questions: Child's Name, Age, Date of Birth, Health Maintenance Organization, Method of Payment, Developmental Milestones, and Relevant Medical History. Permission was given to access the Cyber Pediatric Center's records for Andrea's medical history, including the brain scans that were completed on all newborns. Ten minutes later, the form was completed, and she clicked "Submit."

From her fifth-floor office in the modern-looking steel building, Angela, a certified speech–language pathologist, sat at her computer station. The morning had been typical, at least thus far. There had been the usual delays with public transportation, but she had managed to arrive at work on time. After her usual cup of coffee, she had consulted her computerized secretary to see what the rest of the day would bring. There would be four new evaluations, which had been scheduled in advance. Today, she was responsible for walk-ins. Walk-ins was an old term used to describe evaluations done without an appointment. The term originated from days of yore where patients physically came to speech and hearing clinics for unannounced evaluations. Of course, nowadays, it was rare that a clinician physically saw a patient either for an evaluation or therapy. It wasn't necessary. The computer had extended the clinician's eyes and ears and could reach around the world, in an instant, to evaluate and treat a patient.

Angela preferred to wear the virtual reality headset. It was better than watching the large computer screen because she could walk around her office or sit comfortably in the soft reclining chair. The only disadvantage to the headset is that it always mussed her hair. Technology had come so far, yet the problem of mussed hair—or "virtual hair," as the teenagers were calling it—persisted. After getting comfortable, Angela commanded the computer to begin the new evaluation. The intake form, on a child by the name of Andrea, flashed on her big screen. Highlighted were certain terms the computer deemed salient. As Angela reviewed the form, she began the process of knowing this child's speech and language development. Then, the computer announced, "Beginning synchronsis viewing."

Immediately, the screen zoomed in on Jennifer, a woman in her early 20s. In the lower left part of the screen, a data frame listed the results of the intake questions for easy reference. Angela introduced herself and paused while a recorded message immediately provided her qualifications, license information, areas of specialty, continuing education credits, and other relevant professional information. Angela first engaged in the usual "chewing gum conversation" with the parent, remarking about the weather and current events. She also told the woman her physical location. Cyber clinics could be in any part of the country or the world for that matter.

As Jennifer spoke, the professional information provided by Angela was displayed in written form, in the lower left part of her screen. For future reference, it was automatically saved under the category of "Medical: Professional Information" in Andrea's health and medical files. There was never a need to delete information because storage memory was unlimited. A recent development went beyond the silicon chip and stored memory at the atomic level.

Angela listened intently as Jennifer discussed Andrea's development. Each statement spoken by Jennifer was automatically evaluated for its truthfulness and arousal quotient. Keywords spoken by her were selected and presented in the ever-changing data frames. Words such as *delayed, slow in development, immature*, and *unusual* were spoken with a high emotional content and identified in shades of red. After the initial conversation with Jennifer, Angela was aware of the distress that this young mother was feeling over her child's communication abilities. She made a mental note to include intensive parental counseling and education modules as a part of the treatment program.

Jennifer was impressed with Angela and the way that the interview was being conducted. After Angela had logged off, the formal evaluation began. On the screen, an older man with a pleasant voice appeared. He was a computer-generated composite face and voice found to be comforting and professional. He asked Jennifer detailed questions about Andrea's cognitive, linguistic, and social–communication development. At the end of the parental interview, the completed form and its profile charts with accompanying norms were presented in a data frame and merged into the appropriate section of the diagnostic report, which was constantly under construction.

The hearing evaluation was completed in less than a minute. As Jennifer held Andrea in her lap, with the brightly colored headset and earphones snugly in place, the function and status of the external, middle, inner, and central hearing processes were tested. Clicks, tones, and buzzing sounds were the only things heard by Andrea. On a data frame, the completed hearing evaluation report was created, including colorful graphic charts of her brain and cranial nerve VIII. Andrea's hearing was tracked and evaluated from external ear to temporal lobe, and she passed with flying colors. Angela remembered that in the past a hearing test of this complexity would have taken hours and involved soundproof booths and complicated testing protocols; even then, its accuracy was sometimes suspect.

The direct speech and language evaluation tests were automatically chosen by the computer, and they were adapted to Andrea's interests. The interactive tests used colorful cartoon characters who playfully asked questions of Andrea. As the talking dogs, cats, and chipmunks had Andrea remember, repeat, name, discuss, describe, and point, the computer analyzed and categorized each response. Andrea's cognitive, linguistic, and social–communication abilities were assessed using the latest tests. Phonological process were identified, as was the speed of motor responses and visual scanning times. Her length of utterances and vocabulary was computed in every possible way and charted in bar, pie, and line graphs. Everything from Andrea's cognitive–linguistic functioning to her metalinguistic awareness was assessed by fun-loving cartoon characters. In the past, these types of tests were conducted by professionally dressed people, with test stimuli formally placed in front of the child, and each response carefully noted with pencil and paper. Young children, like Andrea, were frequently intimidated by the strangers, and sometimes it was a crapshoot whether the final results actually reflected the child's communication abilities. Some children had even refused to talk and clung to their mother's leg, with tears flowing from their eyes. Angela chuckled to herself when she thought of the countless frustrated graduate students who had been required to write a diagnostic report based on the responses from a crying, nonverbal child.

Andrea's articulation was acoustically analyzed, and each sound compared to norms for intelligibility and precision for her particular language. It had taken years of research, but each sound produced by humans had been carefully analyzed by powerful acoustic instruments. The international project had finally listed each sound in the 10,000 languages and dialects of the world and provided their specific acoustic parameters. Now, each sound spoken by a person was instantly analyzed and compared to norms, and a deficiency value was given. The scores were provided for individually produced sounds and for ongoing speech. There were even separate intelligibility scores given when the listeners were family members, friends, and people unfamiliar with the child. The newest technology analyzed the articulation of people suffering from brain damage and neurological diseases, and it not only acoustically determined the precision and intelligibility of their motor speech but also identified the site and nature of the central nervous system damage. Although phonetics courses were still taught in graduate school, clinicians rarely used their ears to make judgments about a patient's articulation. Nowadays, the computer was simply faster and more accurate.

Voice parameters were also automatically profiled by the computer. Andrea's pitch, loudness, emphasis, shimmer, jitter, and voice-onset times were assessed and analyzed in seconds. The computer even noted early signs of progressive neurological diseases such as ALS, MS, and Parkinsonism. Early symptoms of these disorders often showed up in minor voice irregularities, and only the computer could detect them. Fortunately, medicine had powerful treatments that were more successful if they were caught early.

The orofacial evaluation was the final assessment. As the talking chipmunk had Andrea open her mouth wide and put her face close to the screen, the embedded camera noted salient facts about her tongue, lips, teeth, and palatal vault. Everything from tongue tremor to speed of ongoing oral muscular movement was assessed. A three-dimensional picture of Andrea's oral structures was created and added to the ongoing report. It highlighted structures and functions found to be nonstandard.

While the evaluation was being conducted by the computer, Angela was monitoring the stuttering therapy being provided to Matt, a fourth grader. With sensors attached to his fingers and wearing the EEG and brain-imaging "hat," he was provided with gradually increasing difficult sounds, words, phrases, and situations through computer interactive activities. One minute Matt was presenting a speech to a cyberaudience, and the next, he was ordering a soyburger at the local MacDougal's. The computer evaluated the tension in his voice, and—along with EEG, brain imagery, and galvanic skin responses—it provided visual and graphic feedback about speech-muscle tension and general levels of speaking anxiety. The computer gently guided him into more stressful situations as he learned to maintain proper levels of fluency and remembered to use his tools of fluent speech, which were automatically provided on the screen when appropriate. As Angela completed the minor adjustments of the stuttering program, the computer announced that the evaluation on Andrea was completed.

The evaluation shown on the screen was complete in every detail. As Angela read it, she made minor additions and corrections to the report. Each deficient area of Andrea's speech and language evaluation was noted and the appropriate short- and long-term objectives listed. The objective and treatment plans were detailed and specific and had been chosen from thousands stored in the treatment banks. The report, with the parent's permission, would be automatically sent to Andrea's pediatrician and preschool. The Parent Training and Language Facilitation Program was loaded, and Nick and Jennifer would be educated, trained, and coached in childhood language development. The program chosen by the computer was specifically adapted to Nick's and Jennifer's ages, education levels, and interests.

A simple click of the computer loaded the appropriate therapy program for each objective and merged them into a comprehensive treatment protocol. Andrea's preferred television and cartoon characters would be used as cyberfacilitators, and her favorite "great adventures" computer game would provide the theme for all therapies. Andrea's language development would improve as she played, talked, and interacted with the colorful cartoon characters. Daily suggestions would be sent to her parents and preschool teacher for their assistance in meeting the goals. Periodic reassessments were automatically given to the youngster, and adjustments made to the individualized education plan. Angela would regularly review improvement with parents and teachers and adjust the treatment programs when required.

Eight months later, Nick and Jennifer again sat at the dinner table, this time trying to converse over Andrea's chatter. The sweet sound of little Andrea's normal speech and language was music to their ears. They talked about the improvement she had made in her ability to communicate as she talked on and on about the great adventure she and the fun-loving chipmunk had taken through the oak grove in the Cyberpark.

Literature, Media, and Personality

Home Pages, Suggested Readings, References, and Resources

Between the time Website information is gathered and then published, it is not unusual for some sites to have closed. Also, the transcription of URLs can result in unintended typographical errors. Students are encouraged to perform online searches through reliable search engines.

CHAPTER 1 • *Communication Disorders, Literature, Media, and Society*

Rowling, J. K. (1997). Harry Potter and the sorcerer's stone (p. 288). New York: Scholastic.

CHAPTER 2 • *Stuttering and Cluttering*

Pearl Harbor

Retrieved from the World Wide Web:
http://www.upcomingmovies.com/pearlharbor.html

Retrieved from the World Wide Web:
http://preview.hollywood.com/sites/pearlharbor

Retrieved from the World Wide Web:
http://www.cinemenium.com/pearlharbor

Howard Stern

Brooks, T., & Marsh, E. (1999). *The complete directory to prime time network and cable TV shows: 1946–present* (pp. 472–473). New York: Ballantine.

Retrieved from the World Wide Web:
http://www.cam.org/~howardg/crew.html

One Flew Over the Cuckoo's Nest

Retrieved from the World Wide Web:
http://movies.yahoo.com/shop?d=1800103151&cf=info

Nichols, P. (Ed.). (1999). *The New York Times guide to the best 1,000 movies ever made* (p. 620). New York: Random House.

My Cousin Vinny

Retrieved from the World Wide Web:
http://www-tech.mit.edu/V112/N13/vinny.13a.html

Retrieved from the World Wide Web:
http://www.currentfilm.com/dvdreviews/mycousinvinnydvd.html

Retrieved from the World Wide Web:
http://www.suntimes.com/ebert_reviews/1992/03/745904.html

Warner Bros. Cartoon Characters: Porky Pig

Brooks, T., & Marsh, E. (1999). *The complete directory to prime time network and cable TV shows: 1946–present* (p. 141). New York: Ballantine.

Retrieved from the World Wide Web:
http://members.aol.com/EO Costello/p.html

Maltin, L. (1987). *Of mice and magic: A history of American animated cartoons.* New York: New American Library.

The Cowboys

French, P. (1977). *Westerns: Aspects of a movie genre* (pp. 181, 183). New York: Oxford.

Retrieved from the World Wide Web:
http://www.amazon.com/exec/obidos/...f=pm_ dp_ln_v_5/103-3342460-0473405

Retrieved from the World Wide Web:
http://amazon.imdb.com/Plot/ASIN=6304457278?0068421

Mel Tillis

Retrieved from the World Wide Web:
Mel Tillis Theater, http://www.nefsky.com/tillis.htm

The Sixth Sense

Maltin, L. (2000). *Leonard Maltin's movie and video guide: 2001 edition.* New York: Signet.

Retrieved from the World Wide Web:
http://mrshowbiz.go.com/reviews/mo...ews/movies/TheSixthSense_1999.html

CHAPTER 3 • *The Voice and Its Disorders*

Julie Andrews

Retrieved from the World Wide Web:
http://theage.com.au/entertainment/20001101/A19065-2000Oct31.html

Retrieved from the World Wide Web:
http://www3.newstimes.com/archive99dec1599/naf.htm

Retrieved from the World Wide Web:
http://mrshowbiz.go.com/celebrities/people/julieandrews/bio.html

Retrieved from the World Wide Web:
http://www.angelfire.com/la2jandrews/bio.html

William Jefferson Clinton

Retrieved from the World Wide Web:
http://www.infoplease.com/ipa/A0760626.html

Jack Klugman

Retrieved from the World Wide Web:
http://us.imdb.com/M/person.biography?Jack+Klugman

Retrieved from the World Wide Web:
http://odd_couple.tripod.com/faq.html

Brooks, T., & Marsh, E. (1999). *The complete directory to prime time network and cable TV shows: 1946–present* (p. 750). New York: Ballantine.

Kenny Rogers

Retrieved from the World Wide Web:
http://rollingstone.netscape.com/artist/artist.btq?aid=3467

Retrieved from the World Wide Web:
http://www.rollingstone.com/sections/artists/text/bio.asp?afl=nscp&LookUpString=3467

Stacy Keach

Retrieved from the World Wide Web:
http://us.imdb.com/Bio?Keach,+Stacy

Retrieved from the World Wide Web:
http://www.compaqsolutions.com/keach.html

Retrieved from the World Wide Web:
http://www.StacyKeach.com/bio.htm

The Godfather

Maltin, L. (2000). *Leonard Maltin's movie and video guide: 2001 edition* (pp. 536–537). New York: Signet.
Mottram, J. (1998). *Public enemies: The gangster movie A–Z* (pp. 79–82). London: B. T. Batsford.
Neale, S. (2000). *Genre and Hollywood* (pp. 80–81). New York: Routledge.

Randy Travis

Retrieved from the World Wide Web:
http://www.randytravis.com/about/content.html

Retrieved from the World Wide Web:
http://imusic.com/showcase/country/randytrav.html

Retrieved from the World Wide Web:
http://www.vicsurf.com/business/oakee/randy/default.htm

CHAPTER 4 • *Articulation and Phonological Disorders*

Barbara Walters

Retrieved from the World Wide Web:
http://mrshowbiz.go.com/people/barbarawalters/Index.html

Retrieved from the World Wide Web:
http://www.wif.org/yearbook/lucy_walters_bio.html

Retrieved from the World Wide Web:
http://abcnews.go.com/onair/2020/b...ails/walters_barbara_bio_2020.html

Warner Bros. Cartoon Characters

Retrieved from the World Wide Web:
http://www.voicechasers.org/Actors/M_Blanc.html

Retrieved from the World Wide Web:
http://www.throttlebox.com/Box/reload?Page=http://www.throttlebox.com/Content/1027.shtml

Brooks, T., & Marsh, E. (1999). *The complete directory to prime time network and cable TV shows: 1946–present.* New York: Ballantine.

Maltin, L. (1987). *Of mice and magic: A history of American animated cartoons.* New York: New American Library.

Retrieved from the World Wide Web:
http://members.aol.com/EOCostello/t.html

Sean Connery

Retrieved from the World Wide Web:
http://search.biography.com/print_record.pl?id=4609

Retrieved from the World Wide Web:
http://mrshowbiz.go.com/people/seanconnery/content/Bio.html

Retrieved from the World Wide Web:
http://www.kcweb.com/superm/s_connery.htm

The World According to Garp

Retrieved from the World Wide Web:
http://www.gumbopages.com/gradual.html

Retrieved from the World Wide Web:
http://mrshowbiz.go.com/reviews/mo.../TheWorldAccordingtoGarp_1982.html

Maltin, L. (2000). *Leonard Maltin's movie and video guide: 2001 edition* (p. 1585). New York: Signet.

My Fair Lady

Maltin, L. (2000). *Leonard Maltin's movie and video guide: 2001 edition* (p. 967). New York: Signet.

Retrieved from the World Wide Web:
http://www.ravecentral.com/myfairlady.html

Canby, V., & Maslin, J. (1999). *The New York Times guide to the best 1,000 movies ever made* (pp. 587–588). New York: Times Books.

The Ladies Man

Retrieved from the World Wide Web:
http://www.saturday-night-live.com/snl/cast-bios/meadows.html

Retrieved from the World Wide Web:
http://movies.yahoo.com/shop?d=hv&cf=info&id=1802956640

Retrieved from the World Wide Web:
http://upcomingmovies.com/ladiesman.html

That '70s Show

Retrieved from the World Wide Web:
http://www.fox.com/70sshow/bios/bio04.html

Retrieved from the World Wide Web:
http://www.teenhollywood.com/celebs/wilmer/getpersonal.asp

Retrieved from the World Wide Web:
http://home.mho.net/newville/fez/information.html

Passions

Gloeckler, A. (2001). Personal correspondence. Flagstaff, Arizona.

Retrieved from the World Wide Web:
http://redrival.com/jumper/bio.htm

Retrieved from the World Wide Web:
http://nbctv.nbci.com/passions/bios/pgv_passions_bios_evans.html

Retrieved from the World Wide Web:
http://redrival.com/jumper/facts.htm

CHAPTER 5 • *Language Development and Disorders*

What's Eating Gilbert Grape?

Retrieved from the World Wide Web: http://ellis.nebbadoon.com/docs/joined_reviewfiles/WHAT'S_EATING_GILBERT_GRAPE.html

Retrieved from the World Wide Web: http://www.dicaprio.net/filmography/gg.html

Maltin, L. (2000). *Leonard Maltin's movie and video guide: 2001 edition.* New York: Signet.

Nichols, P. (Ed.) (1999). *The New York Times guide to the best 1,000 movies ever made.* New York: Times Books.

Nell

Retrieved from the World Wide Web: http://www.prairienet.org/ejahiel/nell.htm

Retrieved from the World Wide Web: http://jinx.sistm.unsw.edu.au/~greenlft/1995/177/177p26.htm

Maltin, L. (2000). *Leonard Maltin's movie and video guide: 2001 edition.* New York: Signet.

Chris Burke

Retrieved from the World Wide Web: http://www.arcark.org/burke.html

Retrieved from the World Wide Web: http://www.arcark.org/drbethinterview.html

Retrieved from the World Wide Web: http://home.earthlink.net/~tvman/lifegoes.html

Rain Man

Retrieved from the World Wide Web: http://www.flickfilosopher.com/oscars/bestpix/rainman.html

Retrieved from the World Wide Web: http://www.wismed.com/foundation/rainman.htm

Maltin, L. (2000). *Leonard Maltin's movie and video guide: 2001 edition.* New York: Signet.

Canby, V., & Moslin, J. (1999). *The New York Times guide to the best 1,000 movies ever made.* New York: Times Books.

Sling Blade

Retrieved from the World Wide Web: http://www.rialto.co.nz/archive/slingblade.html

Retrieved from the World Wide Web: http://www.filmgeek.com/pages/slingblade.htm

Retrieved from the World Wide Web:
http://www.palace.net.au/slingb/review.htm

Maltin, L. (2000). *Leonard Maltin's movie and video guide: 2001 edition.* New York: Signet.

Forrest Gump

Retrieved from the World Wide Web:
http://www.twisted-helices.com/ramblings/movies/forrest_gump.html

Retrieved from the World Wide Web:
http://www.time.com/time/magazine/archive/1994/940801/940801.showbusiness.html

Retrieved from the World Wide Web:
http://www.generationterrorists.com/quotes/gump.html

Maltin, L. (2000). *Leonard Maltin's movie and video guide: 2001 edition.* New York: Signet.

Of Mice and Men

Retrieved from the World Wide Web:
http://www.jdlh.palo-alto.ca.us/pr/micemen_floyd/

Retrieved from the World Wide Web:
http://www.ac.wwu.edu/~stephan/Steinbeck/mice.html

Retrieved from the World Wide Web:
http://www.amazon.com/exec/obidos/ASIN/087891997X/002-6893282-7660865

Retrieved from the World Wide Web:
http://www.steinbeck.org/world/biograph.html

CHAPTER 6 • *Hearing Loss and Deafness*

Children of a Lesser God

Retrieved from the World Wide Web:
http://mrshowbiz.go.com/reviews/mo...ies/ChildrenofaLesserGod_1986.html

Retrieved from the World Wide Web:
http://movies.yahoo.com?d=hv&cf=info&id=1800046832

Maltin, L. (2000). *Leonard Maltin's movie and video guide: 2001 edition.* New York: Signet.

Arnold Palmer

Retrieved from the World Wide Web:
http://www.pgatour.com/players/bios/1910.html

Retrieved from the World Wide Web:
http://web2.sandhillsonline.com/golf/plantation/palmer.htm

Retrieved from the World Wide Web:
http://www.icast.com/movies/1,4003,1042-216274,00.html

Heather Whitestone McCallum

Retrieved from the World Wide Web:
http://www.pressplus.com/missam/pastwinners/pw_1995

Retrieved from the World Wide Web:
http://www.wpsd.org/deafawareness/hwhitestone.html

Retrieved from the World Wide Web:
http://www.al.com/south/celebs3.html

The Heart Is a Lonely Hunter

Maltin, L. (2000). *Leonard Maltin's movie and video guide: 2001 edition.* New York: Signet.

Retrieved from the World Wide Web:
http://mrshowbiz.go.com/reviews/mo.../TheHeartIsaLonelyHunter_1968.html

Retrieved from the World Wide Web:
http://www.mta.link75.org/english/heart/about.htm

Nanette Fabray

Retrieved from the World Wide Web:
http://www.hei.org/htm/srnanett.htm

Retrieved from the World Wide Web:
http://us.imdb.com/Bio?Fabray,+Nanette

Retrieved from the World Wide Web:
http://www.wic.org/bio/nfabray.htm

Leslie Nielsen

Retrieved from the World Wide Web:
http://www.amiamsterdam.on.ca/ln/bio.htm

Retrieved from the World Wide Web:
http://www.betterhearing.org/leslie.htm

Florence Henderson

Retrieved from the World Wide Web:
http://www.bradyworld.com/sketch/flobio.html

Retrieved from the World Wide Web:
http://www.flohome.com/flofaq.html

Rush Limbaugh

Retrieved from the World Wide Web:
http://www.time.com

Retrieved from the World Wide Web:
http://www.rushlimbaugh.c...te_100801/contentlucky.guest.html

Brooks, T., & Marsh, E. (1999). *The complete directory to prime time network and cable TV shows: 1946–present* (p. 878). New York: Ballantine.

The Miracle Worker

Maltin, L. (2000). *Leonard Maltin's movie and video guide: 2001 edition.* New York: Signet.

Canby, V., & Moslin, J. (1999). *The New York Times guide to the best 1,000 movies ever made.* New York: Times Books.

Retrieved from the World Wide Web: http://www.afb.org/helen.html

Box 6.5 Retrieved from the World Wide Web: http://www.hearnet.com/about/about_hearstory.htm

Retrieved from the World Wide Web: http://www.hearnet.com/hear_records/hear_records_index.html

Retrieved from the World Wide Web: http://www.hearnet.com/text/tinnitus.html

CHAPTER 7 • *Motor Speech Disorders and Dysphagia*

Annette Funicello

Retrieved from the World Wide Web: http://people.aol.com/people/pprofiles/afunicello/vital.htm

Retrieved from the World Wide Web: http://www.biography.com/features/sweethearts/afunicello.htm

Retrieved from the World Wide Web: http://us.imdb.com/M/person-biography?Annette+Funicello

Stephen William Hawking

Retrieved from the World Wide Web: http://www.damtp.cam.ac.uk/user/hawking/disability.html

Retrieved from the World Wide Web: http://www.hawking.org.uk/text/disable/disable.html

Retrieved from the World Wide Web: http://www.hawking.org.uk/text/about/about.html

Retrieved from the World Wide Web: http://www.physics.gmu.edu/classinfo/astr103/CourseNotes/ECText/Bios/hawking.htm

Muhammad Ali

Retrieved from the World Wide Web: http://www.nationalgeographic.com/faces/ali/bio.html

Retrieved from the World Wide Web: http://mrshowbiz.go.com/people/Muhammadali/

Retrieved from the World Wide Web:
http://www.danorthside.f2s.com/ali/alibio2.html

Anywhere But Here

Retrieved from the World Wide Web:
http://www.foxmovies.com/anywherebuthere/story/story.html

Retrieved from the World Wide Web:
http://www.weeklywire.com/ww/11-22-99/austin_screens_film3.html

Maltin, L. (2000). *Leonard Maltin's movie and video guide: 2001 edition.* New York: Signet.

Janet Reno

Retrieved from the World Wide Web:
http://www.usdoj.gov/ag/jreno.html

Retrieved from the World Wide Web:
http://www.wic.org/bio/jreno.htm

Retrieved from the World Wide Web:
http://www.usis.usemb.se/cabbio/jreno.html

Deuce Bigalow: Male Gigolo

Retrieved from the World Wide Web:
http://www.eopinions.com/mvie_mu_1093556

Retrieved from the World Wide Web:
http://us.imdb.com/Plot?0205000

Maltin, L. (2000). *Leonard Maltin's movie and video guide: 2001 edition.* New York: Signet.

Kirk Douglas

Retrieved from the World Wide Web:
http://www.onwis.com/letsgo/movies/1013kirkdouglas.stm

Retrieved from the World Wide Web:
http://us.imdb.com/Bio?Douglas,+Kirk

Retrieved from the World Wide Web:
http://www.onwis.com/letsgo/movies/1013kirkdouglas.stm

Malcolm in the Middle

Retrieved from the World Wide Web:
http://us.imdb.com/Name?Traylor,+Craig+Lamar

Montel Williams

Retrieved from the World Wide Web:
http://www.cnn.com/SHOWBIZ/TV/9908/23/montel.williams

CHAPTER 8 • *Aphasia in Adults*

Patricia Neal

Retrieved from the World Wide Web:
http://www.icast.com/movies/1,4003,1043-83055,00.htm

Retrieved from the World Wide Web:
http://covenanthealth.com/aboutus/prnc/patneal.htm

Retrieved from the World Wide Web:
http://www.wic.org/bio/pneal.htm

Regarding Henry

Retrieved from the World Wide Web:
http://movies.yahoo.com/shop?d=hv&id=1800163421&cf=info

Maltin, L. (2000). *Leonard Maltin's movie and video guide: 2001 edition.* New York: Signet.

Wings

Kopit, A. (1978). *Wings: A Play.* New York: Hill & Wang.

The New Twilight Zone: "Word Play"

Retrieved from the World Wide Web:
http://www.geocites.com/john_75915/links/tzonenew.html

Retrieved from the World Wide Web:
http://tnt.turner.com/scifi/zone/main.html

Brooks, T., & Marsh, E. (1999). *The complete directory to prime time network and cable TV shows: 1946–present.* New York: Ballantine.

Legends of the Fall

Retrieved from the World Wide Web:
http://movies.yahoo.com/shop?d=hv&cf=info&id=1800227783

Retrieved from the World Wide Web:
http://www.film.com/film-review/1994/8977/109/default-review.html

Maltin, L. (2000). *Leonard Maltin's movie and video guide: 2001 edition.* New York: Signet.

CHAPTER 9 • *Communication Disorders Resulting from Dementia*

Ronald Wilson Reagan

Box 9.1   Retrieved from the World Wide Web:
http://www.reagan.com/plate.main/ronald/speeches/rrspeech05.html

Abraham "Grampa" Simpson

Retrieved from the World Wide Web:
http://synergizedsolutions.com/simpsons/profiles/abe/

Retrieved from the World Wide Web:
http://grampa.sweeetnet.com/profile.shtml

Retrieved from the World Wide Web:
http://members.tripod.com/~adhuff/residents.html

Retrieved from the World Wide Web:
http://www.angelfire.com/vt/VortexTom/Infinite.Abraham.html (quotes)

Nash Bridges

Retrieved from the World Wide Web:
http://www.lowtek.com/nash/faq/

Brooks, T., & Marsh, E. (1999). *The complete directory to prime time network and cable TV shows: 1946–present.* New York: Ballantine.

Age Old Friends

Retrieved from the World Wide Web:
http://www.library.unt.edu/owl/aging.html

Retrieved from the World Wide Web:
http://sagesite.utmb.edu/coa/FilmLibrary.asp

Maltin, L. (2000). *Leonard Maltin's movie and video guide: 2001 edition.* New York: Signet.

CHAPTER 10 • *Communication Disorders Resulting from Head and Neck Injuries*

James Brady

Retrieved from the World Wide Web:
http://people.aol.com/people/25years/pic/pic3.html

Retrieved from the World Wide Web:
http://www.law.umke.edu/faculty/projects/ftrials/hinckley/brady.html

Christopher Reeve

Retrieved from the World Wide Web:
http://www.geocities.com/Hollywood/Studio/4071/biography.html

Jan Berry

Retrieved from the World Wide Web:
http://www.jananddean.com/bio.html

Gary Busey

Retrieved from the World Wide Web:
http://www.eonline.com/Facts/People/Bio/0,128,2430,00.html

Retrieved from the World Wide Web:
http://www.homegame.org/HG/spotlight/gary/

Retrieved from the World Wide Web:
http://www.connectionmagizine.org/badboy.htm

Retrieved from the World Wide Web:
http://www.hollywoodjesus.com/gary_busey.htm

Awakenings

Retrieved from the World Wide Web:
http://www.michaeldvd.melb.net/Reviews/Awakenings.html

Retrieved from the World Wide Web:
http://www.oliversacks.com/bio.html

Retrieved from the World Wide Web:
http://www.oliversacks.com/awakenings.html

The Bone Collector

Retrieved from the World Wide Web:
http://mrshowbiz.go.com/reviews/moviereviews/movies/TheBoneCollector_1999.html

Retrieved from the World Wide Web:
http://www.ultimate-movie.com/bonecollector.html

Memento

Retrieved from the World Wide Web:
http://www.washington...ent/movies/reviews/mementohowe.htm

Retrieved from the World Wide Web:
http://www.nydailynews...6new_York_Now/Movies/a-103464.asp

Academic References

Alvarez, L., & Kolker, A. (1987). *American tongues* [a film]. New York: Center for New American Media.

American Psychiatric Association. (1994). *Diagnostic and statistical manual of mental disorders* (4th ed.—Rev.) (pp. 133–155). Washington, DC: Author.

American Psychiatric Association. (1996). *Diagnostic and statistical manual of mental disorders* (4th ed.). Washington, DC: Author.

American Speech-Language-Hearing Association. (1988, March). The role of speech-language pathologists in the identification, diagnosis, and treatment of individuals with cognitive-communicative impairments. *ASHA, 30:* 79.

Andrews, B. (1992). Initial management of head injury. In G. Kraft & S. Berrol (Eds.), *Traumatic brain injury: Physical medicine and rehabilitation clinics of North America, 3*(2): 249–258. Philadelphia: Saunders.

Aronson, A. (1990). *Clinical voice disorders: An interdisciplinary approach* (3rd ed.). New York: Thieme.

ASHA. *See* American Speech-Language-Hearing Association.

Bayles, K. (1994). Management of neurogenic communication disorders associated with dementia. In R. Chapey (Ed.), *Language intervention strategies in adult aphasia* (3rd ed.). Baltimore: Williams & Wilkins.

Bello, J. (1995). Hearing loss and hearing aid use in the United States. In *Communication facts*. Rockville, MD: American Speech-Language-Hearing Association.

Benson, D., & Ardila, A. (1996). *Aphasia*. New York: Oxford University Press.

Benton, A. (1981). Aphasia: Historical perspectives. In M. Sarno (Ed.), *Acquired aphasia*. New York: Academic Press.

Benton, A., & Joynt, R. (1960). Early descriptions of aphasia. *Archives of Neurology, 3:* 205–221.

Bess, F., & Humes, L. (1995). *Audiology: The fundamentals* (2nd ed.). Baltimore: Williams & Wilkins.

Billings, K., & Kenna, M. (1999). Causes of pediatric sensorineural hearing loss: Yesterday and today. *Archives of Otolaryngology Head and Neck Surgery, 125:* 517–521.

Bloodstein, O. (1995). *A handbook on stuttering* (5th ed.). San Diego: Singular.

Booth, S. J. (1999). Contemporary issues in communication science and disorders. *National Student Speech-Language-Hearing Association, 26:* 101–105.

Brauner, D. J., Muir, C. J., & Sachs, G. A. (2000). Treating nondementia illnesses in patients with dementia. *Journal of the American Medical Association, 283*(24): 3230–3235.

Brutten, G. J., & Shoemaker, D. (1967). *The modification of stuttering.* Englewood Cliffs, NJ: Prentice Hall.

Catts, H. (1996). Defining dyslexia as a developmental language disorder: An expanded view. *Topics in Language Disorders, 16*(2): 14–29.

Christoffel, K. (1990). Violent death and injury in U.S. children and adolescents. *American Journal of Diseases of Children, 144:* 697–706.

Chui, H. C., Mack, W., Jackson, J. E., Mungas, D., Reed, B. R., Tinklenberg, J., Chang, F-L., Skinner, K., Tasaki, C., & Jagust, W. J. (2000). Clinical criteria for the diagnosis of vascular dementia. *Archives of Neurology, 57:* 191–196.

Code, C., Hemsley, G., & Herrmann, M. (1999). The emotional impact of aphasia. *Seminars in Speech and Language, 20*(1): 19–31.

Corrigan, P., & Jakus, M. (1994). Behavioral treatment. In J. Silver, S. Yudofsky, & R. Hales (Eds.), *Neuropsychiatry of traumatic brain injury*. Washington, DC: American Psychiatric Press.

Culbertson, W. (2001). Personal correspondence. Northern Arizona University, Flagstaff.

Culbertson, W., & Tanner, D. (2001a). Clinical comparisons: Phonological processes and their relationship to traditonal phoneme norms. *Infant-Toddler Intervention, 11*(1): 15–25.

Culbertson, W., & Tanner, D. (2001b). Dependency of neuromotor oral maturation on phonological development. The Ninth Manchester phonology meeting. Manchester, England.

Culbertson, W., Tanner, D., Peck, A., & Hooper, A. (1998). Orientation testing and responses of brain injured subjects. *Journal of Medical Speech-Language Pathology, 6*(2): 93–103.

Curran, C. A., Ponsford, J. L., & Crowe, S. (2000). Coping strategies and emotional outcome following traumatic brain injury: A comparison with orthopedic patients. *Journal of Head Trauma Rehabilitation, 15*(6): 1256–1274.

Dalston, R. M. (2000). Cleft lip and palate. In R. Gillam, T. Marquardt, & F. Martin (Eds), *Communication sciences and disorders*. San Diego: Singular.

Daniels, S., McAdam, C., Brailey, K., & Foundas, A. (1997). Clinical assessment of swallowing and prediction of dysphagia severity. *American Journal of Speech-Language Pathology, 6:* 17–24.

Darley, F. (1982). *Aphasia*. Philadelphia: Saunders.

Darley, F., Aronson, A., & Brown, J. (1975). *Motor speech disorders*. Philadelphia: Saunders.

Davis, B. L., & Bedore, L. M. (2000). Articulatory and phonological disorders. In R. Gillam, T. Marquardt, & F. Martin (Eds.), *Communication sciences and disorders*. San Diego: Singular.

Dodd, B., & Bradford, A. (2000). A comparison of three therapy methods for children with different types of developmental phonological disorder. *International Journal of Language and Communication Disorders, 35*(2): 198–209.

Duffy, J. (1995). *Motor speech disorders*. St. Louis: Mosby.

Durrant, J., & Lovrinic, J. (1995). *Bases of hearing science* (3rd ed.). Baltimore: Williams & Wilkins.

Emilien, G., Maloteaux, J. M., Beyreuther, K., & Masters, C. L. (2000). Alzheimer disease: Mouse models pave the way for therapeutic opportunities. *Archives of Neurology, 57:* 176–181.

Fey, M. (1986). *Language intervention with young children*. Austin: Pro-Ed.

Ghajar, J. (2000). Traumatic brain injury. *Lancet, 356:* 923–929.

Gillam, R. (2000). Fluency disorders. In R. Gillam, T. Marquardt, & F. Martin (Eds.), *Communication sciences and disorders*. San Diego: Singular.

Gillam, R., Marquardt, T., & Martin, F. (Eds.). (2000). *Communication sciences and disorders*. San Diego: Singular.

Gillis, R. (1996). *Traumatic brain injury rehabilitation for speech-language pathologists*. Boston: Butterworth-Heinemann.

Gillis, R., & Pierce, J. (1996). Mechanism of traumatic brain injury and the pathophysiologic consequences. In R. Gillis (Ed.), *Traumatic brain injury rehabilitation for speech-language pathologists*. Boston: Butterworth-Heinemann.

Goldenberg, G., & Hagmann, S. (1998). Tool use and mechanical problem solving in apraxia. *Neuropsychologia, 36*(7): 581–589.

Gonzalez, C., & Calia, F. (1975). Bacteriologic flora of aspiration-induced pulmonary infection. *Archives of Internal Medicine, 135:* 711–714.

Groenen, P., Maassen, B., Crul, T., & Thoonen, G. (1996, June). The specific relation between perception and production errors for place of articulation in developmental apraxia of speech. *Journal of Speech and Hearing Research, 39:* 468–482.

Grossman, H. (1983). *Classification in mental retardation*. Washington, DC: American Association on Mental Deficiency.

Guitar, B. (1998). *Stuttering: An integrated approach to its nature and treatment.* Philadelphia: Lippincott, Williams & Wilkins.

Hagen, C. (1981). Language disorders secondary to closed head injury: Diagnosis and management. *Top Language Disorders, 1:* 73–87.

Hall, B. J., Oyer, H. J., & Haas, W. H. (2001). *Speech, language, and hearing disorders: A guide for the teacher.* Boston: Allyn & Bacon.

Hart, B., & Risley, T. (1995). *Meaningful differences in the everyday experience of young American children.* Baltimore: Brookes.

Hartke, R. J. (1991). *Psychological aspects of geriatric rehabilitation.* Gaithersburg, MD: Aspen.

Harvey, A., & Bryant, K. (2000). Two-year prospective evaluation of the relationship between acute stress disorder and posttraumatic stress disorder following mild traumatic brain injury. *American Journal of Psychiatry, 157*(4): 626–628.

Haynes, W., & Shulman, B. (1998). *Communication development.* Baltimore: Williams & Wilkins.

Herman, C. D. (2000). Post traumatic stress disorder after severe traumatic brain injury. *Journal of Head Trauma Rehabilitation, 15*(5): 1190.

Hertrich, I., & Ackermann, H. (1999). Temporal and spectral aspects of coarticulation in ataxic dysarthria: An acoustic analysis. *Journal of Speech, Language, and Hearing Research, 42:* 367–381.

Hirsch, D. (1998). Ask the doctor: Pervasive developmental disorders. In *Exceptional parent.* Oradell, NJ.

Hopper, T., & Bayles, K. (2001). Management of neurogenic communication disorders associated with dementia. In R. Chapey (Ed.), *Language intervention strategies in aphasia and related neurogenic communication disorders* (4th ed.). Philadelphia: Lippincott, Williams & Wilkins.

Huttlinger, K., & Tanner, D. (1994). The peyote way: Implications for culture care nursing. *Journal of Transcultural Nursing, 5*(2).

Johnson, W. (1938). The role of evaluation in stuttering behavior. *Journal of Speech Disorders, 3:* 85–89.

Johnson, W. (1955). A study of the onset and development of stuttering. In W. Johnson & R. R. Leutennegger (Eds.), *Stuttering in children and adults.* Minneapolis: University of Minnesota.

Katz, W. F., Bharadwaj, S. V., & Carstens, B. (1999). Electromagnetic articulography treatment for an adult with Broca's aphasia and apraxia of speech. *Journal of Speech, Language, and Hearing Research, 42:* 1355–1366.

Kennedy, W. Z. (1999). Delirium, dementia, amnesia, and other cognitive disorders. In P. G. O'Brien, W. Z. Kennedy, & K. A. Ballard (Eds.), *Psychiatric nursing: An integration of theory and practice.* New York: McGraw-Hill.

Kent, R. D. (1997). *The speech sciences.* San Diego: Singular.

Kopit, A. (1978). *Wings* [a play]. New York: Hill & Wang.

Kraus, J., & Sorenson, S. (1994). Epidemiology. In J. Silver, S. Yudofsky, & R. Hales (Eds.), *Neuropsychiatry of traumatic brain injury.* Washington, DC: American Psychiatric Press.

Kreisler, A., Godefory, O., Delmaire, C., Debachy, B., Leclercq, M., Pruvo, J. P., & Leys, D. (2000). The anatomy of aphasia revisited. *Neurology, 54:* 1117–1123.

Kübler-Ross, E. (1969). *On death and dying.* New York: Macmillan.

Kuipers, P., & Lancaster, A. (2000). Developing a suicide prevention strategy based on the perspectives of people with brain injuries. *Journal of Head Trauma Rehabilitation, 15*(6): 1275–1284.

Ladefoged, P., & Maddieson, I. (1988). *Language, speech and mind: Studies in honour of Victoria Fromkin* (pp. 49–61). London: Routledge.

Larkin, M. (2000). Can lost hearing be restored? *Lancet, 356:* 744.

Lawrence, M., & Barclay, D. M. (1998). Stuttering: A brief review. *American Family Physician, 57*(9): 2175–2178.

Lazar, R. M., Marshall, R. S., Prell, G. D., & Pile-Spellman, J. (2000). The experience of Wernicke's aphasia. *Neurology, 55:* 1222–1224.

Lewis, B. A., & Freebairn, L. (1997). Speech production skills of nuclear family members of children with phonology disorders. *Language and Speech, 41*(1): 45–61.

Lezak, M. (1982). The problem of assessing executive functions. *International Journal of Psychology, 17:* 281–297.

Lezak, M. (1983). *Neuropsychological assessment* (2nd ed.). New York: Oxford.

Linn, G. W., & Caruso, A. J. (1998). Perspectives on the effects of stuttering on the formation and maintenance of intimate relationships. *Journal of Rehabilitation, 64*(3): 12–14.

Logemann, J. A. (1998). *Evaluation and treatment of swallowing disorders.* Austin, TX: Pro-Ed.

Lovell, M., & Franzen, M. (1994). Neuropsychological assessment. In J. Silver, S. Yudofsky, & R. Hales (Eds.), *Neuropsychiatry of traumatic brain injury.* Washington, DC: American Psychiatric Press.

Mackay, L., Chapman, P., & Morgan, A. (1997). *Maximizing brain injury recovery: Integrating critical care and early rehabilitation.* Gaithersburg, MD: Aspen.

Martin, F. (1997). *Introduction to audiology* (6th ed.). Boston: Allyn & Bacon.

McAllister, T. (1994). Mild traumatic brain injury and the postconcussive syndrome. In J. Silver, S. Yudofsky, & R. Hales (Eds.), *Neuropsychiatry of traumatic brain injury.* Washington, DC: American Psychiatric Press.

Mesulam, M. (1985). *Principles of behavioral neurology.* Philadelphia: Davis.

Miller, M. K., & Verdolini, K. (1995). Frequency and risk factors for voice problems in teachers of singing and control subjects. *Journal of Voice, 9:* 348–362.

Miniutti, A. (1991). Language deficiencies in inner-city children with learning and behavioral problems. *Language, Speech and Hearing Services in the Schools, 22:* 31–38.

Munson, B. (1999). Myths and facts about deafness. *Nursing99, 29*(12): 84.

Nabokov, V. (1955). *Lolita.* New York: Knopf.

Nathan, L., Stackhouse, J., & Goulandris, N. (1998). Speech processing abilities in children with speech vs. speech and language difficulties. *International Journal of Language and Communication Disorders, 33:* 457–462, supplement.

National Center for Health Statistics. (1988). Current estimates from the National Health Interview Survey, United States, 1988. *Vital and health statistics*, Series 10, No. 173 DHHS Publication No. (PHS) 89-1501.

National Institute of Neurological and Communicative Disorders and Stroke. (1988). *Developmental speech and language disorders: Hope through research.* Bethesda, MD: National Institutes of Health.

NCHS. *See* National Center for Health Statistics.

Neergaard, L. (2000, July 10). Alzheimer's epidemic looming. Associated Press. *The Arizona Republic.*

Nicolosi, L., Harryman, E., & Kresheck, J. (1996). *Terminology of communication disorders* (4th ed.). Baltimore: Williams & Wilkins.

Norris, J. A. (1998). Psycholinguistic foundations of communication development. In W. Haynes & B. Shulman (Eds.), *Communication development: Foundations, processes, and clinical applications.* Baltimore: Williams & Wilkins.

Northern, J., & Downs, M. (1991). *Hearing in children* (4th ed). Philadelphia: Lippincott, Williams & Wilkins.

O'Shanick, G., & O'Shanick, A. (1994). Personality and intellectual changes. In J. Silver, S. Yudofsky, & R. Hales (Eds.), *Neuropsychiatry of traumatic brain injury.* Washington, DC: American Psychiatric Press.

Owens, R. (1995). *Language disorders: A functional approach to assessment and intervention* (2nd ed.). Boston: Allyn & Bacon.

Owens, R. (1998). Development of communication, language, and speech. In G. Shames, E. Wiig, & W. Secord (Eds.), *Human communication disorders: An introduction* (5th ed). Boston: Allyn & Bacon.

Owens, R., Metz, D. E., & Haas, A. (2000). *Communication disorders: A life span perspective.* Boston: Allyn & Bacon.

Perlman, A. L., & Christensen, J. (1997). Topography and functional anatomy of the swallowing structures. In A. L. Perlman & K. S. Schulze-Delrieu (Eds.), *Deglutition and its disorders: Anatomy, physiology, clinical diagnosis, and management*, 15–42). San Diego: Singular.

Pickett, J. M. (1999). *The acoustics of speech communication: Fundamentals, speech perception theory, and technology*. Boston: Allyn & Bacon.

Pimental, P., & Kingsbury, N. (1989). *Neuropsychological aspects of right brain injury*. Austin: ProEd.

Public Health Service. (1994). Vital and health statistics: Prevalence and characteristics of persons with hearing trouble: United States 1990–91. Series 10: Data from the National Health Survey No. 188. DHHS Publication No. 94: 1516.

Ramig, L. O., & Verdolini, K. (1998). Treatment efficacy: Voice disorders. *Journal of Speech, Language, and Hearing Research, 41:* S101–S116.

Ripich, D., & Ziol, E. (1998). Dementia: A review for the speech-language pathologist. In A. Johnson & B. Jacobson (Eds.), *Medical speech-language pathology: A practitioner's guide*. New York: Thieme.

Ruben, R. J. (2000). Redefining the survival of the fittest: Communication disorders in the 21st century. *Laryngoscope, 110:* 241–245.

Sapir, S., Keidar, A., & Mathers-Schmidt, B. (1993). Vocal attrition in teachers: Survey findings. *European Journal of Disorders of Communication, 27:* 129–135.

Sattler, J. (1988). *Assessment of children* (3rd ed.). San Diego: Singular.

Schmidt, D., Holas, M., Halvorson, K., & Reding, M. (1994). Videofluoroscopic evidence of aspiration predicts pneumonia and death but not dehydration following stroke. *Dysphagia, 9:* 7–11.

Shprintzen, R. J. (1997). *Genetics, syndromes, and communication disorders*. San Diego: Singular.

Smeltzer, D., Nasrallah, H., & Miller, S. (1994). Psychotic disorders. In J. Silver, S. Yudofsky, & R. Hales (Eds.), *Neuropsychiatry of traumatic brain injury*. Washington, DC: American Psychiatric Press.

Smith, E., Verdolini, K., Gray, S., Nichols, S., Lemke, J., Barkmeier, J., Dove, H., & Hoffman, H. (1996). Effects of voice disorders on quality of life. *Journal of Medical Speech Language Pathology, 4:* 223–224.

Snow, J., & Hooper, S. (1994). *Pediatric traumatic brain injury*. Thousand Oaks, CA: Sage.

Spahr, F., & Malone, R. (1998). The profession of speech–language pathology and audiology. In G. Shames, E. Wiig, & W. Secord (Eds.), *Human communication disorders: An introduction* (5th ed.). Boston: Allyn & Bacon.

Stothard, S., Snowling, M., Bishop, D. V. M., Chipchase, B. B., & Kaplan, C. A. (1998). Language-impaired preschoolers: A follow-up into adolescence. *Journal of Speech, Language, and Hearing Research, 41:* 407–418.

Stuss, D., & Benson, D. (1986). *The frontal lobes*. New York: Raven Press.

Swindell, C., Holland, A., & Reinmuth, O. (1998). Aphasia and related adult disorders. In G. Shames, E. Wiig, & W. Secord (Eds.), *Human communication disorders: An introduction* (5th ed.). Boston: Allyn & Bacon.

Tanner, D. (1977). Differential diagnosis of organic brain syndrome. A paper presented to the Annual Convention of the Arizona Speech and Hearing Association, Tucson.

Tanner, D. (1978). An overview of communication disorders of the elderly. A paper presented to the Regional Convention of the Western Gerontological Society, Tucson.

Tanner, D. (1980). Analysis of the effects of speech communication courses on selected college students. *Journal of the Arizona Communication and Theatre Association, XI*(2): 44–50.

Tanner, D. (1990a). *Assessment of stuttering behaviors*. Oceanside, CA: Academic Communication Associates.

Tanner, D. (1990b). *Tanner muscular relaxation program for voice disorders*. Oceanside, CA: Academic Communication Associates.

Tanner, D. (1991). *Relaxation training for stutterers*. Oceanside, CA: Academic Communication Associates.

Tanner, D. (1994). *Pragmatic stuttering intervention for children* (2nd ed.). Oceanside, CA: Academic Communication Associates.

Tanner, D. (1997). *Handbook for the speech–language pathology assistant*. Oceanside, CA: Academic Communication Associates.

Tanner, D. (1999a). *The family guide to surviving stroke and communication disorders*. Boston: Allyn & Bacon.

Tanner, D. (1999b). *Understand stuttering: A guide for parents*. Oceanside, CA: Academic Communication Associates.

Tanner, D. (2001a). Hooray for Hollywood: Communication disorders and the motion picture industry. *ASHA Leader, 6*(6): 10.

Tanner, D. (2001b). The brave new world of the cyber speech and hearing clinic. *ASHA Leader, 6*(22): 6–7.

Tanner, D. (2003). *The psychology of neurogenic communication disorders: A primer for health care professionals*. Boston: Allyn & Bacon.

Tanner, D., Belliveau, W., & Siebert, G. (1995). *Pragmatic stuttering intervention for adults*. Oceanside, CA: Academic Communication Associates.

Tanner, D., & Culbertson, W. (1999). *Quick assessment for dysphagia*. Oceanside, CA: Academic Communication Associates.

Tanner, D., Culbertson, W., & Secord, W. (1997). *The developmental articulation and phonology profile* (DAPP). Oceanside, CA: Academic Communication Associates.

Tanner, D., & Gerstenberger, D. (1996). Clinical Forum 9: The grief model in aphasia. In C. Code (Ed.), *Forums in clinical aphasiology*. London: Whurr.

Tanner, D., & Lafferty, H. (2001). Singing about stuttering. *ASHA Leader, 6*(9).

Tanner, D., & Lamb, W. (1984). *The cognitive, linguistic, and social–communicative scales*. Tulsa: Modern Education Corporation.

Tanner, D., Lamb, W., & Secord, W. (1997). *The cognitive, linguistic and social–communicative scales* (2nd ed.). Oceanside, CA: Academic Communication Associates.

Teasdale, G., & Jennett, B. (1974). Assessment of coma and impaired consciousness: A practical guide. *Lancet, 13:* 81–84.

Van Gent, T., Heijnen, C., & Treffers, P. (1997). Autism and the immune system. *Journal of Child Psychology and Psychiatry, 38*(3): 337–349.

Van Mourik, M., Catsman-Berrevoets, C. E., Yousef-Bak, E., Paquier, P. F., & Van Dongen, H. R. (1998). Dysarthria in children with cerebellar or brainstem tumors. *Pediatric Neurology, 18*(5): 411–414.

Van Riper, C. (1973). *The treatment of stuttering*. Englewood Cliffs, NJ: Prentice Hall.

Van Riper, C. (1992). *The nature of stuttering* (2nd ed.). Englewood Cliffs, NJ: Prentice Hall. (Reissued by Waveland Press, Prospect Heights, Illinois).

Van Riper, C., & Erickson, R. (1996). *Speech correction* (9th ed). Boston: Allyn & Bacon.

Vellutino, F. (1979). *Dyslexia: Theory and research*. Cambridge, MA: MIT Press.

Ward, S. (1998). An investigation into the effectiveness of an early intervention method for delayed language development in young children. *International Journal of Language and Communication Disorders, 34*(3): 243–264.

Weber, C., & Smith, A. (1990). Autonomic correlates of stuttering and speech assessed in a range of experimental tasks. *Journal of Speech and Hearing Research, 33:* 690–706.

Weiss, C. E., Gordon, M. E., & Lillywhite, H. S. (1987). *Clinical management of articulatory and phonologic disorders* (2nd ed.). Baltimore: Williams & Wilkins.

Wetherby, A. (2000). *Understanding and enhancing communication and language for young children with autism spectrum disorders*. Flagstaff: Northern Arizona University.

Wiig, E., & Secord, W. (1998). Language disabilities and school-age children and youth. In G. Shames, E. Wiig, & W. Secord (Eds.), *Human communication disorders: An introduction* (5th ed). Boston: Allyn & Bacon.

Williams, A. C., Sandy, J. R., Thomas, S., Sell, D., & Sterne, J. A. C. (1999). Influence of surgeon's experience on speech outcome in cleft lip and palate. *Lancet, 354:* 1697–1698.

Wise, R. J. S., Greene, J., Büchel, C., & Scott, S. K. (1999). Brain regions involved in articulation. *Lancet, 353:* 1057–1061.

Yavas, M. (1998). *Phonology: Development and disorders.* San Diego: Singular.

Yeates, K. (2000). Closed-head injury. In K. Yeates, M. Ris, & H. Taylor (Eds.), *Pediatric neuropsychology.* New York: Guilford Press.

Yellin, M., Culbertson, W., Tanner, D., & Adams, T. (2000). Gender differences in transient evoked otoacoustic emissions (TEOAEs) of newborns. *Infant-Toddler Intervention, 10*(3): 177–200.

Yeoman, B. (1998). Wrestling with words. *Psychology Today, 31*(6): 42–47.

Ylvisaker, M. (1998). Traumatic brain injury in children and adolescents: Introduction. In M. Ylvisaker (Ed.), *Traumatic brain injury rehabilitation* (2nd ed.). Boston: Butterworth-Heinemann.

Ylvisaker, M., & Feeney, T. (1998). *Collaborative brain injury intervention.* San Diego: Singular.

Ylvisaker, M., & Szekeres, S. (1994). Communication disorders associated with closed head injuries. In R. Chapey (Ed.), *Language intervention strategies in adult aphasia* (3rd ed.). Baltimore: Williams & Wilkins.

Zemlin, W. (1998). *Speech and hearing science* (4th ed.). Boston: Allyn & Bacon.

Index